Neurorhinology: Complex Lesions

Guest Editors

RICHARD J. HARVEY, MD
CARL H. SNYDERMAN, MD

OTOLARYNGOLOGIC CLINICS OF NORTH AMERICA

www.oto.theclinics.com

October 2011 • Volume 44 • Number 5

SAUNDERS an imprint of ELSEVIER, Inc.

W.B. SAUNDERS COMPANY
A Division of Elsevier Inc.

1600 John F. Kennedy Boulevard • Suite 1800 • Philadelphia, Pennsylvania 19103-2899

http://www.theclinics.com

OTOLARYNGOLOGIC CLINICS OF NORTH AMERICA Volume 44, Number 5
October 2011 ISSN 0030-6665, ISBN-13: 978-1-4557-2389-8

Editor: Joanne Husovski

Developmental Editor: Donald Mumford

Otolaryngologic Clinics of North America (ISSN 0030-6665) is published bimonthly by Elsevier, Inc., 360 Park Avenue South, New York, NY 10010-1710. Months of issue are February, April, June, August, October, and December. Business and Editorial Offices: 1600 John F. Kennedy Blvd., Suite 1800, Philadelphia, PA 19103-2899. Customer Service Office: 6277 Sea Harbor Drive, Orlando, FL 32887-4800. Periodicals postage paid at New York, NY and additional mailing offices. Subscription prices is $310.00 per year (US individuals), $590.00 per year (US institutions), $149.00 per year (US student/resident), $409.00 per year (Canadian individuals), $741.00 per year (Canadian institutions), $459.00 per year (international individuals), $741.00 per year (international institutions), $230.00 per year (international & Canadian student/resident). Foreign air speed delivery is included in all *Clinics*' subscription prices. All prices are subject to change without notice. **POSTMASTER:** Send address changes to *Otolaryngologic Clinics of North America*, Elsevier Health Sciences Division, Subscription Customer Service, 3251 Riverport Lane, Maryland Heights, MO 63043. **Telephone: 1-800-654-2452 (U.S. and Canada); 314-447-8871 (outside U.S. and Canada). Fax: 314-447-8029. E-mail: journalscustomerservice-usa@elsevier.com (for print support); journalsonlinesupport-usa@elsevier.com (for online support).**

Reprints. For copies of 100 or more of articles in this publication, please contact the Commercial Reprints Department, Elsevier Inc., 360 Park Avenue South, New York, NY 10010-1710. Tel.: 212-633-3812; Fax: 212-462-1935; E-mail: reprints@elsevier.com.

Otolaryngologic Clinics of North America is also published in Spanish by McGraw-Hill Interamericana Editores S.A., P.O. Box 5-237, 06500 Mexico D.F., Mexico.

Otolaryngologic Clinics of North America is covered in *MEDLINE/PubMed (Index Medicus), Current Contents/Clinical Medicine, Excerpta Medica, BIOSIS, Science Citation Index,* and *ISI/BIOMED.*

Printed and bound by CPI Group (UK) Ltd, Croydon, CR0 4YY

Transferred to Digital Print 2011

Contributors

GUEST EDITORS

CARL H. SNYDERMAN, MD
Professor, Departments of Otolaryngology and Neurological Surgery, University of Pittsburgh School of Medicine; Co-Director, Center for Cranial Base Surgery, University of Pittsburgh Medical Center, Pittsburgh, Pennsylvania

RICHARD J. HARVEY, MD
Associate Professor, University of New South Wales/Macquarie University, Department of Otolaryngology/Skull Base Surgery, St Vincent's Hospital, Sydney, Australia

AUTHORS

MICHELLE ALONSO-BASANTA, MD, PhD
Helene Blum Assistant Professor, Department of Radiation Oncology, University of Pennsylvania Health System, Perelman School of Medicine of the University of Pennsylvania, Philadelphia, Pennsylvania

JOHN R. DE ALMEIDA, MD, MSc, FRCS(C)
Department of Otolaryngology-Head and Neck Surgery, University of Toronto, Toronto, Canada

CHARLES S. EBERT, MD, MPH
Assistant Professor, Department of Otolaryngology-Head and Neck Surgery, University of North Carolina at Chapel Hill, Chapel Hill, North Carolina

IVAN H. EL-SAYED, MD, FACS
Department Neurological Surgery; Minimally Invasive Skull Base Program, Department of Otolaryngology-Head and Neck Surgery, University California San Francisco, San Francisco, California

JUAN FERNANDEZ-MIRANDA, MD
Assistant Professor, Department of Neurological Surgery, University of Pittsburgh School of Medicine, Pittsburgh, Pennsylvania

PAUL A. GARDNER, MD
Assistant Professor, Department of Neurological Surgery, University of Pittsburgh School of Medicine; Co-Director, Center for Cranial Base Surgery, University of Pittsburgh Medical Center, Pittsburgh, Pennsylvania

MITCHELL R. GORE, MD, PhD
Assistant Professor, Department of Otolaryngology/ Head and Neck Surgery, University of North Carolina at Chapel Hill, Chapel Hill, North Carolina

RICHARD J. HARVEY, MD
Associate Professor, University of New South Wales/Macquarie University, Department of Otolaryngology/Skull Base Surgery, St Vincent's Hospital, Sydney, Australia

DAVID W. KENNEDY, MD
Professor, Department of Otorhinolaryngology-Head and Neck Surgery, Perelman School of Medicine of the University of Pennsylvania, Philadelphia, Pennsylvania

MARIA KOUTOUROUSIOU, MD
Visiting Research Fellow, Department of Neurological Surgery, University of Pittsburgh School of Medicine, Pittsburgh, Pennsylvania

STEVE LEE, MD, PhD
Assistant Professor, Department of Otolaryngology-Head and Neck Surgery, Loma Linda University Medical Center, Loma Linda, California

VALERIE LUND, MD
Professor of Surgery, Professional Unit, Royal National Throat Nose and Ear Hospital, London, United Kingdom

ROBERT A. LUSTIG, MD, FACR
Professor of Clinical Radiation Oncology, Department of Radiation Oncology, Perelman School of Medicine of the University of Pennsylvania, Philadelphia, Pennsylvania

PRAVEEN V. MUMMANENI, MD
Department Neurological Surgery, University California San Francisco, San Francisco, California

YEW KWANG ONG, MD
Consultant, Department of Otolaryngology-Head and Neck Surgery, National University Hospital, Singapore

PRISCILLA PARMAR, MD
Department of Otolaryngology and Skull Base Surgery, St Vincent's Hospital, Sydney, New South Wales, Australia

BRENT A. SENIOR, MD
Professor and Vice Chair, Department of Otolaryngology-Head and Neck Surgery, University of North Carolina at Chapel Hill, Chapel Hill, North Carolina

CARL H. SNYDERMAN, MD
Professor, Departments of Otolaryngology and Neurological Surgery, University of Pittsburgh School of Medicine; Co-Director, Center for Cranial Base Surgery, University of Pittsburgh Medical Center, Pittsburgh, Pennsylvania

C. ARTURO SOLARES, MD
Assistant Professor, Department of Otolaryngology-Head and Neck Surgery, Medical College of Georgia, Augusta, Georgia

BRIAN D. THORP, MD
Department of Otolaryngology-Head and Neck Surgery, University of North Carolina at Chapel Hill, Chapel Hill, North Carolina

ROWAN VALENTINE, MBBS
Department of Surgery-Otorhinolaryngology, Head and Neck Surgery, University of Adelaide, Adelaide; The Queen Elizabeth Hospital, Woodville, South Australia, Australia

ALLAN D. VESCAN, MD, FRCS(C)
Department of Otolaryngology-Head and Neck Surgery, Mount Sinai Hospital, Toronto, Ontario, Canada

MARK WINDER, MD
Department of Neurosurgery, St Vincent's Hospital, Sydney, New South Wales, Australia

IAN J. WITTERICK, MD, MSc, FRCS(C)
Department of Otolaryngology-Head and Neck Surgery, Mount Sinai Hospital, Toronto, Ontario, Canada

PETER-JOHN WORMALD, MD
Department of Surgery-Otorhinolaryngology, Head and Neck Surgery, University of Adelaide, Adelaide; The Queen Elizabeth Hospital, Woodville, South Australia, Australia

JAU-CHING WU, MD
Department Neurological Surgery, University California San Francisco, San Francisco, California; Department of Neurosurgery, Neurological Institute, Taipei Veterans General Hospital; Institute of Pharmacology, School of Medicine, National Yang-Ming University, Taipei, Taiwan, Republic of China

ADAM M. ZANATION, MD
Assistant Professor, Department of Otolaryngology-Head and Neck Surgery, University of North Carolina at Chapel Hill, Chapel Hill, North Carolina

Contents

Surgical approaches to the craniovertebral junction (CVJ) can result in dysfunction of the upper aerodigestive tract. However, few data are available regarding the incidence of complications after such surgery. Evaluation of a CVJ lesion for treatment must establish the biology, transverse and longitudinal extent of the lesion, and the preoperative and postoperative stability of the spine. Endoscopic approaches to the CVJ, which should reduce the expected morbidity of an open transoral approach, have been described recently. This article reviews common pathologies of the CVJ and surgical approaches, and provides an evidence-based analysis of whether endoscopic approaches reduce velopharyngeal insufficiency.

The traditional approaches to symptomatic cholesterol granuloma (CG), the most common benign pathologic lesion of the petrous apex, have historically been transotic, including middle fossa, translabyrinthine, retrocochlear, or infra- or retrolabyrinthine approaches. These approaches were often fraught with risk to the vestibular or cochlear apparatus, the need for brain retraction, or lack of a natural drainage pathway after marsupialization of the granuloma. This article reviews the literature on the transnasal approach to petrous apex CGs, including medial, medial with carotid medialization, and transpterygoid approaches. Of the 19 reported CGs treated with endoscopic drainage, only one recurrence was noted.

Carotid artery injury during endonasal surgery is the most feared and catastrophic complication. Internal carotid artery injury is more frequent during skull base surgery, and risk factors include acromegaly, previous revision surgery, and prior radiotherapy and bromocriptine therapy. Nasal packing is frequently used to gain hemostasis, often resulting in vascular occlusion. Recent research recommends the crushed muscle patch treatment as an effect hemostat that maintains vascular patency. Endovascular techniques are recommended for vascular control and complication management. Coil or balloon embolization is preferred in patients with adequate collateral cerebral blood flow, and stent-graft placement or bypass surgery is indicated in those who do not.

article evaluates whether proton therapy is still superior to other radiation techniques in the treatment of chordomas.

The goals of treatment of skull base neoplasms are to maximize oncologic outcomes and optimize functional outcomes. Several studies have investigated the former, but fewer examine the latter. This article reviews the available evidence for several functional outcomes, including endocrine, nasal, neurologic, visual, and quality of life outcomes for both endoscopic and open approaches. The quality of evidence for each outcome is compared for endoscopic and open approaches using the Oxford Centre for Evidence-based Medicine guidelines, and recommendations are made. Future longitudinal comparative outcome studies are needed to better delineate the functional status of patients undergoing skull base surgery.

This review describes the sequential learning from initial free tissue grafting reconstructive techniques to the current use of vascularized flaps. Outcomes and limitations of current endoscopic reconstructive techniques are discussed, including a systematic review of the outcomes of endoscopic endonasal techniques to reconstruct large skull base defects (ESBR). The various endoscopic techniques for local and regional flaps in skull base reconstruction are described. Additionally, EMBASE (1980-December 7, 2010) and Medline (1950 – November 14, 2010) were searched using a search strategy designed to include any endoscopic endonasal reconstruction of the skull base. The manuscripts selected were subject to full text review to extract data on perioperative outcomes for ESBR. Surgical technique was used for sub-group analysis.

This article presents a current view of training in neurorhinology and focuses on the level of evidence for the clinical question of "how many cases are needed to achieve proficiency in endoscopic endonasal skull base surgery?" The authors discuss what defines surgical proficiency, what makes up the learning curve and how it shifts with increasing experience, comparisons of learning curves for different skull base surgeries, and conclude with a discussion and recommendations for achieving high-level proficiency.

THE CLINICS ARE NOW AVAILABLE ONLINE!

Access your subscription at:
www.theclinics.com

Skull Base: Meeting Place for Multidisciplinary Collaboration

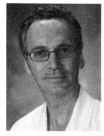 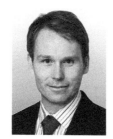

Carl H. Snyderman, MD   Richard J. Harvey, MD
Guest Editors

The skull base is at a crossroads. It is a meeting point for anatomical regions, surgical specialties, and surgical philosophies. Skull base surgery is a dynamic subspecialty and the last decade has witnessed the application of endoscopic techniques to the ventral skull base using an endonasal corridor. The transition from external approaches to an endonasal corridor has not been without controversy. In this volume, we explore the nascent field of *neurorhinology*, a term that emphasizes the multidisciplinary collaboration between neurosurgeons and rhinologic head and neck surgeons. A wide variety of topics are covered, demonstrating the breadth of skull base surgery.

This issue of *Otolaryngologic Clinics*, focusing on *neurorhinology*, has been separated into two volumes. The first volume broadly touches on the common pathologies encountered and the second volume focuses on more complex lesions. There is a contribution by endocrinologists and radiation oncologists in each issue, respectively. Skill acquisition and training are addressed in the second volume.

We confront the controversies head on, asking the authors to apply evidence-based medicine techniques to critically evaluate the literature and attempt to answer some of the most important clinical questions. We further hope that the questions raised here will identify areas in need of better data and stimulate new investigations.

Otolaryngol Clin N Am 44 (2011) xi–xii
doi:10.1016/j.otc.2011.08.025
0030-6665/11/$ – see front matter © 2011 Elsevier Inc. All rights reserved.

oto.theclinics.com

As always, we wish to acknowledge our spouses and families, whose support has been an integral part of our careers.

Carl H. Snyderman, MD
Departments of Otolaryngology and Neurological Surgery
University of Pittsburgh School of Medicine
Center for Cranial Base Surgery
University of Pittsburgh Medical Center
200 Lothrop Street, Pittsburgh, PA 15213, USA

Richard J. Harvey, MD
University of New South Wales/Macquarie University
Department of Otolaryngology/Skull Base Surgery
St Vincent's Hospital
354 Victoria Street
Sydney, NSW 2010, Australia

E-mail addresses:
snydermanch@upmc.edu (C.H. Snyderman)
richard@sydneyentclinic.com (R.J. Harvey)

Diseases of the Odontoid and Craniovertebral Junction with Management by Endoscopic Approaches

Jau-Ching Wu, MD[a,b,c], Praveen V. Mummaneni, MD[a],
Ivan H. El-Sayed, MD[a,d],*

KEYWORDS

- Carniovertebral junction • Craniocervical junction • Odontoid
- Endoscopic surgery • Velopharyngeal insufficiency

EBM Question	Level of Evidence	Grade of Recommendation
Is endoscopic surgery associated with decreased velopharyngeal insufficency?	3b	D

DISEASES OF THE ODONTOID AND CRANIOCERVICAL JUNCTION
Anatomy

The craniovertebral junction (CVJ) is a funnel-shaped region consisting of the upper 2 cervical vertebrae inferiorly and the clivus and foramen magnum superiorly. The upper spine consists of the C1 ring and body of C2 along with odontoid process. The first

[a] Department of Neurological Surgery, University of California San Francisco, 505 Parnassus Avenue, Room M779, San Francisco, CA 94143-0112, USA
[b] Department of Neurosurgery, Neurological Institute, Taipei Veterans General Hospital, Room 509, 17F, No. 201, Shih-Pai Road, Sec 2, Beitou, Taipei 11217, Taiwan, Republic of China
[c] Institute of Pharmacology, School of Medicine, National Yang-Ming University, 3rd Floor, Medical Hall, #155, Sec 2, Linong Street, Beitou, Taipei, Taiwan
[d] Department of Otolaryngology-Head and Neck Surgery, University of California San Francisco, 2233 Post Street, 3rd Floor, San Francisco, CA 94115, USA
* Corresponding author. Department of Otolaryngology-Head and Neck Surgery, University of California San Francisco, 2233 Post Street, 3rd Floor, San Francisco, CA 94115.
E-mail address: Ielsayed@ohns.ucsf.edu

Otolaryngol Clin N Am 44 (2011) 1029–1042
doi:10.1016/j.otc.2011.06.013
0030-6665/11/$ – see front matter © 2011 Elsevier Inc. All rights reserved.

cervical vertebra, the atlas, forms an osseous ring anteriorly and articulates laterally with the occiput condyles to support the cranial skull. Instead of a spinous process, the atlas forms an osseous ring projecting anteriorly and lacks a vertebral body. Through this ring projects the odontoid process of C2 vertebra. A wide range of movement is made possible by the lack of a C1 spinous process. The odontoid process is joined by the apical dental ligament superiorly. The clivus projects inferiorly toward the tip of the odontoid. The craniocervical junction is supported laterally by articulation of the occiput and atlas at the condyles, which are wrapped in dense ligaments (**Fig. 1**).[1]

The anterior longitudinal ligament extends along the ventral vertebral surface, attaching to the anterior arch of the atlas, and forms the anterior atlanto-occipital membrane, which connects the clivus. The posterior longitudinal ligament extends cephalad along the posterior vertebral surface and forms the tectorial membrane at the foramen magnum. The posterior atlanto-occipital membrane is the anatomic equivalent of the interspinous ligament of the subaxial spine, and connects the posterior margin of the foramen magnum to the posterior arch of the atlas. The alar ligaments connect the odontoid to the occipital condyles and the lateral masses of the atlas bilaterally. The apical ligament connects the odontoid tip to the lower end of the clivus. The transverse ligament, dorsal to the odontoid process, forms a strong connection between the two lateral masses of the atlas and holds the odontoid pressed anteriorly.[2]

The foramen magnum is formed within the occipital bone, which is composed anteriorly of the clivus and laterally of the occipital condyles. The clivus is a midline bone that joins the sphenoid bone superiorly and forms a portion of the posterior and inferior walls of the sphenoid sinus. Cranial nerve 12 emerges lateral to the clivus, at the anterior edge of the occipital condyle extracranially through the hypoglossal canal. The vertebral arteries course within the transverse process of the cervical vertebrae to the level of C1 and then project posteriorly across the posterior arch of the atlas. The vertebral arteries enter the foramen magnum laterally and join to form the basilar artery along the anterior face of the brainstem. The angle of the clivus in relation to the skull base can vary, and normally averages 134° to 137°.[3,4] Angles greater than 143° are associated with the diagnosis of platybasia, a flattened skull base.[5] Anomalies of the occiput,

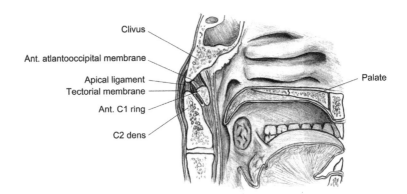

Fig. 1. Craniovertebral junction (CVJ). Ant, anterior. The odontoid joins the clivus at the cranial cervical junction and is attached by dense ligaments. The ring of C1 protrudes anterior to the odontoid. Lesions in this region can project posteriorly into the brainstem and spinal cord. Instability can allow the odontoid to project posteriorly-superiorly, while fractures of the odontoid can displace. (*Courtesy of* Belinda Hahn.)

including condylar hypoplasia, basiocciput hypoplasia, and atlanto-occipital assimilation, are often associated with decreased skull base height and basilar invagination.[6]

PATHOLOGY OF CRANIOCERVICAL JUNCTION

A wide range of pathology occurs at the craniocervical junction, such as congenital malformation, trauma, malignancy, benign neoplasms, and autoimmune diseases. Tumors can arise primarily in the region of the craniocervical junction, or secondarily as hematologic, lymphatic, or metastatic deposits. Goals of care should be tailored to the tumor pathology.

Anatomic Disorders Affecting the Craniocervical Junction

In general, congenital or acquired anatomic lesions causing defects that need surgical intervention all cause their effect through basilar impression of the odontoid onto the brainstem and spinal cord. The pressure results in neurologic dysfunction experienced by the patient as early numbness and tingling in the limbs, and later as motor nerve weakness and anesthesia. Surgical intervention is necessary to relieve pressure and preserve neuronal function.

A range of malformations can affect the craniocervical junction, such as odontoid malformations, primary basilar invagination syndromes, secondary acquired basilar impression syndromes due to softening of the bone, and several anomalies of the skull base. Whereas primary lesions can cause basilar invagination, secondary lesions are considered to cause basilar impression. McGregor's line is drawn from the posterior hard palate to the base of the occiput. Chamberlain's line is drawn from the posterior hard palate to the anterior lip of the foramen magnum. In about 50% of individuals the tip of the odontoid is at or below this line. Basilar invagination or impression is considered present when the tip of the dens is more than 4.5 mm above McGregor's line and 6 mm above Chamberlain's line (**Fig. 2**).

Several congenital lesions are associated with pathology of the craniocervical junction, such as Klippel-Feil syndrome, Down syndrome, osteogenesis imperfecta, achondroplasia, and mucopolysaccharide diseases.[7] Rare disorders can also cause basilar impression including cloverleaf skull, Hajdu-Cheney syndrome, bathrocephaly (an

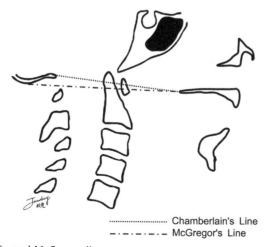

.... Chamberlain's Line
– · – · – · – · – McGregor's Line

Fig. 2. Chamberlain and McGregor lines.

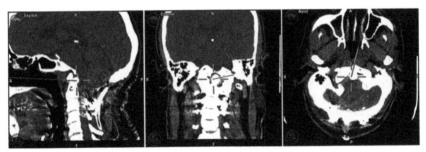

Fig. 3. Anatomic disorders affecting the CVJ. A case of platybasia with basilar invagination underwent posterior suboccipital decompression and fixation followed by anterior decompression. Lesion rest superior to the endoscopic transnasal approach was performed under guidance of computed image navigation.

unusual protuberance of the occipital bone), basilar invagination with unusual facial and extremity abnormalities, Sjögren-Larsson syndrome, and pyknodysostosis (**Fig. 3**).[1]

Acquired cranial disorders can result in bone softening with resultant basilar invagination, and can occur in diseases such as osteomalacia, osteogenesis imperfecta, cretinism, parathyroid disorder, and rickets. The weight of the head over time may result in inferior displacement of the skull and apparent odontoid elevation.[1]

Odontoid malformation can result from a few diseases such as Aarskog syndrome, Morquio syndrome (mucopolysaccharide type IVB), Dyggve-Melchior-Clausen syndrome, spondylometaphyseal dysplasia, congenital spondyloepiphyseal dysplasia, and cartilage-hair hypoplasia.

Trauma

Trauma of the craniocervical junction requiring surgical management is rare. Odontoid fractures account for 9% to 15% of cervical spine fractures, and are the most common cervical spine fracture in individuals older than 70 years. Such fractures result from overextension or hyperflexion of the neck. Three types of odontoid fracture can occur depending on the location: at the tip (Type I), between the inferior aspect of the anterior C1 ring and lacking extension into the superior articular facets (Type II), and at the junction with the body of C2 with extension into the superior articular facets of C2 (Type III). In general, Types I and III are considered stable and can be treated with collar immobilization. If a Type III fracture is combined with a C2-C3 fracture dislocation, it may be very unstable. Type II factures are generally less stable, and immobilization with a halo vest still results in a 26% to 80% nonunion rate. Stabilization may be achieved through a posterior approach, or at times through an anterior approach with screw fixation.[8]

Infectious Disease

Infections can afflict the spine and require surgery for culture and/or debridement. Infections typically occur through direct extension or hematologic seeding and cause prevertebral, intraspinal, and epidural abscess. Retropharyngeal abscess, a well-known otolaryngic infection, rarely causes an intraspinal infection. Of the 14 cases reported in the literature due to retropharyngeal origin, all were due to *Staphylococcus aureus*.[9]

Spinal epidural abscess can be associated with intravenous drug use, a history of diabetes mellitus or human immunodeficiency virus (HIV) infection, multiple medical illnesses, trauma, prior spine surgery, morbid obesity, prior spinal nerve block, and end-stage renal disease.[10] Other sources include hematogenous spread associated with dental extractions or endocarditis. The traditionally defined classic triad of clinical manifestations is localized pain, progressive neurologic deficit, and fever, but has been reported to occur concurrently in as low as 40% of patients.[10] The most common organisms cultured are *S aureus* or *Streptococcus*, while tuberculosis is a rare but known entity. Infections can progress to a spinal epidural abscess, which can be associated with a rapid decline and high morbidity. Clinical findings include developing neurologic deficits with decreased motor strength, and an elevated white blood cell count and erythrocyte sedimentation rate. Imaging with computed tomography (CT) and enhanced magnetic resonance imaging can accurately diagnose these entities, but culture and surgical decompression may be required. Surgical management consists of decompression with drainage of pus, removal of granulation tissue, and irrigation. In the cervical region, lesions are addressed aggressively because of the relatively small space within the spinal cord.

Autoimmune: Rheumatoid Pannus

Rheumatoid arthritis incites an inflammatory condition known as a rheumatoid pannus that requires surgical decompression. The developing pannus causes ligamentous laxity, bone erosion, and brainstem compression due to either direct pressure from the pannus, or a static or dynamic subluxation of the cervical spine.[11] These patients also typically have advanced rheumatoid conditions with many peripheral joints severally afflicted. Access via the transoral route may be impeded if the temporal mandibular joint is involved, causing trismus of the oral cavity (inability to open jaw more than 4 cm), and creating the need for a mandibulotomy. Preliminary reports suggest infliximab, a monoclonal antibody against tumor necrosis factor α and a successful a medical therapy, may reduce the inflammatory pannus size and avoid surgery.[12]

Neoplasms

A range of hematologic, lymphatic, and solid malignancies have been found in the craniocervical junction, which can arise primarily or seed it secondarily from a distant source. Surgical intervention may be necessary to obtain an adequate biopsy, for extirpation, or for decompression. A CT-guided fine-needle aspiration can be considered for soft-tissue lesions in this region. However, lesions occurring within the bone cannot be accessed by the needle and require a surgical approach. When in doubt, it is reasonable to attempt a fine-needle aspiration first.

Hematologic spread of tumor can seed the craniocervical junction with lymphoma, myeloma, or metastatic tumors, which can produce lytic lesions of the bone or infiltrate the marrow. Radiographic evaluation of the osseous skeleton can be performed to identify the easiest site for biopsy.

Solid tumors may arise from the overlying epithelium, such as nasopharyngeal carcinoma, salivary gland tissue such as adenocarcinoma or adenoid cystic carcinoma, mesenchymal tissue such hemangiomas and sarcomas, or cartilaginous/osseous tissue of the spine. A range of tumors of the bone can affect the cervical spine, including chordoma, chondroma, chondrosarcoma, osteosarcoma, and fibrous dysplasia. Other lesions can involve the CVJ including eosinophilic granuloma, aneurysmal bone cyst, schwannoma, neurenteric cyst, meningioma, and neurofibromas.[13] In one series[14] a single vertebra was affected in 75% of benign and 40% of malignant lesions, with more than one vertebra affected in 25% of benign and 60% of malignant lesions.

Nasopharyngeal Carcinoma

The most common tumor of the nasopharynx is nasopharyngeal squamous cell carcinoma (NPC). NPC is a rare tumor with an incidence of 0.2 to 1 per 100,000 in North America and Europe, and 25 per 100,000 in South-East Asia. NPC is classified into World Health Organization Type I (keratinizing), Type II (differentiated), and Type III (undifferentiated). In endemic areas Type III is associated with Epstein-Barr virus, infection, a genetic predisposition, and dietary intake of preserved food. The tumor starts in the epithelial lining of the nasopharynx and can spread laterally via the Eustachian tube, intracranially via cranial foramen, or posteriorly into the CVJ. Erosion into the spine is delayed until the late stages due to the dense fibrous tissue of the pharyngobasilar fascia. Given the need to manage the lymphatic spread in the neck and the excellent response rates, these lesions are typically managed with combined cisplatin-based chemotherapy and radiation regimens. The 5-year overall survival rate is 90% and 84% for stage I and IIA disease, respectively.[15] Stage IIB has an increased rate for distant disease. However, recurrences isolated to the nasopharynx may be appropriate for surgery in selected cases.[16] Long-term effects of radiation may result in osteoradionecrosis that may require surgical debridement.[17]

Osseous Lesions: Chordoma

Chordomas, the most common tumor of the mobile spine, are rare tumors that arise from the remnants of the notochord, a structure that induces formation of the vertebral column. While chordomas do not usually metastasize, they are locally aggressive, causing local bone erosion and neurologic dysfunction. In the largest current series over a 25-year period, 5-year and 10-year survival rates are reported at 55% and 36%, respectively.[18]

En bloc resection of chordoma is considered the key to long-term survival in patients with chordoma to prevent tumor seeding and dissemination. Survival rates in patients with chordoma of the thoracolumbar spine and appendicular musculoskeletal system demonstrate improved survival when an en bloc resection with wide margins is achieved.[19] However, to date only 6 cases have been published describing an en bloc resection of the C2 vertebra, only one of which included the C1 vertebra.[20] Due to the intricate anatomic relations of the vertebral arteries, basilar artery, brainstem, and important cervical rootlets of the upper extremities, and limited exposure in this region, few cases are amenable to an en bloc resection. Thus resection of the craniocervical junction is often performed as a piecemeal resection, with high recurrence rates (**Fig. 4**).

Osseous Lesions: Chondrosarcoma

Chondrosarcomas are a heterogeneous group of malignant tumors of cartilaginous origin, comprising rare and usually slow-growing malignancies of cartilage. In the skull base a chondrosarcoma may arise from remnant cartilage elements after ossification. It can rarely metastasize. The most common cause of death is due to local invasion of the base of skull. The diagnosis and treatment is similar to chordoma based on its origin, location, and growth. Both lesions are similar on radiographic imaging, and histopathology and may require immune-histochemical staining to distinguish them. In the skull base the most common tumor site is in the petroclival junction, but it is also found to occur in the jugular foramen, clivus, sphenoid bone, and retro-orbital region. The primary treatment paradigm is surgical resection when possible, followed by postoperative radiation.[21] In a meta-analysis of the American College of Surgeons

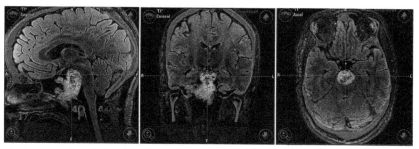

Fig. 4. An example of chordoma at the CVJ. The lesion extends posterior-superior to the pituitary gland and invades the clivus inferiorly. The lesion lies superior to the palatal line and was approached with a transnasal endoscopic approach. The hard palate obstructs access via the transoral corridor. The lesion was resected in piecemeal fashion, working inferior to the pituitary gland and decompressing the brainstem posteriorly.

National Cancer database of 400 patients with chondrosarcoma of the head and neck, there was a 70% 10-year survival rate.[22]

SURGICAL APPROACHES OF ODONTOID AND CRANIOCERVICAL JUNCTION
Traditional Transoral

The transoral approach has been accepted as a standard procedure over the past several decades for anterior decompression at the craniocervical junction (**Table 1**).[23–31] In general, approach via this corridor involves distraction of the jaw, retraction of the tongue as well as surrounding structures, and an incision over the oral pharyngeal mucosa. Through improved anatomic studies of the craniocervical junction and refinement of instruments and surgical techniques, the mortality and morbidity rates of the standard approach have been significantly reduced.[32–36] However, there are still some drawbacks, including traversing the oral cavity and the risk of contamination by bacterial flora with subsequent infection, prolonged postoperative intubation, need for gastric tube feeding after surgery, and possible adverse effects on phonation due to soft palate splitting or hard palate resection in selected cases. The standard transoral approach remains the approach of choice for pathologies involving the region of the craniocervical junction, because it offers a wider operative field from the lower clivus down to C3 by a direct route and is relatively less technically demanding as compared with endoscopic approaches.

Endoscopic Transcervical Approach

In 2007, Wolinsky and colleagues[37] reported 3 patients who underwent odontoidectomy by endoscopic transcervical approach. These investigators modified the standard neurosurgical approach for anterior cervical discectomy and fusion into an upward extension to reach the anterior surface of C2 vertebra. With the aid of a tubular metallic retractor, image-guided navigation, and endoscopes, decompression of the ventral spinal cord and brainstem was achieved effectively in a caudal to rostral fashion. The advantage of this approach is to preserve the integrity of the pharyngeal mucosa, which greatly minimizes the risk of contamination by bacterial flora. The limitation of the transcervical approach is its longer working distance, and the difficulty of performing the procedure in obese patients and those with a barrel-chest or kyphotic cervical spine.[38] This approach has also been shown to be effective for pediatric patients.[39]

Table 1
Comparison of different surgical approaches to the craniocervical junction from anterior route

Approach	Advantages	Disadvantages
Standard open transoral	1. Wide exposure 2. 3-Dimensional visualization 3. Well-accepted standard procedure	1. Prolonged intubation or need of a feeding tube 2. Risk of contamination by oral bacterial flora 3. Possible need of palate splitting
Endoscopic transcervical	1. No mucosal incision	1. 2-Dimensional visualization 2. Extraordinarily long working distance 3. Limited exposure 4. Limitation in kyphotic neck, obesity, or barrel chest 5. Difficulty in reaching high-lying lesions
Endoscopic transnasal	1. Avoidance of palate split, prolonged intubation and feeding tube	1. 2-Dimensional visualization 2. Long working distance 3. Limited exposure 4. Difficulty in reaching low-lying lesions 5. Chronic nasal hygiene
Combined endoscopic transnasal/transoral	1. Avoidance of prolonged intubation and feeding tube 2. Wider exposure than purely transnasal approach 3. Possible decreased nasal morbidity	1. 2-Dimensional visualization 2. Risk of contamination by oral bacterial flora 3. Possible nasal morbidity

Endoscopic Transnasal Approach

The feasibility of endoscopic transnasal odontoidectomy was first demonstrated by the anatomic study by Alfieri and Jho in 2002.[40] Kassam and colleagues[41] reported a case of endoscopic transnasal resection of the odontoid process in 2005. These investigators used an expanded endonasal approach for resection of the odontoid process, compressing the craniocervical spinal cord in a 73-year-old woman with rheumatoid arthritis. This expanded approach consists of a resection of the middle turbinate, ethmoidectomy, sphenoidotomy, and posterior septectomy. Wu and colleagues[42] reported 3 cases of odontoidectomy achieved via a transnasal approach in 2008. Decompression was achieved through a linear mucosa incision over the nasopharynx using an endoscope through the nostril, without resection of the middle turbinate. This approach was subsequently reported for use in Down syndrome and after posterior occipitocervical fusion.[43,44]

Use of endoscopes for transnasal decompression does have some advantages, including an adjustable, panoramic, and wider surgical view (using angled scopes) throughout the procedure. Greater magnification and higher resolution of visualization are also achieved by endoscopes than by microscopes. However, the endoscope per se only provides 2-dimensional images, which inherently makes it more technically demanding and thus may require a longer learning curve. Furthermore, the substantially smaller incision in the nasopharynx created during the endoscopic approach rather than the more caudally located incision made via the open transoral approach also avoids the need for temporary feeding-tube placement postoperatively. It is also postulated that the transnasal approach can minimize the chances of upper airway swelling the early postoperative period, as well as dysphonia or velopharyngeal insufficiency (VPI) for the later postoperative period.

Combined Endoscopic Transnasal and Transoral Approach

Using endoscopes for a transoral approach to the craniocervical junction has been reported in the past decade.[45–47] El-Sayed and colleagues[48] published a series of patients who underwent combined transoral and transnasal endoscopic approaches to address the pathologies at the ventral craniocervical junction. These investigators claimed combination of an endoscopic transnasal and transoral route to be a pragmatic way to conserve the advantages of endoscopic visualization via different corridors, while minimizing procedure-related morbidity due to splitting of the soft palate. The surgical morbidity created by the expanded endonasal approach that is caused by resection of the turbinate and posterior septectomy can be avoided in some cases. Further, using an endoscopic transoral corridor has the advantage of allowing extended reach inferiorly and greater manual dexterity by allowing surgical instruments to angle laterally within the oral cavity[42] (**Fig. 5**). Moreover, in standard open transoral approaches with microscope visualization, the hard palate sometimes still obstructs visualization of the upper extent of the compressive lesion. The use of the endoscope overcomes this obstacle with ease, as it can be navigated to look around the palate.

Previously reported endoscopic transnasal odontoidectomy reports mentioned the most caudal limiting extent of the transnasal route to be the C1 rim (due to the position of the hard palate and the size of the nostril).[42,49] By combining the endonasal approach with a transoral endoscopic approach, access to the mid-body of C2 and below is easily achieved. El-Sayed and colleagues[48] divided the craniocervical

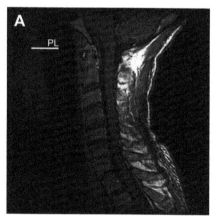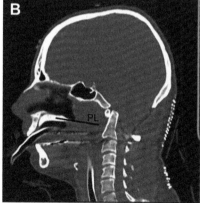

Fig. 5. The endo-oral approach and the combined endonasal endo-oral approach. (*A*) A patient with osteomyelitis of odontoid. The tip of odontoid lies below the palatal line (PL) and the lesion extends into the body of C2. A transoral approach with an endoscope avoids the need for palate split and provides excellent access to debride the infected bone. (*B*) A patient with symptoms attributable to a Chiari malformation and basilar impression. The tip of the odontoid lies nearly in line with the PL. Passing the endoscope through the endonasal corridor allows adequate visualization, while bringing the instrument through the oral corridor allows maneuverability of the instruments. This action avoids the need for extensive resection within the nasal cavity (no middle turbinate resection or posterior septectomy), also avoiding the associated postoperative nasal morbidity.

junction anatomy into 3 types. Types A, B, and C were categorized with regard to a line drawn along the nasal palate, the palatal line (PL). Lesions that extend high above (>1 cm) the PL (Type A) are best approached endonasally, whereas those located near the level of the palate (Type B) could be approached with a combined endonasal/oral route, and those extending far below the PL (>1 cm) could be approached endo-orally (**Fig. 6**).

EVIDENCE-BASED QUESTION: IS ENDOSCOPIC SURGERY ASSOCIATED WITH DECREASED VELOPHARYNGEAL INSUFFICIENCY?

Conventional anterior decompression of the craniocervical junction usually involves a transoral approach. Although the standard open transoral approach has been used for years by neurosurgeons and otolaryngologists for such ventral spinal cord or brainstem compression at the craniocervical junction, splitting of the palate is often required for adequate exposure. Mummaneni and Haid[50] highlighted a modification of the technique to minimize the need of palate split by using a red rubber catheter passed transnasally and secured to the uvula for retraction of the soft palate. Despite the modification, in some circumstances more invasive procedures (ie, splitting the soft palate, resecting the hard palate, glossotomy, or midline mandibulotomy) are still required to provide surgical access to the craniocervical junction. These additional maneuvers may become necessary for access to lesions located higher than the level of the palate, and in patients with difficult oral anatomy or inability to distract the jaw

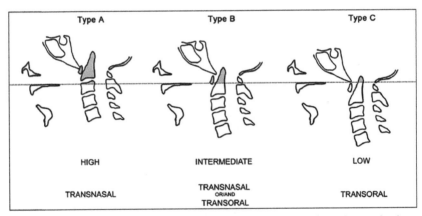

Fig. 6. Approaches used for selected lesions of the CVJ. A line drawn along the nasal palate, the palatal line (PL), defines the default plane of the endoscope entering through the nares. de Al-meida and colleagues[49] defined a line drawn from the nasal dorsum to the posterior hard palate that intersects the spine on average 9 mm below the palate and defines the inferiormost extent of transnasal surgical dissection. El-Sayed and colleagues[48] proposed that the optimal approach to the lesion may be defined by the relation of the lesion to a line drawn along the palate: the PL. Lesions are defined as type A (>1 cm above the PL), B (intermediate location above the PL), or C (>1 cm below the PL). (*Left*) Type A. For lesions located well above the hard palate, an endoscopic transnasal approach is optimal. (*Middle*) Type B. For intermediately located compressive lesions of the CVJ that protrude above the hard palate, either a transnasal or transoral endoscopic route may be used. Also, the authors have found that a combination of both approaches is often help-ful. (*Right*) Type C. For lesions located at the level of the hard palate (or below), an endoscopic oral or standard open, transoral approach is preferred. (*From* El-Sayed IH, Wu JC, Ames CP, et al. Combined transnasal and transoral endoscopic approaches to the craniovertebral junction. J Craniovertebr Junction Spine 2010;1:44–8; with permission.)

open (trismus). Palatal splitting has been reported to increase patient morbidity, especially VPI, dysphonia, and dysphagia.[51,52] VPI occurs when there is incomplete closure of the nasopharynx with resultant escape of air and food into the nose during speech and swallowing. Causes of VPI after a transoral approach can be:

1. Impaired mobility of the palatal muscles due to fibrosis or denervation
2. Disarticulation of the palate muscles of the hard palate preventing appropriate contraction
3. Loss of height of the cervical spine as result of surgical removal of vertebrae, preventing complete closure of the velopharynx
4. Impaired movement of the posterior pharyngeal muscles due to innervation or fibrosis.

Whereas dysphagia often resolves within 12 months following surgery, VPI can persist over the longer term and might require surgical correction.

Endoscopic surgery has been reported to successfully decompress the protruded odontoid process in basilar invagination, trauma, or congenital anomalies.[39,42,45,48] To date, there is only one report that has specifically compared the rate of morbidity and VPI between an endoscopic and open transoral approach. Endoscopic approaches could reduce VPI by preventing disarticulation of the muscles and fibrosis in the soft palate, and by reducing the incision on the posterior pharyngeal wall. El-Sayed and colleagues[48] demonstrated a significantly reduced length of hospital admission and reduced need for prolonged intubation/tracheostomy. In their series they found an overall 45% incidence of VPI developing or lasting more than 2 months after surgery and a statistical trend toward less VPI ($P = .061$) using the endoscopic approach (**Table 2**) [Level III evidence]. The study is limited by its being a retrospective study of 11 patients. Further, some of the patients undergoing endoscopic surgery had previously undergone open palate-splitting surgery. When all patients who had a current or prior palate split were considered, there was a statistical trend toward significance for risk of VPI. Therefore, there is a lack of evidence in the literature to answer whether morbidities are reduced with the endoscopic surgical approaches at the craniocervical junction.

One caveat that needs to be addressed when looking at the complication rates of endoscopic surgery at the craniocervical junction is the variety of endoscopic approaches. For example, transnasal endoscopic odontoidectomy can be achieved

Table 2
Comparison of combined endonasal/endo-oral approach and open transoral approach

	Approach of Craniovertebral Surgery			Even Palate Split		
	Endo (n = 8)	Open (n = 3)	P	Yes (n = 7)	No (n = 4)	P
LOS	7 (7–11)	15 (12–20)	0.014			
Airway	1/8	3/3	0.024	4/7	0/4	.19
VPI	2/8	3/3	0.061	5/7	0/4	.061
Dysphagia >7 days	2/8	3/3	0.061	5/7	0/4	.061
Airway	1/8	3/3	0.024	4/7	0/4	.19
PEG	0/8	1/3	0.061	1/7	0/4	1.0

Abbreviations: Airway, patient required prolonged intubation >24 hours or tracheotomy; Dysphagia, patient required nasogastric of percutaneous gastric feeding tube; LOS, length of stay in hospital (days); PEG, percutaneous endoscopic gastrostomy; VPI, velopharyngeal insufficiency.

From El-Sayed IH, Wu JC, Ames CP, et al. Combined transnasal and transoral endoscopic approaches to the craniovertebral junction. J Craniovertebr Junction Spine 2010;1:44–8; with permission.

via a one nostril or two nostrils, with or without resection of the nasal turbinates.[42–44,48] Transcervical and combined transoral endoscopic odontoidectomy both have achieved adequate odontoidectomy for decompression as well.[37,39,48] The preliminary results demonstrated that patients who underwent transnasal endoscopic odontoidectomy were capable of early extubation and oral intake, which was assumed to be superior to open transoral odontoidectomy requiring a feeding tube[42] [Level IV evidence]. However, the actual incidence of complications and morbidities after each specific endoscopic surgery at the craniocervical junction will require more investigation.

SUMMARY

Choices of surgical approach to the CVJ depend on contemplation of the pathology, anatomy, and surgeon's experience tailored for each patient. The authors' early results of transnasal and/or transoral endoscopic techniques demonstrate excellent access for a range of lesions and offer the possibility of reduced hospital stay and fewer complications. Improvement in technology and expansion of endoscopic surgical experiences may increase the role of minimally invasive approaches to the CVJ for both benign and malignant pathologies.

EBM Question	Author's Reply
Is endoscopic surgery associated with decreased velopharyngeal insufficiency?	Endoscopic approach is associated with less morbidity (Grade C) but only a trend towards less VPI in a small case-control study (Grade D)

REFERENCES

1. Donald PJ. Surgery of the skull base. Philadelphia: Lippincott-Raven; 1998.
2. Martin MD, Bruner HJ, Maiman DJ. Anatomic and biomechanical considerations of the craniovertebral junction. Neurosurgery 2010;66(3 Suppl):2–6.
3. McGreger M. The significance of certain measurements of the skull in the diagnosis of basilar impression. Br J Radiol 1948;21(244):171–81.
4. Poppel MH, Jacobson HG, Duff BK, et al. Basilar impression and platybasia in Paget's disease. Radiology 1953;61(4):639–44.
5. Koenigsberg RA, Vakil N, Hong TA, et al. Evaluation of platybasia with MR imaging. AJNR Am J Neuroradiol 2005;26(1):89–92.
6. Smoker WR. Craniovertebral junction: normal anatomy, craniometry, and congenital anomalies. Radiographics 1994;14(2):255–77.
7. Smoker WR, Khanna G. Imaging the craniocervical junction. Childs Nerv Syst 2008;24(10):1123–45.
8. Maak TG, Grauer JN. The contemporary treatment of odontoid injuries. Spine (Phila Pa 1976) 2006;31(11 Suppl):S53–60 [discussion: S61].
9. Chern SH, Wei CP, Hsieh RL, et al. Methicillin-resistant *Staphylococcus aureus* retropharyngeal abscess complicated by a cervical spinal subdural empyema. J Clin Neurosci 2009;16(1):144–6.
10. Rigamonti D, Liem L, Sampath P, et al. Spinal epidural abscess: contemporary trends in etiology, evaluation, and management. Surg Neurol 1999;52(2): 189–96 [discussion: 197].
11. Robinson AJ, Taylor DH, Wright GD. Infliximab therapy reduces periodontoid rheumatoid pannus formation. Rheumatology (Oxford) 2008;47(2):225–6.
12. Salli A, Sahin N, Paksoy Y, et al. Treatment of periodontoid pannus with infliximab in a patient with rheumatoid arthritis. J Clin Rheumatol 2009;15(5):250–1.

13. Menezes AH. Craniovertebral junction neoplasms in the pediatric population. Childs Nerv Syst 2008;24(10):1173–86.
14. Di Lorenzo N, Delfini R, Ciappetta P, et al. Primary tumors of the cervical spine: surgical experience with 38 cases. Surg Neurol 1992;38(1):12–8.
15. Chan AT. Nasopharyngeal carcinoma. Ann Oncol 2010;21(Suppl 7):vii308–12.
16. Wei WI, Chan JY, Ng RW, et al. Surgical salvage of persistent or recurrent nasopharyngeal carcinoma with maxillary swing approach—critical appraisal after 2 decades. Head Neck 2011;33(7):969–75.
17. Hua YJ, Chen MY, Qian CN, et al. Postradiation nasopharyngeal necrosis in the patients with nasopharyngeal carcinoma. Head Neck 2009;31(6):807–12.
18. Choi D, Melcher R, Harms J, et al. Outcome of 132 operations in 97 patients with chordomas of the craniocervical junction and upper cervical spine. Neurosurgery 2010;66(1):59–65 [discussion: 65].
19. Cloyd JM, Chou D, Deviren V, et al. En bloc resection of primary tumors of the cervical spine: report of two cases and systematic review of the literature. Spine J 2009;9(11):928–35.
20. Chou D, Acosta F Jr, Cloyd JM, et al. Parasagittal osteotomy for en bloc resection of multilevel cervical chordomas. J Neurosurg Spine 2009;10(5):397–403.
21. Oghalai JS, Buxbaum JL, Jackler RK, et al. Skull base chondrosarcoma originating from the petroclival junction. Otol Neurotol 2005;26(5):1052–60.
22. Koch BB, Karnell LH, Hoffman HT, et al. National cancer database report on chondrosarcoma of the head and neck. Head Neck 2000;22(4):408–25.
23. Apuzzo ML, Weiss MH, Heiden JS. Transoral exposure of the atlantoaxial region. Neurosurgery 1978;3(2):201–7.
24. Sakou T, Morizono Y, Morimoto N. Transoral atlantoaxial anterior decompression and fusion. Clin Orthop Relat Res 1984;(187):134–8.
25. Shaha AR, Johnson R, Miller J, et al. Transoral-transpharyngeal approach to the upper cervical vertebrae. Am J Surg 1993;166(4):336–40.
26. Menezes AH, VanGilder JC. Transoral-transpharyngeal approach to the anterior craniocervical junction. Ten-year experience with 72 patients. J Neurosurg 1988;69(6):895–903.
27. Menezes AH, VanGilder JC, Clark CR, et al. Odontoid upward migration in rheumatoid arthritis. An analysis of 45 patients with "cranial settling". J Neurosurg 1985;63(4):500–9.
28. Menezes AH, VanGilder JC, Graf CJ, et al. Craniocervical abnormalities. A comprehensive surgical approach. J Neurosurg 1980;53(4):444–55.
29. Kingdom TT, Nockels RP, Kaplan MJ. Transoral-transpharyngeal approach to the craniocervical junction. Otolaryngol Head Neck Surg 1995;113(4):393–400.
30. Spetzler RF, Hadley MN, Sonntag VK. The transoral approach to the anterior superior cervical spine. A review of 29 cases. Acta Neurochir Suppl (Wien) 1988;43:69–74.
31. Hadley MN, Spetzler RF, Sonntag VK. The transoral approach to the superior cervical spine. A review of 53 cases of extradural cervicomedullary compression. J Neurosurg 1989;71(1):16–23.
32. Messina A, Bruno MC, Decq P, et al. Pure endoscopic endonasal odontoidectomy: anatomical study. Neurosurg Rev 2007;30(3):189–94 [discussion: 194].
33. Hadley MN, Martin NA, Spetzler RF, et al. Comparative transoral dural closure techniques: a canine model. Neurosurgery 1988;22(2):392–7.
34. Husain M, Rastogi M, Jha DK, et al. Endoscopic transaqueductal removal of fourth ventricular neurocysticercosis with an angiographic catheter. Neurosurgery 2007;60(4 Suppl 2):249–53 [discussion: 254].

35. Goel A, Bhatjiwale M, Desai K. Basilar invagination: a study based on 190 surgically treated patients. J Neurosurg 1998;88(6):962–8.
36. Crockard HA. Transoral surgery: some lessons learned. Br J Neurosurg 1995; 9(3):283–93.
37. Wolinsky JP, Sciubba DM, Suk I, et al. Endoscopic image-guided odontoidectomy for decompression of basilar invagination via a standard anterior cervical approach. Technical note. J Neurosurg 2007;6(2):184–91.
38. de Divitiis O, Conti A, Angileri FF, et al. Endoscopic transoral-transclival approach to the brainstem and surrounding cisternal space: anatomic study. Neurosurgery 2004;54(1):125–30 [discussion: 130].
39. McGirt MJ, Attenello FJ, Sciubba DM, et al. Endoscopic transcervical odontoidectomy for pediatric basilar invagination and cranial settling. Report of 4 cases. J Neurosurg Pediatr 2008;1(4):337–42.
40. Alfieri A, Jho HD, Tschabitscher M. Endoscopic endonasal approach to the ventral cranio-cervical junction: anatomical study. Acta Neurochir (Wien) 2002; 144(3):219–25 [discussion: 225].
41. Kassam AB, Snyderman C, Gardner P, et al. The expanded endonasal approach: a fully endoscopic transnasal approach and resection of the odontoid process: technical case report. Neurosurgery 2005;57(1 Suppl):E213 [discussion: E213].
42. Wu JC, Huang WC, Cheng H, et al. Endoscopic transnasal transclival odontoidectomy: a new approach to decompression: technical case report. Neurosurgery 2008;63(1 Suppl 1):ONSE92–4 discussion [discussion: ONSE94].
43. Cornelius JF, Kania R, Bostelmann R, et al. Transnasal endoscopic odontoidectomy after occipito-cervical fusion during the same operative setting-technical note. Neurosurg Rev 2011;34(1):115–21.
44. Magrini S, Pasquini E, Mazzatenta D, et al. Endoscopic endonasal odontoidectomy in a patient affected by Down syndrome: technical case report. Neurosurgery 2008;63(2):E373–4 [discussion: E374].
45. Frempong-Boadu AK, Faunce WA, Fessler RG. Endoscopically assisted transoral-transpharyngeal approach to the craniovertebral junction. Neurosurgery 2002;51(5 Suppl):S60–6.
46. Pillai P, Baig MN, Karas CS, et al. Endoscopic image-guided transoral approach to the craniovertebral junction: an anatomic study comparing surgical exposure and surgical freedom obtained with the endoscope and the operating microscope. Neurosurgery 2009;64(5 Suppl 2):437–42 [discussion: 442–4].
47. Welch WC, Kassam A. Endoscopically assisted transoral-transpharyngeal approach to the craniovertebral junction. Neurosurgery 2003;52(6):1511–2.
48. El-Sayed I, Wu J-C, Ames C, et al. Combined transnasal and transoral endoscopic approaches to the craniovertebral junction. J Craniovertebr Junction Spine 2010;1(1):44–8.
49. de Almeida JR, Zanation AM, Snyderman CH, et al. Defining the nasopalatine line: the limit for endonasal surgery of the spine. Laryngoscope 2009;119(2):239–44.
50. Mummaneni PV, Haid RW. Transoral odontoidectomy. Neurosurgery 2005;56(5): 1045–50 [discussion: 1045–50].
51. Jones DC, Hayter JP, Vaughan ED, et al. Oropharyngeal morbidity following transoral approaches to the upper cervical spine. Int J Oral Maxillofac Surg 1998;27(4):295–8.
52. Cantarella G, Mazzola RF, Benincasa A. A possible sequela of transoral approach to the upper cervical spine. Velopharyngeal incompetence. J Neurosurg Sci 1998;42(1):51–5.

Cholesterol Granuloma of the Petrous Apex

Mitchell R. Gore, MD, PhD, Adam M. Zanation, MD,
Charles S. Ebert, MD, MPH, Brent A. Senior, MD*

KEYWORDS

- Petrous apex • Cholesterol granuloma
- Endoscopic • Endonasal

Key Points: CHOLESTEROL GRANULOMA OF THE PETROUS APEX

1. Cholesterol granuloma is the most common benign petrous apex lesion

2. Cholesterol granulomas have a characteristic appearance on magnetic resonance imaging (MRI) that is hyperintense on both T1-weighted and T2-weighted sequences, owing to the fat and fluid content of these lesions

3. The endonasal, endoscopic approach is safe, providing a low rate of recurrence and durable marsupialization of these lesions

4. The medial endonasal approach is the most frequently used approach described in the literature.

EBM Question	Level of Evidence	Grade of Recommendation
What is rate of clinical and radiographic recurrence following endoscopic transnasal drainage of cholesterol granuloma?	4	C

EPIDEMIOLOGY OF CHOLESTEROL GRANULOMA

Cholesterol granuloma is the most common benign pathologic lesion of the petrous apex, the most medial portion of the temporal bone. Cholesterol granulomas typically arise from

---

The authors have no conflicts of interest.
Department of Otolaryngology/Head and Neck Surgery, University of North Carolina at Chapel Hill, CB 7070, Physicians Office Building Manning Drive, Chapel Hill, NC 27599, USA
* Corresponding author.
E-mail address: brent_senior@med.unc.edu

Otolaryngol Clin N Am 44 (2011) 1043–1058
doi:10.1016/j.otc.2011.06.005
0030-6665/11/$ – see front matter © 2011 Elsevier Inc. All rights reserved.

a pneumatized petrous apex, with about 10% of the population showing pneumatization of the petrous apex . Primary petrous apex lesions are those that arise from the central petrous apex or the anatomic boundaries of the region, and account for approximately 40% of petrous apex lesions.[1-6] Secondary lesions impinge on the petrous apex from an outside source, which may derive from invasion from a bordering region or from a metastatic lesion; secondary lesions account for the remaining 60% of petrous apex lesions.

Clinical

Cholesterol granulomas are typically symptomatic or present with subtle symptoms such as headache. Larger lesions may present with hearing loss and cranial neuropathies.

Investigation

Computed tomography (CT) and MRI are typically used to characterize cholesterol granuloma. CT will typically show an expansive lesion of the petrous apex with bony erosion and scalloping. Thinning of the posterior wall of the sphenoid and petrous carotid artery dehiscence may also be seen.

MANAGEMENT OF CHOLESTEROL GRANULOMA

The traditional approaches to cholesterol granulomas have historically been transotic, including middle fossa, translabyrinthine, retrocochlear, or infralabyrinthine or retrolabyrinthine approaches. These approaches were often fraught with risk to the vestibular or cochlear apparatus, the need for brain retraction, or the lack of a natural drainage pathway after marsupialization of the granuloma. Since the early 1990s endoscopic transsphenoidal drainage and marsupialization of petrous apex cholesterol granulomas has been described. This approach avoids potential risk to the auditory and vestibular organs, and provides a natural drainage pathway into the sinuses. In this article the authors review the literature on the transnasal approach to petrous apex cholesterol granulomas and the described approaches, including medial, medial with carotid medialization, and transpterygoid approaches.

Prognosis and Natural History

Slow-growing cholesterol granulomas or small lesions may remain asymptomatic for many years. Larger lesions left untreated may continue to expand and cause increasing signs and symptoms with progressive hearing loss, vertigo, facial weakness, and lower cranial nerve neuropathies. The endoscopic transnasal transsphenoid approaches offer a low recurrence rate, with low risk to inner ear structures and a natural drainage pathway into the sinonasal cavity.

Anatomy and Epidemiology

The petrous apex is a pyramidal structure comprising the most medial portion of the temporal bone. The base of the pyramid is the bony labyrinth including the semicircular canals and cochlea. Anteriorly, the base of the pyramid is partly formed by the tensor tympani and internal carotid artery. The superior petrous apex makes up a large portion of the middle cranial fossa floor, extending from the superior semicircular canal and arcuate eminence to the ascending portion of the internal carotid artery and the Gasserian ganglion situated in Meckel's cave. The superior surface extends from the superior petrosal sinus posteriorly to the petrosphenoid suture line anteriorly. The posterior surface of the petrous apex forms the anterolateral wall of the posterior cranial fossa, and extends medially from the posterior semicircular canal and the endolymphatic sac to the petroclinoid ligament and Dorello's canal containing the abducens nerve. This posterior surface then extends from the petro-occipital suture line inferiorly to the superior petrosal sinus superiorly. Inferiorly, the petrous pyramid is bounded by the jugular bulb and the inferior petrosal sinus. The inferior surface also has a foramen for the entry of the internal carotid artery. Medial to the jugular fossa is a depression that is associated with the cochlear aqueduct (perilymphatic duct). The petrous bone articulates with the greater wing of the sphenoid anteriorly. The foramen lacerum is found between the petrous apex and the sphenoid bone and contains, but does not transmit, the internal carotid artery.

The posteroinferior margin of the temporal bone articulates with the occipital bone. Laterally, the petrous temporal bone fuses with the squamous portion of the temporal bone at the petrosquamosal fissure. The transverse portion of the internal carotid artery and the internal auditory canal traverse the petrous pyramid. The petrous apex can be divided into anterior and posterior areas by a vertical plane through the modiolus of the cochlea and the internal auditory canal. The posterior petrous apex, located between the internal auditory canal and the vestibular apparatus, is usually composed of compact bone and is rarely involved by disease processes. The petrous bone may be pneumatized, diploic (marrow-filled), or sclerotic. About 10% of the population has pneumatization of the petrous apex. Primary petrous apex lesions are those that arise from the central petrous apex or the anatomic boundaries of the region. Secondary lesions are those that impinge on the petrous apex from an outside source, possibly from invasion from a bordering region or from a metastatic lesion. Primary lesions account for approximately 40% of petrous apex lesions.[1–6]

PATHOPHYSIOLOGY OF CHOLESTEROL GRANULOMA

Cholesterol granuloma of the petrous apex forms as a result of foreign-body giant-cell reaction to cholesterol crystals. The poor ventilation, interference with drainage, and hemorrhage in a usually pneumatized space are predisposing factors leading to the formation of the cyst. Negative pressure from air resorption leads to the degradation of the blood and formation of cholesterol crystals. These crystals initiate a foreign-body reaction that results in granuloma or cyst formation. The cyst wall is made up of fibrous connective tissue and lacks the keratinizing squamous epithelium seen in cholesteatoma. Foreign-body giant cells, hemosiderin-laden macrophages, and cholesterol crystals are seen on pathologic evaluation.[7]

Clinical

Cholesterol granulomas are often asymptomatic and may be discovered incidentally on imaging for other reasons. When symptoms are present they may be subtle, such as headache or hearing loss. Cholesterol granulomas of the petrous apex can be dangerous, due to their proximity to the inner and middle ear structures and their proximity to the seventh, eighth, and lower cranial nerves, and more overt signs and symptoms such as permanent hearing loss, cranial neuropathies, and osseous destruction can occur if the cholesterol granuloma is left untreated and continues its expansile growth.

Investigation

Both CT and MRI are valuable in the workup of petrous apex cholesterol granuloma. A characteristic finding on CT of a cholesterol granuloma is a sharply marginated expansile lesion with bony erosion (**Fig. 1**). The lesions are avascular and therefore do not enhance with contrast, and are isodense with brain tissue. A thin, peripheral calcified rim may be noted as well as pneumatization of the contralateral petrous apex. The MRI findings of cholesterol granuloma are unique. The lesions demonstrate high signal intensity on

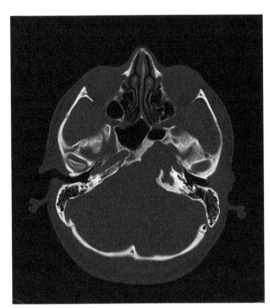

Fig. 1. Coronal computed tomography (CT) image showing a left petrous apex cholesterol granuloma with bony erosion and expansion into the posterior sphenoid bone.

both T1-weighted and T2-weighted images (**Figs. 2** and **3**). The unique increased signal intensity on the T1-weighted image may be due to the combination of cholesterol crystals, chronic hemorrhage, and proteinaceous crystals. Occasionally it may be difficult to distinguish a small cholesterol granuloma from normal marrow because both may demonstrate increased signal intensity on T1-weighted images; however, they may be differentiated by examining the T2-weighted images. Marrow fat will exhibit a progressive decrease in signal intensity with increasing T2 weighting (fat saturation). Cholesterol granulomas maintain their high signal intensity on T2-weighted images.

Specialized MRI pulse sequences may sometimes be needed to evaluate these lesions. Partial saturation gradient recalled echo (GRE) sequences may be employed instead of the usual spin-echo sequences. GRE imaging demonstrates an enlarging peripheral ring of decreased signal intensity as the echo time is lengthened. This ring indicates a peripheral magnetic susceptibility effect, suggesting that hemosiderin-laden macrophages are present on the wall of the lesion. Whereas this pattern may be possible in a thrombosed aneurysm, it is unlikely in vestibular schwannomas, cholesteatomas, or mucoceles. Protein chemical shift imaging may also be used to evaluate these lesions. The mixed population of aliphatic (CH2) and water protons produces a cyclic pattern of signal intensity in the center of the lesion. A cholesteatoma may produce this pattern but typically a thrombosed aneurysm, schwannoma, or mucocele would not. Because of this unique ability to evaluate cholesterol granulomas, MRI is now used both for preoperative evaluation and to follow the patient postoperatively for recurrence.[8]

MANAGEMENT OF CHOLESTEROL GRANULOMAS
Surgical Indications and Approaches

Treatment of cholesterol granulomas is based on presentation and progression of symptoms. The usual presentation is unilateral headaches; however, cranial nerve

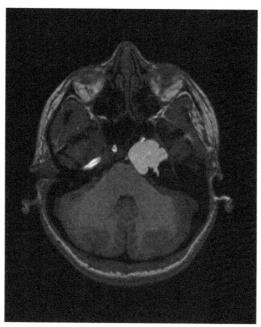

Fig. 2. Coronal T1-weighted magnetic resonance (MR) image of a left petrous apex cholesterol granuloma. Note that it is hyperintense and abuts the left internal carotid artery.

symptoms such as diplopia, hearing loss, or facial anesthesia can also occur.[9,10] CT and MRI will reveal either an expanded or nonexpanded petrous apex. For nonexpanded lesions, it is at times difficult to know how much of the patient's symptoms are a result of the petrous apex disease. In this situation, observation and serial imaging can be helpful in ensuring optimal selection of medically recalcitrant patients for surgical treatment.

The key to successful petrous apex cholesterol granuloma surgery is surgical drainage and aeration. Complete surgical removal is rarely performed because the lesion lacks an epithelial lining. Multiple surgical approaches have been described for treating these lesions, including infralabyrinthine, transcanal infracochlear, transsphenoidal, middle cranial fossa, and retrosigmoid approaches. The approach taken depends on the patient's hearing and the site and extent of the lesion.

Traditional approaches to the petrous apex include transtemporal and middle fossa approaches. For the drainage of cystic lesions such as cholesterol granulomas, approaches to the petrous apex include infralabyrinthine, infracochlear, middle cranial fossa, and transsphenoidal approaches for ears with serviceable hearing. In patients with minimal residual hearing without the need for hearing preservation, translabyrinthine approaches can be used. In poorly pneumatized temporal bones transtemporal approaches to the petrous apex may not be feasible, and continuous drainage and aeration of the petrous apex may be difficult to maintain. Transtemporal approaches pose a potential risk to hearing and balance function as well as to facial nerve function. The transcranial middle fossa approach is technically difficult, and suffers from the lack of a permanent drainage pathway. Some degree of brain retraction is necessary, which carries the risk of brain injury.

The retrosigmoid and middle cranial fossa approaches are designed for hearing preservation but do not provide for permanent drainage or aeration. Chemical

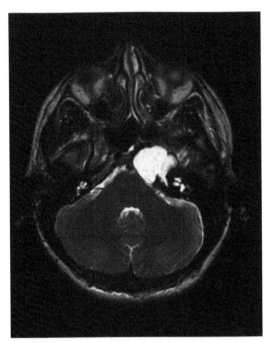

Fig. 3. Coronal T2-weighted MR image of a left petrous apex cholesterol granuloma. Note that it is hyperintense and can be seen abutting the posterior surface of the flow void representing the left internal carotid artery.

meningitis from subarachnoid space contamination by the contents of the cholesterol granuloma is also a risk. Drainage, aeration, and hearing preservation are the goals of the infralabyrinthine, transcanal infracochlear, and transsphenoidal approaches. Detailed analysis of the preoperative CT scan to define the jugular bulb, facial nerve, sigmoid sinus, bony labyrinth, and posterior wall of the sphenoid is mandatory before surgery.

The infralabyrinthine approach shares the same goals as the other transtemporal approaches. Thedinger and colleagues[9] reported on 3 patients who underwent this approach for cholesterol granuloma. Two required surgery for recurrence. By contrast, Goldofsky and colleagues[7] reported on 9 patients followed from 1 to 10 years who underwent such a procedure, with only one recurrence. Hearing results from 14 patients showed 7 improved with 7 remaining the same. The infralabyrinthine approach involves a simple mastoidectomy then removal of the air cells in Trautmann's triangle. The sigmoid sinus is followed until the jugular bulb is identified: this represents the inferior margin of the approach. The semicircular canals are skeletonized and the infralabyrinthine air cell tract is developed anteriorly. Once the lesion is identified, it is evacuated and the opening is enlarged. A stent may be placed to prevent stenosis of the opening. This approach is limited if the patient has a high jugular bulb that limits access to the infralabyrinthine air cell tract.

The transcanal infracochlear approach involves a postauricular incision and reflection of the ear anteriorly. Typanomeatal flaps are developed, and the external auditory canal is enlarged anteriorly and inferiorly to expose the hypotympanum. The chorda tympani is followed inferoposteriorly to define the extent of posterior dissection possible without injury to the facial nerve. The air cell tract below the cochlea is developed in the hypotympanum to expose the course of the carotid artery and the jugular bulb. The round window provides the superior line of dissection, and Jacobson's nerve leads to the "crutch" of the carotid and jugular bulb. If the plane of dissection remains below the round window, the internal auditory canal structures will not be at risk. Once the lesion is entered, it is drained and a catheter may be placed. A high jugular bulb does not block access via this route as it does with the infralabyrinthine approach, and provides more dependent drainage for the cyst.

The retrosigmoid approach is performed through a craniotomy posterior to the sigmoid sinus. The cerebellum is retracted posteromedially, allowing for access to the cerebellopontine angle. This procedure has been of limited usefulness because of the location of most petrous apex cholesteatomas anterior of the internal auditory canal. The interposition of the cerebellum, as well as brainstem and cranial nerves, makes total extirpation of these tumors extremely difficult. This approach may be useful for removal of petrous apex cholesteatomas with significant intracranial extension.

If the lesion does make a significant impression on the sphenoid, a transsphenoidal approach may be used. The approach has excellent panoramic endoscopic exposure but risks the optic nerve and internal carotid artery. The transsphenoidal approach is useful when the cholesterol granuloma forms a large surface area against the posterior/lateral wall of the sphenoid sinus. Multiple approaches may be used toward the sphenoid, including external ethmoidectomy sphenoidotomy, intranasal sphenoethmoidectomy, intranasal sphenoidotomy, transseptal sphenoidotomy, or transpalatal approaches. The lateral and superior walls of the sphenoid sinus must be closely examined to locate indentations of the pituitary gland, optic nerve, maxillary nerve, carotid artery, and cavernous sinus. Once the wall of the cyst is identified, it can be opened and drained. A large opening should be created to decrease the chance of postoperative stenosis.

Literature Review of Endoscopic Approaches

Endoscopic endonasal approaches to the ventral skull base have been used increasingly over the past 10 to 15 years, and are generally categorized based on their orientation in coronal and sagittal planes. For all of these approaches, the sphenoid sinus is the starting point and provides orientation to important vascular and neural structures.

In 1994 Fucci and colleagues[11] described endoscopic drainage of a 2.5-cm giant cholesterol granuloma of the petrous apex. Their patient was a 36-year-old woman with a chief complaint of headache, with a CT scan showing a 2.5-cm lytic lesion in the left petrous apex, the anteromedial extent of which abutted the posterior wall of the sphenoid sinus. Their procedure took down the anterior wall of the sphenoid sinus, and exposed the posterior wall of the sphenoid sinus and the crest of bone along the posterolateral wall of the sphenoid sinus, identifying the carotid artery. The posterior wall of the sphenoid sinus was removed and a Hardy pituitary dissector was used to remove the bone of the posterior wall of the sphenoid sinus over the cholesterol granuloma. The cyst was exposed and opened from medial to lateral, the fluid was evacuated, and the anterior wall was marsupialized. A T-shaped silicone stent was placed into the cyst to maintain a tract between the cyst and the nasal cavity. Follow-up nasal endoscopy showed the stent to be open and in place at 3 months after surgery.

Michaelson and colleagues[12] reported endoscopic management of a petrous apex cholesterol granuloma in a 13-year-old African American girl presenting with a 2-month history of intermittent right-sided, retro-orbital headaches and diplopia. MRI scan showed a large petrous apex mass abutting the sphenoid sinus. Endoscopic drainage of the granuloma was performed using a Messerklinger approach with a right

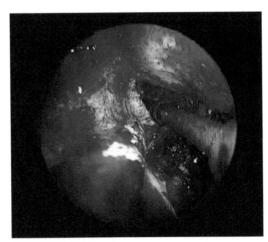

Fig. 4. Drilling in the clival recess medial to the left internal carotid artery, exposing the anterior wall of the cholesterol granuloma cavity. Note that the drill is directly under and posterior to the second genu of the carotid artery seen in the superior right quadrant of the endoscopic picture.

sphenoidotomy. The inferior posterolateral wall of the sphenoid sinus was removed revealing a large, dark, fluid-filled cyst in the petrous apex (see **Fig. 3**; **Fig. 4**). The cyst was opened, drained, and widely marsupialized. Headaches were immediately relieved and sixth nerve function returned within 1 week. Six months after surgery, she remained asymptomatic with a widely patent posterior sphenoid sinus drainage port on office endoscopy.

DiNardo and colleagues[13] described endoscopic drainage of a left petrous apex cholesterol granuloma in a 62 year-old woman with several months of disequilibrium and headaches. The approach was performed through the right side of the sphenoid sinus, allowing for extensive access to the cyst cavity through the right posterior medial wall of the sphenoid sinus. The left sphenoid was not used because of the proximity of the left internal carotid artery to the posterior wall of the left sphenoid. Golden-brown fluid and debris were drained and the cyst was widely marsupialized. Pathologic evaluation confirmed a cholesterol granuloma. The patient's imbalance and headache resolved within 1 week of the procedure, and she remained asymptomatic 12 months after surgery with a narrowed but patent cyst tract.

Oyama and colleagues[14] reported a 28-year-old woman with left-sided hemifacial pain. MRI showed hyperintense lesions of the left petrous apex on T1-weighted and heterogeneous intensity on T2-weighted images, consistent with cholesterol granuloma. The left trigeminal nerve was compressed upward by the lesion, separated from the posterior sphenoid sinus by a thin layer of bone with the left carotid canal adjacent to the lesion. Endoscopic transsphenoidal surgery was performed through the right nostril to allow for wide access to the cyst cavity and to avoid injury to the left internal carotid artery. The eroded petrous bone was easily removed. After cutting the cyst wall, brownish fluid typical of granulomas flowed out, and the cyst cavity was opened wide. Her left trigeminal neuralgia improved within a few days after surgery. She remained asymptomatic during the course of 24-month outpatient follow-up, and MRI confirmed collapse of the left cyst cavity.

In 2007 Chatrath and colleagues[15] undertook an anatomic study to investigate the surgical anatomy of the petrous apex through an endonasal endoscopic approach, to investigate its feasibility and to characterize clear and consistent surgical landmarks for transsphenoidal access to the area. Cadaveric dissections were performed on 5 heads. The landmark for entry into the petrous apex was determined to be the intersection of a vertical line halfway between the medial surface of the internal carotid artery and the midline, with a horizontal line one-third of the way up from the posteroinferior floor of the sphenoid sinus. The dimensions of the posterosuperior sphenoid sinus were characterized by the intercarotid distance, pituitary to sphenoid floor distance, and the width of the sphenoid sinus floor, which were 15 ± 3 mm, 16 ± 3 mm, and 26 ± 1.6 mm, respectively. The surface area of surgical access was 193 ± 28 mm^2, increasing to 316 ± 39 mm^2 after drilling of the sphenoid rostrum (P<.001).

Georgalas and colleagues[16] reported 4 cases of petrous apex cholesterol granulomas drained via a transsphenoidal approach over a 10-year period. The first case was a man with vertigo, facial palsy, and sensorineural hearing loss. CT scan showed a large, erosive lesion of the petrous apex, while MRI confirmed a large, cystic lesion that was hyperintense on T1-weighted and T2-weighted images, abutting the posterolateral wall of the sphenoid sinus. The lesion was drained via an endoscopic transsphenoid approach. The middle turbinate was resected, a posterior ethmoidectomy and wide sphenoidotomy were performed, and the cyst was opened and marsupialized with pathologic examination of the cyst wall showing cholesterol granuloma. Following surgery, the facial palsy resolved and hearing returned to normal. Repeat MRI 7 years later showed no evidence of cyst recurrence. The second case was a 13-year-old boy with headache and progressive diplopia. MRI showed a cystic lesion of the lateral sphenoid region, hyperintense on T1-weighted and T2-weighted sequences, abutting the cavernous sinus and the middle cranial fossa, displacing the posterolateral sphenoid sinus wall medially, and nearly obliterating the left sphenoid sinus. A middle fossa approach was used initially by a pediatric neurosurgeon but the patient's symptoms recurred. A large sphenoidotomy was performed, which included the medial pterygoid ala, and the cyst was marsupialized. His diplopia and headache resolved following surgery and 6 years later he remained clinically asymptomatic. The third case involved a 34-year-old woman with a cholesterol granuloma of the petrous apex incidentally found on brain MRI. Initially she was asymptomatic and was observed. Ten years later she developed headaches, and a CT scan demonstrated that the lesion had developed anterior to the internal auditory meatus; medially the tumor was encasing and displacing the vertical part of the internal carotid artery and displacing anteriorly the posterior wall of the sphenoid sinus, eroding the sphenoid sinus septum, and entering the left sphenoid sinus. The posterior part of the vomer was drilled and the perpendicular plate of the ethmoid was removed. A wide sphenoidotomy was made, and adequate access to both sphenoid sinuses was achieved with exposure of both optic nerves and carotid arteries. The anterior wall of the cyst was opened and removed, and widely marsupialized. The carotid as well as the dura of the posterior fossa was visible inside the cyst cavity. The opening of the cyst had closed at 2 years but the patient was without clinical signs of recurrence and remained symptom-free. The fourth case described a 58-year-old man with progressive deterioration of visual acuity on the right. An MRI showed a large cystic lesion filling the entire sphenoid, hyperintense on T1-weighted and isointense on T2-weighted images. During surgery, it was noted that the anterior wall of the sphenoid was displaced anteriorly and the sphenoethmoidal recess was obliterated. After sphenoidotomy, drainage of a characteristic oily material was obtained. The cavity of the cyst was explored and noted to be lined with granulomatous tissue that was excised from the sella turcica, the dura of the posterior cranial fossa, and the underlying carotid arteries and optic nerves. Histology confirmed a cholesterol granuloma of the petrous apex. The patient's visual acuity improved progressively and he remained stable postoperatively.

Samadian and colleagues[17] described a case of a cholesterol granuloma in the left petrous apex occurring in a 28-year-old woman with a 6-month history of intermittent left hemicranial headache and diplopia. CT scan of the petrous bone and skull base showed an expansile left petrous apex mass, and MRI revealed a large left petrous apex mass abutting the sphenoid sinus. The mass was hyperintense on both T1-weighted and T2-weighted images, consistent with cholesterol granuloma. For surgical removal a transrostral transsphenoid approach was used. Her headache and diplopia resolved within 2 days after surgery. She remained asymptomatic 4 years after surgery. Follow-up MRI confirmed drainage of lesion without any mass effect, and outpatient endoscopy confirmed patent cyst marsupialization.

Haginomori and colleagues[18] reported a 21-year-old woman with a 10-year history of left hearing impairment and aural fullness. Pure tone audiometry showed conductive hearing loss in the left ear. CT revealed a round lesion in the petrous apex with bony dehiscence of the carotid canal. MRI showed a lesion in the petrous apex, tympanic cavity, antrum, and mastoid cavity, which was hyperintense on T1-weighted and heavily-weighted T2 images, consistent with cholesterol granuloma of the petrous apex and middle ear.

The MRI also indicated that the cholesterol granuloma in the petrous apex was distinct from the lesion in the middle ear cavity. An endoscope-assisted combined approach was used for the petrous apex cholesterol granuloma. Tympanotomy with a canal wall take-down procedure and temporary removal of the incus was performed to facilitate access to the middle ear cholesterol granuloma. For drainage of the petrous apex lesion a Lucae's catheter was passed from the left nostril into the nasal cavity, and the tip of the catheter moved toward the pharyngeal orifice of the Eustachian tube under guidance with a flexible endoscope. The cyst wall of the cholesterol granuloma was penetrated using a Rosen needle and the hole enlarged using forceps under the view of the rigid endoscope with guidance from the guidewire, creating a drainage/ventilation route from the nasopharynx to the middle ear. Topical mitomycin, 0.4 mg/mL was used at the edges of the holes penetrating the cholesterol granuloma cyst (the tympanic orifice and cartilaginous portion of the Eustachian tube) to prevent restenosis of the marsupialized cyst cavity. Postoperative CT showed patency of the Eustachian tube. The preoperative hearing impairment recovered with an air-bone gap of 14 dB.

Dhanasekar and Jones[19] reported drainage of a cholesterol granuloma of the petrous apex, which was tackled using an endoscopic transsphenoidal approach The lesion, which abutted the posterior wall of the sphenoid sinus, was approached endoscopically via a bilateral sphenoidotomy, and the large cholesterol granuloma evacuated and marsupialized. The patient made an uneventful recovery.

Zanation and colleagues[20] described endoscopic surgical approaches to the petrous apex including the medial approach, the medial approach with internal carotid artery lateralization, and the transpterygoid infrapetrous approach (inferior to the petrous internal carotid artery). These investigators described treatment of 9 cholesterol granulomas among the 20 petrous apex lesions treated. Cholesterol granulomas all presented with variations of headache symptoms. Two had occasional vertigo. Eight of the 9 cholesterol granuloma cystic lesions were drained endoscopically (one surgery was aborted). Five patients had medial approaches (3 with carotid lateralization) and 3 had infrapetrous approaches. All drained patients had resolution of presenting symptoms. Two patients did not have complete resolution of their entire headache syndromes but described a resolution of the more severe unilateral pressure headaches, with continued occasional bilateral tension headaches that were also present preoperatively. Both of these patients described significant improvement in their quality of life and reductions in severity of pain postoperatively. These 2 patients continued to be treated by Neurology. One patient had closure of the outflow tract at 2 years without return of symptoms, and the other had revision endoscopic medial drainage at 2.5 years for reasons of scarring and neo-osteogenesis as well as return of unilateral headache. After the revision surgery, the patient had resolution of her symptoms.

Endoscopic Medial Transsphenoid Approach

With a bilateral approach, the posterior septum is transected and disarticulated from the rostrum of the sphenoid bone, and the bone of the sphenoid rostrum is removed and wide sphenoidotomies are performed. The posterior edge of the transected nasal septum is resected for approximately 1 cm with back-biting rongeurs to provide more room for instrumentation and augment the angle of approach to the lateral sphenoid.

Within the sphenoid sinus the planum sphenoidale, sella, clival recess, optic canal, medial and lateral optic-carotid recesses, and the carotid canal are identified. Depending on the degree of pneumatization, image guidance may be necessary to define the course of the internal carotid artery. Septations within the sphenoid sinus are removed with the realization that lateral septations lead to the internal carotid artery, which may be dehiscent in some cases. Care is taken during removal of these septations to avoid injury to the internal carotid artery.

If the petrous apex lesion expands into the sinus, the overlying mucosa is stripped and the bone overlying the cyst is thinned with a coarse diamond burr. Drilling starts on the medial surface of the bony deformity and runs along a vertical plane parallel to the course of the internal carotid artery. Once the bone is thin enough to fracture, small pieces of bone are "egg-shelled," then removed with a 1-mm or 2-mm angled Kerrison rongeur, and the lesion is completely unroofed. In the case of a cholesterol granuloma, the cyst wall is opened and the cyst contents are evacuated with suctions, curettes, and irrigation (**Fig. 5**). Wide communication with the cystic cavity is achieved following evacuation of the contents, and a silastic stent or cut silastic pediatric tracheal T-tube

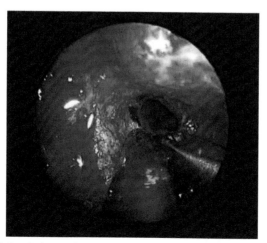

Fig. 5. Opening of the cholesterol granuloma during a medial approach. Note the characteristic yellow/brown fluid and cholesterol crystals spilling from the cavity.

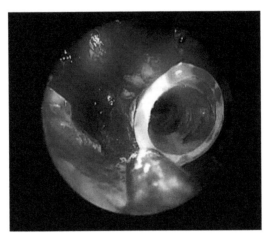

Fig. 6. An 8-mm silastic stent placed in the marsupialized cavity.

may be placed into the opening to maintain patency during the healing process (**Fig. 6**). The stent is removed in the office approximately 3 to 6 months following surgery.

Endoscopic Medial Approach with Internal Carotid Artery Lateralization

When the contour of the petrous apex lesion cannot be appreciated because of poor pneumatization of the sphenoid sinus, minimal medial expansion of the cyst, or a more posterolateral location of the cyst, additional bone removal is necessary. Decompression of the internal carotid artery allows lateral displacement of the artery and creates a larger medial window. Greater access can also be provided by thinning the bone of the clivus overlying the brainstem with the drill until the clival dura is exposed. Key landmarks for locating the internal carotid artery include the vidian artery and nerve. A transpterygoid approach is used to identify the vidian artery and trace its course to the second genu of the internal carotid artery. A middle meatal antrostomy is first performed, and the sphenopalatine artery is located at its exit from the sphenopalatine canal. Overlying bone is removed to expose the medial contents of the pterygopalatine space. The posterior nasal and sphenopalatine arteries are cauterized and transected, and the soft tissues are elevated from the underlying bone to expose the base of the pterygoids. The pterygoid tissues are dissected from medial to lateral until the vidian artery and nerve can be visualized exiting from the pterygoid canal. Bone medial and inferior to the canal is removed with a hybrid diamond drill until the course of the internal carotid artery can be delineated at the second genu. The bone overlying the vertical paraclival segment of the internal carotid artery can then be thinned and elevated to completely unroof this segment of the carotid canal. This maneuver widens the exposure by several millimeters by allowing lateral displacement of the paraclival vertical carotid segment. The petrous apex is then approached via this expanded medial corridor as described for the medial approach.

Endoscopic Transpterygoid Infrapetrous Approach

In some cases, the petrous apex lesion is not accessible via the sphenoid and is best approached inferior to the petrous internal carotid artery. This procedure requires a transpterygoid infrapetrous approach as well as dissection of the Eustachian tube and the foramen lacerum. The vidian artery and nerve are transected and

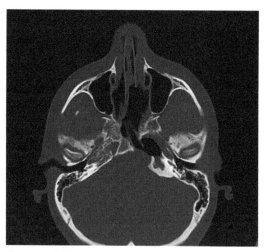

Fig. 7. Coronal CT after a medial approach and drainage of a left petrous apex cholesterol granuloma, showing complete granuloma decompression and a silastic stent in place to maintain patency.

pterygopalatine soft tissues are elevated from the base of the pterygoids in a medial to lateral direction until the second division of the trigeminal nerve is identified, where it exits the foramen rotundum. The vidian artery is traced back to the second genu of the internal carotid artery at the junction of the paraclival vertical segment and the petrous horizontal segment. Additional bone is removed from the base of the

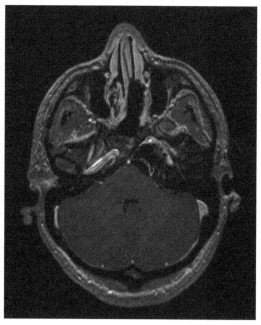

Fig. 8. Coronal T1-weighted MR image after a medial approach and drainage of a left petrous apex cholesterol granuloma, showing complete granuloma decompression.

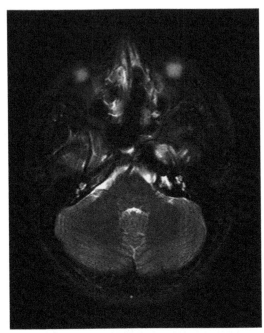

Fig. 9. Coronal T2-weighted MR image after a medial approach and drainage of a left petrous apex cholesterol granuloma, showing complete granuloma decompression.

pterygoids and the superior aspect of the medial and lateral pterygoid plates. The cartilaginous segment of the Eustachian tube is resected for approximately 1 cm. Dissection along the posterior edge of the lateral pterygoid plate exposes the third division of the trigeminal nerve. The inferior surface of the petrous apex is reached by drilling the bone between the horizontal segment of the petrous internal carotid artery and the Eustachian tube, medial to the third division of the trigeminal nerve. Once the vertical and horizontal segments of the internal carotid artery are visualized, drilling proceeds inferior to the petrous carotid into the petrous apex. Here the cyst cavity is evaluated and opened. In the case of a cholesterol granuloma, a silastic stent or cut silastic pediatric tracheal T-tube (see **Fig. 6**) is placed into the opening to maintain patency during the healing process.

The majority of cases described in the literature use a medial transsphenoid approach. Of the 19 petrous apex cholesterol granulomas described in the aforementioned case reports and case series that were drained endoscopically, 13 of 19 were approached using the medial approach; 3 of 19 were drained using the medial approach with carotid artery lateralization, and the remaining 3 drained using the infrapetrous transpterygoid approach. This variation is likely due to the majority of these lesions following a pattern of expansion that involves growth out of the petrous apex and into the posterior wall of the sphenoid sinus. Only one recurrence was reported, although several articles reported some asymptomatic narrowing of the marsupialization tract.

SUMMARY

Cholesterol granuloma is the most common benign pathologic lesion of the petrous apex, characteristically hyprintense on T1-weighted and T2-weighted MRI sequences.

These lesions can be approached via an endonasal approach using either a medial, medial with carotid lateralization, or infrapetrous transpterygoid approach. Due to the characteristic growth pattern of cholesterol granulomas, the medial approach is most frequently used. In experienced hands and with adequate drainage and marsupialization, the rate of recurrence reported in the literature is low. The transnasal, transsphenoid approach offers the advantage of no external incisions as well as a natural drainage pathway into the sinonasal cavity (**Figs. 7–9**, which match preoperative **Figs. 1–3**). Compared with traditional routes to the petrous apex including transmastoid approaches that must navigate around the facial nerve and otic capsule, or middle fossa approaches that involve brain retraction and craniotomy, the transsphenoidal approach can be faster and safer in selected cases.

EBM Question	Author's Reply
What is rate of clinical and radiographic recurrence following endoscopic transnasal drainage of cholesterol granuloma?	Endoscopic approach is associated with a 5% recurrence compared to 14.7% managed transotic. For anatomically favourable CG, the endoscopic approach is favoured (Grade C).

EVIDENCE-BASED QUESTION: WHAT IS RATE OF CLINICAL AND RADIOGRAPHIC RECURRENCE FOLLOWING ENDOSCOPIC TRANSNASAL DRAINAGE OF CHOLESTEROL GRANULOMA?

Of the 19 cholesterol granulomas reported in the literature treated with endoscopic drainage only one recurrence was noted, giving a recurrence rate of approximately 5%, as compared with a recurrence rate of 14.7% (5/34) noted in the series of transotic drainage procedures by Brackmann and Toh.[21] Thus for cases with favorable anatomy, the endoscopic transsphenoid approaches offer a low recurrence rate with minimal risk of hearing loss or damage to inner ear structures. The risk of injury to the petrous carotid or of cerebrospinal fluid leak is inherent to transotic or transsphenoid approaches; however, pneumatization along with the location of the cholesterol granuloma and the carotid should be used to guide the approach (see **Figs. 1–3, 7–9**).[22]

REFERENCES

1. Chole RA. Petrous apicitis: surgical anatomy. Ann Otol Rhinol Laryngol 1985;94: 251–7.
2. Fisch U. Infratemporal fossa approach to tumours of the temporal bone and base of skull. J Laryngol Otol 1978;92:969–77.
3. Franklin DJ, Jenkins HA, Horowitz BL, et al. Management of petrous apex lesions. Arch Otolaryngol Head Neck Surg 1989;115:1121–5.
4. Ghorayeb BY, Jahrsdoerfer RA. Subcochlear approach for cholesterol granulomas of the inferior petrous apex. Otolaryngol Head Neck Surg 1990;103:60–5.
5. Giddings NA, Brackmann DE, Kwartler JA. Transcanal infracochlear approach to the petrous apex. Otolaryngol Head Neck Surg 1991;104:29–36.
6. Glasscock ME, Woods CI, Poe DS, et al. Petrous apex cholesteatoma. Otolaryngol Clin North Am 1989;22:981–1002.
7. Goldofsky E, Hoffman RA, Holliday RA, et al. Cholesterol cysts of the temporal bone diagnosis and treatment. Ann Otol Rhinol Laryngol 1991;100:181–7.
8. Greenberg JJ, Oot RF, Wismer GL, et al. Cholesterol granuloma of the petrous apex: MR and CT evaluation. AJNR Am J Neuroradiol 1988;9:1205–14.

9. Thedinger BA, Montgomery WW, Nadol JB, et al. Radiographic diagnosis, surgical treatment, and long-term follow-up of cholesterol granulomas of the petrous apex. The Laryngoscope 1989;99(9):896–907.

10. Gianoli GJ, Amedee RG. Hearing results in surgery for primary petrous apex lesions. Otolaryngol Head Neck Surg 1993;109(2):271.

11. Fucci MJ, Alford EL, Lowry LD, et al. Endoscopic management of a giant cholesterol cyst of the petrous apex. Skull Base Surg 1994;4(1):52–8.

12. Michaelson PG, Cable BB, Mair EA. Image-guided transsphenoidal drainage of a cholesterol granuloma of the petrous apex in a child. Int J Pediatr Otorhinolaryngol 2001;57(2):165–9.

13. DiNardo LJ, Pippin GW, Sismanis A. Image-guided endoscopic transsphenoidal drainage of select petrous apex cholesterol granulomas. Otol Neurotol 2003;24(6): 939–41.

14. Oyama K, Ikezono T, Tahara S, et al. Petrous apex cholesterol granuloma treated via the endoscopic transsphenoidal approach. Acta Neurochir (Wien) 2007;149(3): 299–302.

15. Chatrath P, Nouraei SA, De Cordova J, et al. Endonasal endoscopic approach to the petrous apex: an image-guided quantitative anatomical study. Clin Otolaryngol 2007;32(4):255–60.

16. Georgalas C, Kania R, Guichard JP, et al. Endoscopic transsphenoidal surgery for cholesterol granulomas involving the petrous apex. Clin Otolaryngol 2008;33(1): 38–42.

17. Samadian M, Vazirnezami M, Moqaddasi H, et al. Endoscopic transrostral-transsphenoidal approach to petrous apex cholesterol granuloma: case report. Turk Neurosurg 2009;19(1):106–11.

18. Haginomori S, Mori A, Kanazawa A, et al. Endoscopy-assisted surgery with topical mitomycin for a cholesterol granuloma in the petrous apex. Laryngoscope 2009; 119(12):2437–40.

19. Dhanasekar G, Jones NS. Endoscopic trans-sphenoidal removal of cholesterol granuloma of the petrous apex: case report and literature review. J Laryngol Otol 2010;26:1–4.

20. Zanation AM, Snyderman CH, Carrau RL, et al. Endoscopic endonasal surgery for petrous apex lesions. Laryngoscope 2009;119(1):19–25.

21. Brackmann DE, Toh EH. Surgical management of petrous apex cholesterol granulomas. Otol Neurotol 2002;23(4):529–33.

22. Lee SC, Senior BA. Endoscopic skull base surgery. Clin Exp Otorhinolaryngol 2008; 1(2):53–62.

Carotid Artery Injury After Endonasal Surgery

Rowan Valentine, MBBS[a,b], Peter-John Wormald, MD[a,b],*

KEYWORDS

- Carotid artery injury • Hemostasis • Endoscopic
- Transphenoidal • Pseudoaneurysm

EBM Question	Level of Evidence	Grade of Recommendation
What factors contribute to ICA injury and what is best management of ICA injury?	4	C

Over the past 2 decades a paradigm shift has occurred from traditional external approaches to the skull base, paranasal sinuses, and intracranial cavities, to the completely endonasal surgical approach. Endonasal microscopic techniques to the sella turcica rapidly became the preferred approach after the introduction of the operating microscope in 1951. The introduction of the surgical endoscope has seen a rejuvenated interest into the paranasal sinus and endonasal skull base anatomy. The endoscopic resection of pituitary and other skull base tumors is rapidly being adopted as the standard of care by otolaryngologists and neurosurgeons worldwide.[1] The popularity of endonasal techniques is largely because of the well-recognized advantages, including the avoidance of external skin incisions, minimal sacrifice of intervening structures, improved visualization, reduced postoperative pain, and shorter hospital admissions.[2]

Rupture of the internal carotid artery (ICA) is the most feared and devastating complication of endoscopic sinus and skull base surgery, and may result in death.[3] Injury to the cavernous ICA most commonly results in rupture and overwhelming

Disclosures and Conflicts of interest: Dr Wormald receives royalties from Medtronic ENT for instruments designed and is a consultant for Neilmed Pharmaceuticals. Dr Valentine has nothing to disclose.

[a] Department of Surgery-Otorhinolaryngology, Head and Neck Surgery, University of Adelaide, North Terrace, Adelaide 5000, Australia

[b] Department of Surgery-Otorhinolaryngology, Head and Neck Surgery, The Queen Elizabeth Hospital, 28 Woodville Road, Woodville, South Australia 5011, Australia

* Corresponding author. Department of Surgery-Otorhinolaryngology, Head and Neck Surgery, The Queen Elizabeth Hospital, 28 Woodville Road, Woodville, South Australia 5011, Australia.
E-mail address: Peter.Wormald@adelaide.edu.au

Otolaryngol Clin N Am 44 (2011) 1059–1079
doi:10.1016/j.otc.2011.06.009
0030-6665/11/$ – see front matter. Crown Copyright © 2011 Published by Elsevier Inc. All rights reserved.

hemorrhage, with the frequent formation of a pseudoaneurysm.[3,4] Injury may also cause spasm, thrombosis, embolism, or the formation of a caroticocavernous fistula (CCF)[4] with significant associated morbidity.

Injury to the cavernous ICA is a rare event during endoscopic sinus surgery (ESS). May and colleagues[5] reviewed their experience with ICA injury during ESS and only found 1 case among 4691 patients. Despite the frequency of ESS within the community, a review of the English literature shows a total of only 28 case reports of ICA injury since the advent of the endoscopic approach to the paranasal sinuses (**Table 1**). The frequency of cavernous ICA injury is much more significant during endonasal, transphenoidal skull base surgery. Raymond and colleagues[3] and Ciric and colleagues[54] showed a 1.1% incidence of ICA injury after the microscopic transphenoidal pituitary approach. More extended endonasal approaches (EEA) center around the management of the internal carotid artery, and not surprisingly have a much higher incidence of ICA injury. Frank and colleagues,[7] Gardner and colleagues,[9] and Couldwell and colleagues[22] reviewed their experience with consecutive EEA resections of craniopharyngiomas, clival chordomas, and chondrosarcomas, showing a 5% to 9% incidence of ICA rupture.

Although experience and knowledge of the relevant anatomy can prevent many potential complications associated with transphenoidal surgery, ICA injury cannot be completely eliminated considering the frequency of these procedures and the increasing complexity of the skull base pathologies encountered. Through review of the endonasal surgical literature, this article focuses on the risk factors for an ICA injury during endonasal surgery, the management of an ICA injury and the complications of this catastrophic surgical event.

PATIENTS AT RISK

Prevention of the catastrophic bleeding scenario is better than treatment. It is important to recognize the patient that maybe at risk of an ICA injury. The anatomic relationship between the ICA and the sphenoid sinus makes it particularly vulnerable. Fujii and colleagues[55] demonstrated that the bony wall overlying the ICA is not sufficient to protect the artery, at less than 0.5 mm thick. Additionally, in 4 to 22% of cases the lateral sphenoid wall is dehiscent over the carotid with only dura and the sphenoid sinus mucosa separating the ICA from the sphenoid.[15,55] Renn and Rhoton also found that the ICA bulges into the sphenoid sinus in 71% of cases, and that the artery maybe located as close as 4 mm from the midline.[56] Some authors have found that the distance between the internal carotid arteries within the sphenoid maybe as little as 4 mm,[57] and that the boney sphenoid septum inserts on to the ICA canal wall 16.3%[58] of occasions.

Cavernous ICA anomalies are also not infrequent, with cavernous ICA aneurysm making up 12.8% of all intracranial aneurysms. Some authors have shown an increased incidence of aneurysms in patients with pituitary adenomas,[59,60] leading some to suggest mechanisms such as mechanical influence, infiltration by the tumor, growth hormone and an IGF-1 effect on the arterial wall.[29,59] There have been numerous reports of unrecognized pre-operative cavernous ICA aneurysms resulting in ICA rupture. When reviewing all 111 case reports of endonasal cavernous ICA ruptures (see **Table 1**), there are a total of 6 patients that had a pre-operative unrecognized ICA aneurysm. In the 3 patients reported by Koitschev and colleagues,[10] all 3 patients died as a result of uncontrolled hemorrhage, perhaps as a result of a larger defect of the vessel wall with a consecutively higher blood loss.

Table 1
Case reports and case series of ICA rupture events following endonasal surgery

				English Literature Case Reports of ICA Rupture Following Endonasal Surgery				
Article	ESS	S.B.	Pres.	Management	Out.	Patency	Comp.	Risk F.
Chen[6]	—	*	I + D	packing/balloon	-	✗	PA	-
		*	I + D	packing/balloon	✓	✗	PA	-
		*	I + D	packing/conservative	-	✓	PA	-
		*	I + D	packing/coil	✓	✓	PA	R
Frank et al[7]	—	*	—	packing/unknown	✗	-	PA	R
Fukushima[8]	—	*	—	bipolar + surgicel packing	✓	-	✗	-
		*	—	bipolar + surgicel packing	✓	-	✗	-
		*	—	teflon + m. methacrylate	✓	✓	✗	-
		*	—	teflon + m. methacrylate	✓	✓	✗	-
		*	—	teflon + m. methacrylate	✓	✓	✗	-
		*	—	teflon + m. methacrylate/surgery	-	-	PA/CCF	-
Gardner et al[9]	—	*	—	syvek patch	✗	-	-	-
Koitschev[10]	*	—	—	packing + balloon	✓	✗	✗	-
	*	—	—	packing + balloon	✓	✗	✗	-
Laws[4]	—	*	—	exanguination	✢	-	-	-
		*	—	direct suture repair	-	-	-	-
		*	—	direct suture repair	-	-	-	-
		*	—	sundt-type clip graft	-	-	-	-
		*	—	balloon	-	-	-	-
		*	—	balloon	-	-	-	-
Lippert[11]	—	*	D	rubber foam + stent	✓	✓	PA	-
	*	—	—	stent/stent	✓	✓	PA	-
Park[12]	*	—	—	carotid tie off + packing + coil	✓	✗	-	-
Pepper[13]	—	*	—	packing/balloon	✓	✗	PA	-
	*	—	—	packing + balloon	✗	✗	✗	-

(continued on next page)

Table 1
(continued)

				English Literature Case Reports of ICA Rupture Following Endonasal Surgery				
Article	ESS	S.B.	Pres.	Management	Out.	Patency	Comp.	Risk F.
Raymond[3]	-	*	D	surgicel ± muscle ± glue/balloon	✓	✗	PA	-
		*	-	surgicel ± muscle ± glue	✗	s	✗	-
		*	-	surgicel ± muscle ± glue	✓	✗	✗	B
		*	- + D	surgicel ± muscle ± glue/balloon	✗	✗	✗	-
		*	-	surgicel ± muscle ± glue	✗	✗	✗	A
		*	-	surgicel ± muscle ± glue + balloon + bypass	✗	✗	✗	-
		*	-	surgicel ± muscle ± glue	✓✓	✗	✗	R
		*	-	surgicel ± muscle ± glue	✓✓	✗	✗	A
		*	- + D	surgicel ± muscle ± glue/balloon	✗	✗	PA	R
		*	D	exanguination	✛	-	PA	-
		*	-	surgicel ± muscle ± glue	✛	✗	✗	B
		*	D	surgicel ± muscle ± glue	✓✓	✗	✗	A
		*	-	surgicel ± muscle ± glue	✓✓	✗	PA	A, R, RT, B
		*	-	surgicel ± muscle ± glue	✓	-	-	B
		*	-	surgicel ± muscle ± glue/balloon	✗	✗	✗	-
		*	- + D	surgicel ± muscle ± glue/ exanguination	✛	-	PA	R
		*	-	surgicel ± muscle ± glue + balloon	✗	✗	✗	-
Stippler[14]	-	*	-	unknown	✗	-	-	R, RT
Weidenbecher[15]	*	-	-	packing	✛	-	-	-
	*			muscle	✓	-	✗	-
	*			muscle/surgical clipping	✓✓	-	PA	-
	*			muscle/balloon occlusion	✓✓	-	PA	-
Ahuja[16]	-	*	-	packing	✓✓	✓	CCF	-
		*	- + D	muscle + fibrin glue/balloon	✓✓	✗	PA/CCF	-
		*	-	gelfoam + surgicel pack/balloon	✓	✗	PA	A
Cappabianca[17]	-	*	-	packing/coil	-	✗	PA	R, A

Study				Treatment			PA	A
Fatemi[18]	—	*	I	packing/balloon	✓	✗		R
			I	packing	✓	✗	x	-
			I	packing	✓	✗	x	-
			I	packing	✓	✓	x	-
Zhao[19]	—	*	I	packing	✗	-	-	-
			I + D	packing + stent	✗	-	x	-
Lister[20]	*	—	I	packing/surgical	✗	✗	PA/CCF	R, RT
Kaptain[21]	—	*	I	unknown	✗	✗	-	-
Couldwell[22]	—		I	unknown	✗	-	-	-
			I	unknown	-	-	-	-
			I	unknown	-	-	-	-
			I	unknown	-	-	-	-
Maniglia[23]	*	—	I	unknown	⊕	-	PA	-
Bavinzski[24]	—	*	D	balloon	✓	x	PA	-
Cappabianca[25]	—		I	floseal/coil	-	-	CCF	-
Weber[26]	*		I	Packing	-	-	-	-
	*		I	unknown	⊕	-	-	-
	*		I	unknown	⊕	-	-	-
Park[27]	—	*	I	fleece coated fibrin glue/stent/coil	✓	✓	-	-
Reddy[28]	—	*	I + D	packing/surgical	✓	x	PA	A
Berker[29]	—	*	I	packing/stent	✓	-	PA	R
Biswas[30]	—	*	D	surgical/coil	x	-	PA	-
Kocer[31]	—	*	I	packing/stent	-	-	CCF	-
Kadyrov[32]	—	*	I	packing/coil/stent	✓	x	PA	-
Zada[33]	—	*	I	muslin gauze + glue + fat/coil	✓	✓	PA	A

(continued on next page)

Table 1
(continued)

English Literature Case Reports of ICA Rupture Following Endonasal Surgery

Article	ESS	S.B.	Pres.	Management	Out.	Patency	Comp.	Risk F.
Kim[34]	—	*	—	cottonoid pressure/coil	✓	✗	PA	R
Isenberg[35]	*	—	—	packing/balloon	✓	✗	PA	-
Hudgins[36]	*	—	—	packing/balloon	✓	✗	PA	-
Wigand[37]	*	—	—	unknown	±	-	-	-
De Souza[38]	—	*	—	unknown/stent	-	✓	PA	A
Leung[39]	*	—	—	packing + stent	-	✓	✗	-
Keerl[40]	*		—	unknown	±	-	-	-
	*		—	unknown	±	-	-	-
	*		—	unknown	±	-	-	-
	*		—	unknown	✓	-	-	-
	*		—	unknown	✓	-	-	-
	*		—	unknown	✗	-	-	-
	*		—	unknown	✗	-	-	-
	*		—	unknown	✗	-	-	-
Charalampaki[41]	—	*	—	packing + stent	✓	-	-	-
Ghatge[42]	—	*	—	packing/Amplazt embolization	✓	✗	✗	-
	—	*	—	packing/stent	±	✗	-	R, RT
Crowley[43]	—	*	D	packing + coil	✗	✗	PA	-

Study				Technique				
Cathelinaud[44]	*	—	I + D	packing/coil/stent	✓	✓	PA	-
Ciceri[45]	—	*	D	no management	✓	✓	PA	-
			I	bipolar	-	-	PA	-
			D	stent/coil	-	✓	PA	-
				coil/balloon	-	✗	PA	-
Vanninen[46]	—	*	I + D	Oxygel + glue/stent	✓	✓	PA	-
Dolenc[47]	—	*	I	surgicel packing/surgery	✓	✓	PA/CCF	-
Pigott[48]	—	*	I + D	packing/balloon	✗	✓	PA/CCF	-
Dusick[49]	—	*	I	Muslin gauze + fibrin glue/coils	✓	-	PA	A
				Muslin gauze + fibrin glue/coils	✓	✗	PA	-
Lempert[50]	—	*	I	packing + foley balloon/coil	✓	✓	PA	-
			I	unknown/coil	✓	✓	PA	-
			D	unknown/coil	✓	✓	PA	-
Paullus[51]	—	*	I	surgicel packing/surgery	✓	✗	PA/CCF	-
Cabezudo[52]	—	*	I + D	surgicel + gauze packing/surgery	✓	✗	PA/CCF	A
Wilson[53]	—	*	I + D	packing/surgery	-	✗	PA	A

Abbreviations: A, acromegaly; B, bromocriptine; CCF, cartico-cavernous fisula; Comp., complication; D, delayed; I, intraopeative; Out., outcome; PA, pseudoaneurysm; Pres., presentation; R, revision surgery; RT, radiotherapy; S.B., skull base surgery; ✓, no sequalae; ✗, permanent neurologic morbidity or occlusion of ICA; -, unknown; Φ, death.

Numerous authors have linked the association of a number of important patient risk factors associated with a cavernous ICA injury. Raymond and colleagues[3] reviewed their series of 17 ICA injuries showing that 5/17 patients had prior bromocriptine therapy, 5/17 were revision cases, 4/17 had previous radiation therapy and 6/17 pts had acromegaly. Additionally patients with acromegaly tend to have more tortuous and ectatic carotid arteries.[4,61] While most case reports and series do not discuss the specific case risk factors, a review of the literature (see **Table 1**) demonstrates that it is known that these risk factors contributed in 27 ICA injury cases, some cases with multiple risk factors (revision surgery = 13, radiotherapy = 4, acromegaly = 13, bromocriptine therapy = 4). These features may cause more fibrosis and adherence to the carotid artery, or may simply reflect a more aggressive attempt at complete resection of invasive lesions.

Tumors closely adherent to the ICA require close and careful dissection. Bejjani and colleagues[62] demonstrated that vasospasm occurred in 9 of 470 patients undergoing skull base tumor dissection. In this series vasospasm manifested as altered mental status and/or hemiparesis with risk factors including preoperative embolization, tumor size, vessel encasement/narrowing and total operative time. Three of these patients suffered permanent neurologic deficits. Laws[4] also cautions regarding dissection of tumor away for the cavernous ICA, or displacement of the carotid within the cavernous sinus during attempted hemostasis. They describe 1 fatal, and 2 non-fatal cases as a result of carotid spasm and thrombosis following endonasal transsphenoidal surgery.

It is imperative that the 'at risk' patient is identified by a thorough pre-operative assessment so that a cavernous ICA injury can be minimized (**Box 1**). A thorough and careful preoperative assessment of the sella region should be obtained, with the use of a CT scan to help delineate vessel anatomy and its relationship to the sphenoid sinus. MRI scans can demonstrate preoperative ICA aneurysms, with any suspicion confirmed with MRA or digital subtraction angiography.[29,31]

INTRA-OPERATIVE MANAGEMENT OF A CAVERNOUS ICA RUPTURE
Controlling the Surgical Field

Intra-operative ICA rupture creates an immediately challenging surgical field, with a high pressure/high flow bleeding scenario, which may rapidly result in exsanguination of the patient. Massive bleeding leads to a loss of orientation and an obscured surgical field often resulted in the surgeon blindly attempting nasal packing to control the hemorrhage. Additional suction is important to regain orientation of the surgical

---

Box 1
Risk factors for ICA rupture

- Anatomic relationships
  - Carotid dehiscence
  - Sphenoid septal attachment to ICA
  - Midline ICA
- Revision surgery
- Prior radiotherapy
- Prior bromocriptine treatment
- Acromegaly

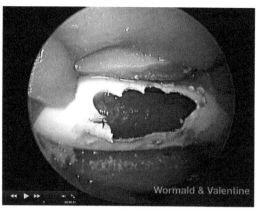

Fig. 1. Animal model of endonasal carotid artery injury, with exposure of the carotid artery within sphenoid sinus.

field. The advantages of the '2 surgeon' skull base team allows for dynamic handling of the endoscope, rather than the single surgeon scenario. Valentine and colleagues have recently developed a reproducible animal model for the carotid artery catastrophe that recreates the intranasal confines of the human nasal cavity, paranasal sinuses and nasal vestibule (**Fig. 1**). The authors describe their experience with 42 carotid artery injuries and this model, and the surgical steps that enable rapid control the surgical field. The authors relied on the surgical cooperation of both surgeons, acting fluently and quickly to navigate the endoscope's tip away from the vascular stream and maintaining vision. Frequently a 'jet of blood' quickly soiled the endoscopes tip, and the authors found it useful to deliberately place the endoscope into the nostril that afforded some protection offered by the posterior septal edge deflecting the vascular stream into the opposite nostril (**Fig. 2**). Two large bore suction systems were particularly useful. If the suction instruments were placed below the endoscope (as is routine during ESS) then it frequently results in blood tracking up

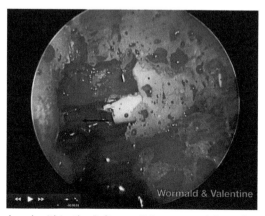

Fig. 2. Endoscope placed within the left nostril is protected from frequent tip soiling by posterior septal edge (*arrow* indicates vascular stream).

the suction and soiling the endoscope tip. This frequent occurrence was prevented by placing the suction in the opposite nasal cavity, and allowed the suction to simultaneously guide the vascular stream away from the endoscope tip (in press, laryngoscope).

Intra-Operative Hemostatic Techniques

Every surgical team should have a plan in place should this unexpected complication occur; formulating and executing a plan of action during a crisis is difficult. Emergency surgical ligation has traditionally been used to treat an ICA injury; however, this treatment is often associated with a high incidence of major complications such as death and stroke,[3,63] and is often an ineffective and harmful treatment. In good collateralization or contralateral compensation the bleeding is likely to still be rapid. Ligation of the internal and external carotid arteries would not only waste time but also block the interventional radiologists' access to the site of injury.

In the event of unexpected massive bleeding during endonasal surgery then immediate packing is required. A number of techniques have been described and advocated in order the aid this. Some authors advocated for head elevation, and controlled hypotension to reduce the hemorrhage.[11] These measures are likely unnecessary considering the immediate and significant hypotension that will result from massive bleeding while the anesthetic team is trying to implement active resuscitation.[34] If large bore suction devices and the immediate state of hypotension are not enough to keep pace with the bleeding and allow nasal packing then ipsilateral common carotid artery compression is frequently advocated to slow the bleeding rate and can aid the accurate placement of nasal packing.[3,8,11,15] Regarding blood pressure control, Kassam and colleagues, Solares and colleagues and Pepper and colleagues all recommend maintaining normotension through resuscitative measures and fluid replacement to maintain contralateral cerebral perfusion.[13,64,65] However, normotension is unlikely to be achieved until the hemorrhage has been controlled. Once vascular control is assured then attention should focus on maintaining adequate cerebral perfusion.

There is a number of different packing agents that have been used during an ICA rupture. A review of the literature demonstrates that gauze packing is overwhelmingly the most frequently used material, likely due to its availability and easy of use. However a number of different agents have been used including Teflon and methyl methacrylate patch,[8] Syvek marine polymer,[9] muscle patch,[3,15,16] fibrin glue,[12,16] gel foam and oxidized cellulose packing,[16,30,47] thrombin-gelatin matrix,[25] Oxygel and glue[46] and muslin gauze.[33,49] Packing materials ideally should be placed with just enough force to control the hemorrhage but not to occlude vascular flow.[4] Absorbable and biocompatible hemostatic agents are advantageous as they don't require subsequent removal, which can result in re-bleeding if no additional endovascular procedures are undertaken. Raymond and colleagues[3] describe their success with oxidized regenerated cellulose, muscle plugs and tissue adhesives. Profuse intra-operative bleeding occurred in 14 patients and was controlled in all cases, however later reoccurred in 3 patients requiring either a return to theater or endovascular balloon occlusion. Packing was the only method of treatment in 9 patients, with no endovascular treatment, however 1 patient died on day 7 from concurrent basilar artery compression, and another from recurrent tumor at 2 mths of follow-up. The other seven patients had no further bleeding events (follow-up 6mths – 10yrs).[3] Recently Valentine and colleagues compared the hemostatic efficacy of various absorbable and biocompatible materials in the endoscopic carotid artery injury scenario. This study investigated the efficacy of a thrombin-gelatin matrix, oxidized

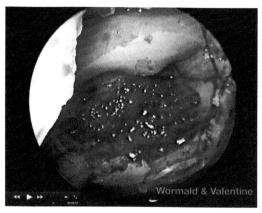

Fig. 3. 'Crushed' muscle patch in situ on carotid injury site. Complete hemostasis has been achieved.

regenerated cellulose and the crushed muscle patch treatment (**Fig. 3**). Hemostats were applied with just enough force to not compress the artery and allowing ongoing vascular flow. Results demonstrated that the muscle patch treatment achieved rapid hemostasis in all cases, with a mean time to hemostasis of 11 minutes 25 secs. Hemostasis was not achieved in all other topical treatment agents. This evidence strongly supports the use of the crushed muscle patch treatment. However, its application requires careful placement without compression of the vessel, and held in direct contact the vessel defect for approximately 12 minutes. Which packing material to use depends on the size of the vascular defect, what is available within the theater environment and also the past experiences of the surgical team.

Over-packing of the injury site can also be a problem. Endonasal packing often can result in occlusion or stenosis of the cavernous ICA and other major vascular structures.[66] Raymond and colleagues[3] reviewed their angiographic data in 12 patients showing that 8 of 12 had ICA occlusion, and 4 of 12 patients had carotid stenosis. They concluded that over-packing can contribute to the morbidity and mortality of the patient. Laws[4] also concedes that while patency of the ICA is preferred, there our some occasions that the only option is to occlude the ICA with packing and raise the blood pressure in the hope that the collateral circulation will prevent stroke formation.

Direct vascular closure has also been used intra-operatively. Laws[4] described the successful use of direct suture repair in 2 cases, and the use of a sundt-type clip graft, however the details and outcomes of these techniques are not described. Valentine and colleagues[67] recently analyzed the hemostatic efficacy the U-Clip anastomotic device (Medtronic, Jacksonville, FL, USA). This is an endoscopic suturing device that has been successfully used for the suturing of coronary artery vascular anastomosis and for dural reconstructions of the skull base. This device was very effective at achieving hemostasis and maintaining vascular patency however the long-term outcomes remain (**Fig. 4**).

Unfortunately it is not always possible to achieve intra-operative hemostasis, and transfer to the angiography suite is needed so that endovascular intervention can be performed while the airway is secured.[30,31] Even though intra-operative hemostasis and vascular control is achieved in most cases, all patients need to have an immediate angiogram so that ICA injury complications can be sought. Angiography should also

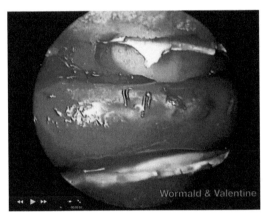

Fig. 4. Four endoscopically place U-clips close the ICA injury site. Hemostasis has been achieved while maintaining vascular patency, and without significant narrowing.

include the external carotid artery if no abnormality is found within the ICA territory. The otolaryngologist should be available and present to loosen the packing if localization of the ICA injury is not possible due to overtight nasal packing.[65] The optimal management is a balloon test occlusion (BTO); however, this requires a cooperative and awake patient to allow for a full neurologic examination. Awaking the patient and removal of a secure airway is unwise in the face of ongoing ICA bleeding, and hemodynamic instability.[12,24,42] Other measures that have been used to determine the presence of adequate collateral flow include analysis of the preoperative MR angiography,[12] transcranial doppler analysis,[44] SPECT imaging[38] and Xenon CT.[11] Even with a well performed and normal BTO there is still a 5–10% risk of delayed infarction after therapeutic carotid artery occlusion.[68]

Endovascular techniques that are available to the interventional radiologist include both balloon and coil embolization, however there are increasing reports of the successful use of endovascular stent-graft placement. Over the last 10yrs transluminal endovascular stent-grafts have increased in popularity, and grafts within the aorta, peripheral vessels and coronary arteries have been reported as safe and effective.[69] Numerous authors recommend the use of endovascular balloon or coil embolization in those patients that have adequate collateral blood flow.[6,27,38,42] Otherwise either an endovascular or surgical bypass procedure is required. Stent-graft placement is advised in those that don't tolerate ICA occlusion.[27,38,42,44] Some have suggested that all patients have a trial of stent placement, but if this is unsuccessful, then those patients should undergo embolization if tolerated, otherwise a extracranial/intracranial bypass procedure is required.[64]

ENDOVASCULAR TECHNIQUES

Endovascular techniques aimed at closing a vascular wall defect can either occlude the parent vessel or maintain vascular flow. When performing endovascular techniques it is important to remember that carotid artery injury most frequently occurs only a few millimeters below the origin of the ophthalmic artery.[3] Both the deployment of a endovascular balloon and coil can be associated with subsequent distal migration and slippage.[27] The main difficulty is deployment in a high-flow vessel where distal migration may occur, resulting in blindness or death.[11] The distal balloon should be detached from the introducer only after the more proximal balloon is inflated (minimizing migration).[27] Regarding the deployment of an endovascular coi, Park and colleagues[12] describe a technique of digital compression of the cervical ICA and creating a angiographically confirmed low-flow system. This enabled more accurate distal and proximal trapping of the injury site.

Balloon occlusion techniques should be performed at the level of the vascular injury, thus preventing ongoing bleeding from both antegrade and retrograde vessel filling. It is also important that a more proximal balloon is placed as balloon deflation can occur.[70] If a balloon cannot be placed at the site of injury, a balloon proximal to the injury and a balloon distal to the injury should be sited. Endovascular coil occlusion uses stainless steel or platinum based material that is helically shaped with multiple attached dacron wool strands that increase its thrombogenicity. As the straightened coil is released into the parent vessel it resumes its spiral shape and wedges against the vessel wall to form a thrombus. This thrombus formation may take a little time and, theoretically, there is an increased risk of thromboembolic events; however, this has not been shown in the literature. Finally, Higashida and colleagues[71] recommends close post-intervention monitoring to keep the blood pressure between 110 to 160 Hg systolic and 60 to 110 mmHg diastolic for a 2 to 3 days post occlusion.

The main technical difficulty associated with stent-graft placement within the cavernous ICA is the limited longitudinal flexibility of the graft. Newer sent grafts have improved significantly and there are 12 successful case reports (see **Table 1**), however 3 of these had poor longitudinal flexibility and poor intravascular seating requiring additional procedures. These 3 cases required further coiling and a novel 'stent-in-stent' technique.[11,27,32] ICA spasm has also been reported as a result of difficult positioning of the stent-graft.[31] The most frequently used stent is the coronary stent-graft, consisting of both sides (luminal and abluminal sides) covered with polytetrafluoroethylene. Stent-graft placement also risks distant migration. In the future improved longitudinal flexibility may see endovascular stent-graft placement become the preferred option of management in all patients regardless of BTO results.

Complications following endovascular occlusion or repair can result in thromboemoblic events or stent-graft thrombsis. A survey performed by Wholey and colleagues[72] showed a 4.4% risk of stroke within the first 30 days following carotid stent placement. However the risk of stroke from the placement on endovascular stent is likely to be significantly less than performing endovascular occlusion in a patient that can't tolerate BTO. Antiplatelet therapy and heparin treatment can provide effective prophylaxis and reversal in cases of TIA or stroke.[6] Regarding the anticoagulation and antiplatelet regimen used, most authors advocate for some preventative treatment. Heparin therapy is recommended before endovascular intervention and before the BTO.[27,39,44] De Souza uses oral ticlopidine for 4 weeks following stent placement,[38] Park and colleagues and Leung and colleagues recommended aspirin and clopidogrel therapy for upto 3 months.[27,39]

DELAYED CAVERNOUS ICA INJURY

It is important to remember that not all ICA injuries manifest during the intra-operative period. The occurrence of vasospasm in the ICA following transphenoidal surgery has been described as early as a few hours following surgery and upto 1 month following,[4] and can be recognized as altered consciouness or stroke formation. Laws[4] also notes 2 cases of carotid artery thrombosis following transphenoidal surgery. Delayed formation of a pseudoaneurysm following uneventful transphenoidal surgery is also well known, with 9 known case reports (see **Table 1**), developing anywhere from 1 week post-operatively to over 20 years later.[24] Perhaps the most surprising, to both the patient and the surgical team, is the delayed presentation of a ruptured pseudoaneurysm in the post-operative period following an uneventful transphenoidal surgical procedure. Raymond and colleagues reported 3 patients that underwent uneventful surgery, with one ruptured pseudoaneurysm presenting on day 9, another on day 12 and the last some 10 years after the surgical procedure. This scenario is likely to present out of the hospital setting, and patients will present in severe haemodynamic comprimise, with a particularly poor prognosis (**Fig. 5**). Review of the literature shows there are 6 case reports of a delayed ruptured pseudoaneurysm following uneventful surgery. Two patients survived without long-term sequelae, 1 patient died, and 3 patients suffered permanent neurologic deficits (see **Table 1**).

COMPLICATIONS OF CAVERNOUS ICA RUPTURE

Following an ICA rupture it is important that all patients receive a post-operative angiogram. If this is normal then all patients should receive a repeat angiogram after the packing has been removed. Iatrogenic ICA injury can create a communicating channel between the sphenoid and/or the cavernous sinus and the sidewall of ICA. This

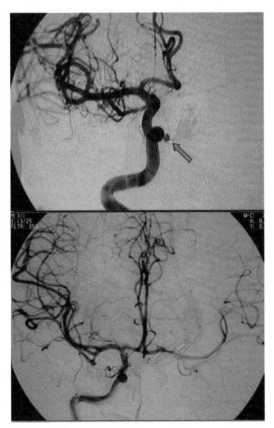

Fig. 5. Angiogram demonstrating a right ICA pseudoaneurysm (*red arrow*) in a 54 yr old male developed following pituitary surgery. Treated with proximal and distal balloon occlusion. (*Courtesy of* Dr Aldo Stamm.)

situation may present as an acute hemorrhage, pseudoaneurysm or a CCF. A CCF can most easily be recognized clinically by the presence of proptosis with opthalmoplegia and an orbital bruit.

The most frequent complication following cavernous ICA rupture is the formation of a pseudoaneurysm. A pseudoaneurysm is a tear through all the layers of the artery with persistent flow outside the vessel into a space contained by surrounding tissue.[73] Pseudoaneurysm formation is a common occurrence following intra-operative rupture and trauma to the cavernous ICA, and hence active followup and regular angiographic screen is recommended in all patients, both postoperatively and following discharge. Pseudoaneurysm as a complication of ICA rupture may present 10 years later.[3] Some authors state that all direct injuries to the ICA repaired by indirect measures will result in a pseudoaneurysm,[4,66] however Laws[4] also concedes that placing muscle as a hemostat offers an opportunity for effective healing without the formation of a pseudoaneurysm. There are a total of 72 reports of intraoperative ICA rupture events (undergoing local packing treatment) where the pseudoaneurysm status is published. A review of these cases demonstrates that 43 subsequently developed a pseudoaneurysm, a 60% incidence (see **Table 1**). A total of 12 of 43 ruptured postoperatively and required subsequent treatment. The other 25/43 were identified at routine angiography and underwent prophylactic treatment. Six cases were managed conservatively. It is interesting to note that only 3/17 patients in Raymond and colleagues[3] series developed a pseudoaneurysm. This maybe to due to the high rate of permanent vascular occlusion during intra-operative packing control.

Pseudoaneurysm's frequently rupture and treatment begins with airway control, rapid resuscitation and local packing measures. Similar hemostatic measures can be performed as described above. While most advocate for prompt neuroradiological intervention, some authors transfered the patient directly to theater for hemorrhage control first.[3] Once again a BTO is preferred, but in the intubated patient this makes neurologic assessment difficult. Ideally, in the patient who is not actively bleeding and where local packing measures are adequate, then the patient should undergo a formal BTO. When a pseudoaneurysm is found at a routine followup angiogram is more easily managed. In this situation a 30-minute BTO is performed, where tolerance is assessed by a complete neurologic examination, with collateral circulation assessed by angiography.[3] This can be performed in conjunction with other neurophysiological techniques. Once again, a number of techniques are described to manage a pseudoaneurysm including endovascular balloon or coil isolation and stent-graft placement. Endovascular isolation techniques are preferred in those patients who can tolerate the BTO. As always, a period of close observation to ensuring normotension/mild hypertension is warranted. In the patient that cannot tolerate BTO there are 3 main treatment options; stent-graft placement, isolated endovascular occlusion of the pseudoaneurysm lumen and surgery (either bypass surgery, or aneurismal clipping). It is well accepted that extracranial/intracranial bypass surgery is associated with a high complication rate and that stent-graft placement represents a safer treatment option.[74]

There is much controversy regarding endovascular coil or balloon occlusion of the pseudoaneurysm lumen while preserving the parent artery in an attempting to maintain parent vessel patency. Most authors state that a pseudoaneurysm is fragile and has no wall to contain the embolus,[4,38,75] and that there is a considerable risk of fatal rebleeding due to compression on the fragile wall.[46,76] Fox and colleagues[77] demonstrated in a series of 68 patients that isolated pseudoaneurysm lumen occlusion was associated with an increased complication profile. Higashida and colleagues[78] have demonstrated an increased morbidity and mortality when treated in this fashion.

This treatment is probably reserved for those patients who cannot tolerate complete occlusion of the cavernous ICA, and in which stent-graft placement is not possible. Despite this, pseudoaneurysm lumen occlusion with preservation of patency of the cavernous ICA has been achieved following transphenoidal injury. A review of the literature demonstrates that there a 7 cases of ICA injury that resulted in the formation of a pseudoaneurysm that was subsequently treated by isolated coiling or balloon therapy of the lumen, with preservation of ICA vascular flow (see **Table 1**).[6,33,48,50] However, 1 case resulted in subsequent migration of the balloon embolus through the wall of the pseudoaneurysm[6] and another resulted in asymptomatic migration of the coil within the pseudoaneurysm necessitating stent-graft placement.[32] CCF is probably the only injury in which treatment with detachable balloons or coils is appropriate, while attempting to preserve the patency of the parent vessel. This situation is more likely to be successful as this injury is somewhat less urgent than other arterial injuries.[31]

OUTCOMES

Rupture of the cavernous ICA represents a significant insult to the hemodynamic stability of the patient and is not surprising associated with a significant morbidity and subsequent mortality. If is difficult to draw any significant conclusions from a comprehensive literature review as these are case reports only. Many cases of intraoperative ICA rupture may not be published, especially as death and neurologic injury are a common endpoint. Reviewing the 111 cases of ICA rupture, there are a total of 89 cases where the endpoint was published. While likely underestimated, there was a mortality rate of 15% (13/89) and a permanent morbidity rate of 26% (23/89). A total of 59% of patients (53/89) that suffered from a ruptured ICA escaped the event without any permanent sequalae (see **Table 1**). This is similar to the series published by Raymond and colleagues[3] that described a 17% mortality and 29% related morbidity.

SUMMARY

Internal carotid artery injury is the most feared and dramatic complication of endonasal skull base surgical approaches with massive bleeding that may result in exanguination of the patient. While ICA injury during endoscopic sinus surgery is a rare event, its frequency during endonasal skull base surgery is much more significant. Prevention is better than cure and surgeons need to be familiar with patients who maybe at risk. Formulating and executing a plan of action during a crisis is difficult and surgeons need to be prepared for this unexpected complication. Nasal packing is often all a surgeon can do to achieve hemostasis, while rapid resuscitation attempts to restore and maintain adequate cerebral perfusion. With the development of live, large vessel vascular injury animal models, training may improve surgeon's confidence and technical skills in the management of an ICA rupture. These vascular workshops teach the use of vascular clamps and the crushed muscle patch and make direct endoscopic repair of vessels a possibility. Immediate angiographic assessment is warranted for hemostasis and/or investigation of pseudoaneurysm/CCF formation. Pseudoaneurysm/CCF treatment should begin with an assessment of collateral vascular flow, with endovascular embolization in those patients that can tolerate it. Otherwise endovascular stent-graft placement is warranted. Some patients may require extracranial/intracranial bypass surgery. All patients require active assessment for delayed pseudoaneurysm formation following an ICA rupture event.

EBM Question	Author's Reply
What factors contribute to ICA injury and what is best management of ICA injury?	Risk factors include: Anatomic relationships (Carotid dehiscence, Sphenoid septal attachment to ICA, Midline ICA), Revision surgery, Prior radiotherapy, Prior bromocriptine treatment and Acromegaly (Grade C).
	Animal models demonstrate the superiority of crushed muscle compared to other hemostatic techniques (Level 2b). Crushed muscle is suggested with followup angiographic intervention or U-clip closure where training and equipment exist (Level C).

REFERENCES

1. Carrau RL, Kassam AB, Snyderman CH. Pituitary surgery. Otolaryngol Clin North Am 2001;34:1143.
2. Casler JD, Doolittle AM, Mair EA. Endoscopic surgery of the anterior skull base. Laryngoscope 2005;115:16.
3. Raymond J, Hardy J, Czepko R, et al. Arterial injuries in transsphenoidal surgery for pituitary adenoma; the role of angiography and endovascular treatment. AJNR Am J Neuroradiol 1997;18:655.
4. Laws ER Jr. Vascular complications of transsphenoidal surgery. Pituitary 1999; 2:163.
5. May M, Levine HL, Mester SJ, et al. Complications of endoscopic sinus surgery: analysis of 2108 patients–incidence and prevention. Laryngoscope 1994;104: 1080.
6. Chen D, Concus AP, Halbach VV, et al. Epistaxis originating from traumatic pseudoaneurysm of the internal carotid artery: diagnosis and endovascular therapy. Laryngoscope 1998;108:326.
7. Frank G, Sciarretta V, Calbucci F, et al. The endoscopic transnasal transsphenoidal approach for the treatment of cranial base chordomas and chondrosarcomas. Neurosurgery 2006;59:ONS50.
8. Fukushima T, Maroon JC. Repair of carotid artery perforations during transsphenoidal surgery. Surg Neurol 1998;50:174.
9. Gardner PA, Kassam AB, Snyderman CH, et al. Outcomes following endoscopic, expanded endonasal resection of suprasellar craniopharyngiomas: a case series. J Neurosurg 2008;109:6.
10. Koitschev A, Simon C, Lowenheim H, et al. Management and outcome after internal carotid artery laceration during surgery of the paranasal sinuses. Acta Otolaryngol 2006;126:730.
11. Lippert BM, Ringel K, Stoeter P, et al. Stentgraft-implantation for treatment of internal carotid artery injury during endonasal sinus surgery. Am J Rhinol 2007;21:520.
12. Park AH, Stankiewicz JA, Chow J, et al. A protocol for management of a catastrophic complication of functional endoscopic sinus surgery: internal carotid artery injury. Am J Rhinol 1998;12:153.
13. Pepper JP, Wadhwa AK, Tsai F, et al. Cavernous carotid injury during functional endoscopic sinus surgery: case presentations and guidelines for optimal management. Am J Rhinol 2007;21:105.
14. Stippler M, Gardner PA, Snyderman CH, et al. Endoscopic endonasal approach for clival chordomas. Neurosurgery 2009;64:268.
15. Weidenbecher M, Huk WJ, Iro H. Internal carotid artery injury during functional endoscopic sinus surgery and its management. Eur Arch Otorhinolaryngol 2005;262:640.

16. Ahuja A, Guterman LR, Hopkins LN. Carotid cavernous fistula and false aneurysm of the cavernous carotid artery: complications of transsphenoidal surgery. Neurosurgery 1992;31:774.

17. Cappabianca P, Briganti F, Cavallo LM, et al. Pseudoaneurysm of the intracavernous carotid artery following endoscopic endonasal transsphenoidal surgery, treated by endovascular approach. Acta Neurochir (Wien) 2001;143:95.

18. Fatemi N, Dusick JR, de Paiva Neto MA, et al. The endonasal microscopic approach for pituitary adenomas and other parasellar tumors: a 10-year experience. Neurosurgery 2008;63:244.

19. Zhou WG, Yang ZQ. Complications of transsphenoidal surgery for sellar region: intracranial vessel injury. Chin Med J (Engl) 2009;122:1154.

20. Lister JR, Sypert GW. Traumatic false aneurysm and carotid-cavernous fistula: a complication of sphenoidotomy. Neurosurgery 1979;5:473.

21. Kaptain GJ, Vincent DA, Sheehan JP, et al. Transsphenoidal approaches for the extracapsular resection of midline suprasellar and anterior cranial base lesions. Neurosurgery 2001;49:94.

22. Couldwell WT, Weiss MH, Rabb C, et al. Variations on the standard transsphenoidal approach to the sellar region, with emphasis on the extended approaches and parasellar approaches: surgical experience in 105 cases. Neurosurgery 2004;55:539.

23. Maniglia AJ. Fatal and major complications secondary to nasal and sinus surgery. Laryngoscope 1989;99:276.

24. Bavinzski G, Killer M, Knosp E, et al. False aneurysms of the intracavernous carotid artery–report of 7 cases. Acta Neurochir (Wien) 1997;139:37.

25. Cappabianca P, Esposito F, Esposito I, et al. Use of a thrombin-gelatin haemostatic matrix in endoscopic endonasal extended approaches: technical note. Acta Neurochir (Wien) 2009;151:69.

26. Weber R, Draf W, Keerl R, et al. Endonasal microendoscopic pansinusoperation in chronic sinusitis. II. Results and complications. Am J Otolaryngol 1997;18:247.

27. Park YS, Jung JY, Ahn JY, et al. Emergency endovascular stent graft and coil placement for internal carotid artery injury during transsphenoidal surgery. Surg Neurol 2009;72:741.

28. Reddy K, Lesiuk H, West M, et al. False aneurysm of the cavernous carotid artery: a complication of transsphenoidal surgery. Surg Neurol 1990;33:142.

29. Berker M, Aghayev K, Saatci I, et al. Overview of vascular complications of pituitary surgery with special emphasis on unexpected abnormality. Pituitary 2010;13:160.

30. Biswas D, Daudia A, Jones NS, et al. Profuse epistaxis following sphenoid surgery: a ruptured carotid artery pseudoaneurysm and its management. J Laryngol Otol 2009;123:692.

31. Kocer N, Kizilkilic O, Albayram S, et al. Treatment of iatrogenic internal carotid artery laceration and carotid cavernous fistula with endovascular stent-graft placement. AJNR Am J Neuroradiol 2002;23:442.

32. Kadyrov NA, Friedman JA, Nichols DA, et al. Endovascular treatment of an internal carotid artery pseudoaneurysm following transsphenoidal surgery. Case report. J Neurosurg 2002;96:624.

33. Zada G, Kelly DF, Cohan P, et al. Endonasal transsphenoidal approach for pituitary adenomas and other sellar lesions: an assessment of efficacy, safety, and patient impressions. J Neurosurg 2003;98:350.

34. Kim SH, Shin YS, Yoon PH, et al. Emergency endovascular treatment of internal carotid artery injury during a transsphenoidal approach for a pituitary tumor–case report. Yonsei Med J 2002;43:119.

35. Isenberg SF, Scott JA. Management of massive hemorrhage during endoscopic sinus surgery. Otolaryngol Head Neck Surg 1994;111:134.
36. Hudgins PA, Browning DG, Gallups J, et al. Endoscopic paranasal sinus surgery: radiographic evaluation of severe complications. AJNR Am J Neuroradiol 1992; 13:1161.
37. Wigand ME, Hosemann W. Paranasal sinus surgery. J Otolaryngol 1991;20:386.
38. de Souza JM, Domingues FS, Espinosa G, et al. Cavernous carotid artery pseudo-aneurysm treated by stenting in acromegalic patient. Arq Neuropsiquiatr 2003;61:459.
39. Leung GK, Auyeung KM, Lui WM, et al. Emergency placement of a self-expandable covered stent for carotid artery injury during trans-sphenoidal surgery. Br J Neurosurg 2006;20:55.
40. Keerl R, Weber R, Drees G, et al. Individual learning curves with reference to endonasal micro-endoscopic pan-sinus operation. Laryngorhinootologie 1996; 75:338 [in German].
41. Charalampaki P, Ayyad A, Kockro RA, et al. Surgical complications after endoscopic transsphenoidal pituitary surgery. J Clin Neurosci 2009;16:786.
42. Ghatge SB, Modi DB. Treatment of ruptured ICA during transsphenoidal surgery. Two different endovascular strategies in two cases. Interv Neuroradiol 2010;16:31.
43. Crowley RW, Dumont AS, Jane JA Jr. Bilateral intracavernous carotid artery pseudoaneurysms as a result of sellar reconstruction during the transsphenoidal resection of a pituitary macroadenoma: case report. Minim Invasive Neurosurg 2009;52:44.
44. Cathelinaud O, Bizeau A, Rimbot A, et al. Endoscopic endonasal surgery complication: new methods of intracavernous internal carotid artery injury treatment. Rev Laryngol Otol Rhinol (Bord) 2008;129:305.
45. Ciceri EF, Regna-Gladin C, Erbetta A, et al. Iatrogenic intracranial pseudoaneurysms: neuroradiological and therapeutical considerations, including endovascular options. Neurol Sci 2006;27:317.
46. Vanninen RL, Manninen HI, Rinne J. Intrasellar iatrogenic carotid pseudoaneurysm: endovascular treatment with a polytetrafluoroethylene-covered stent. Cardiovasc Intervent Radiol 2003;26:298.
47. Dolenc VV, Lipovsek M, Slokan S. Traumatic aneurysm and carotid-cavernous fistula following transsphenoidal approach to a pituitary adenoma: treatment by transcranial operation. Br J Neurosurg 1999;13:185.
48. Pigott TJ, Holland IM, Punt JA. Carotico-cavernous fistula after trans-sphenoidal hypophysectomy. Br J Neurosurg 1989;3:613.
49. Dusick JR, Esposito F, Malkasian D, et al. Avoidance of carotid artery injuries in transsphenoidal surgery with the Doppler probe and micro-hook blades. Neurosurgery 2007;60:322.
50. Lempert TE, Halbach VV, Higashida RT, et al. Endovascular treatment of pseudoaneurysms with electrolytically detachable coils. AJNR Am J Neuroradiol 1998;19:907.
51. Paullus WS, Norwood CW, Morgan HW. False aneurysm of the cavernous carotid artery and progressive external ophthalmoplegia after transsphenoidal hypophysectomy. Case report. J Neurosurg 1979;51:707.
52. Cabezudo JM, Carrillo R, Vaquero J, et al. Intracavernous aneurysm of the carotid artery following transsphenoidal surgery. Case report. J Neurosurg 1981;54:118.
53. Wilson CB, Dempsey LC. Transsphenoidal microsurgical removal of 250 pituitary adenomas. J Neurosurg 1978;48:13.

54. Ciric I, Ragin A, Baumgartner C, et al. Complications of transsphenoidal surgery: results of a national survey, review of the literature, and personal experience. Neurosurgery 1997;40:225.
55. Fujii K, Chambers SM, Rhoton AL Jr. Neurovascular relationships of the sphenoid sinus. A microsurgical study. J Neurosurg 1979;50:31.
56. Renn WH, Rhoton AL Jr. Microsurgical anatomy of the sellar region. J Neurosurg 1975;43:288.
57. Lee KJ. The sublabial transseptal transsphenoidal approach to the hypophysis. Laryngoscope 1978;88(Suppl 10):1.
58. Koitschev A, Baumann I, Remy CT, et al. Rational CT diagnosis before operations on the paranasal sinuses. HNO 2002;50:217 [in German].
59. Imamura J, Okuzono T, Okuzono Y. Fatal epistaxis caused by rupture of an intra-tumoral aneurysm enclosed by a large prolactinoma–case report. Neurol Med Chir (Tokyo) 1998;38:654.
60. Wakai S, Fukushima T, Furihata T, et al. Association of cerebral aneurysm with pituitary adenoma. Surg Neurol 1979;12:503.
61. Hatam A, Greitz T. Ectasia of cerebral arteries in acromegaly. Acta Radiol Diagn (Stockh) 1972;12:410.
62. Bejjani GK, Sekhar LN, Yost AM, et al. Vasospasm after cranial base tumor resection: pathogenesis, diagnosis, and therapy. Surg Neurol 1999;52:577.
63. Chaloupka JC, Putman CM, Citardi MJ, et al. Endovascular therapy for the carotid blowout syndrome in head and neck surgical patients: diagnostic and managerial considerations. AJNR Am J Neuroradiol 1996;17:843.
64. Kassam A, Snyderman CH, Carrau RL, et al. Endoneurosurgical hemostasis techniques: lessons learned from 400 cases. Neurosurg Focus 2005;19:E7.
65. Solares CA, Ong YK, Carrau RL, et al. Prevention and management of vascular injuries in endoscopic surgery of the sinonasal tract and skull base. Otolaryngol Clin North Am 2010;43:817.
66. Oskouian RJ, Kelly DF, Laws ER Jr. Vascular injury and transsphenoidal surgery. Front Horm Res 2006;34:256.
67. Valentine RJ, Boase S, Jervis-Bardy J, et al. The efficacy of hemostatic techniques in the sheep model of carotid artery injury. Allergy and Rhinology 2011;1:118.
68. Segal DH, Sen C, Bederson JB, et al. Predictive value of balloon test occlusion of the internal carotid artery. Skull Base Surg 1995;5:97.
69. Parodi JC. Endovascular repair of abdominal aortic aneurysms and other arterial lesions. J Vasc Surg 1995;21:549.
70. Higashida RT, Halbach VV, Tsai FY, et al. Interventional neurovascular treatment of traumatic carotid and vertebral artery lesions: results in 234 cases. AJR Am J Roentgenol 1989;153:577.
71. Higashida RT, Halbach VV, Dowd C, et al. Endovascular detachable balloon embolization therapy of cavernous carotid artery aneurysms: results in 87 cases. J Neurosurg 1990;72:857.
72. Wholey MH, Jarmolowski CR, Eles G, et al. Endovascular stents for carotid artery occlusive disease. J Endovasc Surg 1997;4:326.
73. Kalapatapu VR, Shelton KR, Ali AT, et al. Pseudoaneurysm: a review. Curr Treat Options Cardiovasc Med 2008;10:173.
74. Fox AJ, Vinuela F, Pelz DM. Results of the international extracranial/intracranial arterial bypass: implications for radiologists. AJNR Am J Neuroradiol 1986;7:736.
75. Kinugasa K, Mandai S, Tsuchida S, et al. Direct thrombosis of a pseudoaneurysm after obliteration of a carotid-cavernous fistula with cellulose acetate polymer: technical case report. Neurosurgery 1994;35:755.

76. Crow WN, Scott BA, Guinto FC Jr, et al. Massive epistaxis due to pseudoaneurysm. Treated with detachable balloons. Arch Otolaryngol Head Neck Surg 1992; 118:321.
77. Fox AJ, Vinuela F, Pelz DM, et al. Use of detachable balloons for proximal artery occlusion in the treatment of unclippable cerebral aneurysms. J Neurosurg 1987; 66:40.
78. Higashida RT, Halbach VV, Dowd CF, et al. Intracranial aneurysms: interventional neurovascular treatment with detachable balloons–results in 215 cases. Radiology 1991;178:663.

Endoscopic Skull Base Surgery for Sinonasal Malignancy

Richard J. Harvey, MD[a],*, Mark Winder, MD[b],
Priscilla Parmar, MD[a], Valerie Lund, MD[c]

KEYWORDS

- Esthesioneuroblastoma • Olfactory neuroblastoma
- Adenocarcinoma • SCC • Adenocystic • Mucosal melanoma
- Sinonasal • Skull base

EBM Question	Level of Evidence	Grade of Recommendation
Are oncological outcomes the same with EES compared to open craniofacial surgery?	4	C

Many of the surgical techniques described endoscopically within the skull base can be applied to malignant sinonasal disease. However, it is the oncological principles of such treatment that must be adhered to when undertaking endoscopic tumor surgery. A focus should be maintained on a surgical philosophy that is driven by the disorder and its staging rather than the available surgical expertise and equipment. The endoscopic tumor surgeon should be equally comfortable in managing the patient by an open craniofacial as well as an endoscopic approach.

There are 3 foundations for successful endoscopic surgery. First, the resection should be defined with frozen section control of surgical margins. Few endoscopic tumor removals are en bloc and thus margin control is essential. Surgical mapping of such margins are advised (**Fig. 1**). This mapping also aids postoperative adjuvant

Conflict of interest statement: No external funding was received. Prof. Harvey has served on an advisory board for Schering Plough and serves on the speaker's bureau for Glaxo Smith Klein. Prof. Lund has served on advisory boards for Bayer, Glaxo Smith Klein, Medtronic, Merck, and Schering Plough. Dr Parmar and Dr Winder have no financial interests to declare.

[a] Department of Otolaryngology/Skull Base Surgery, St Vincent's Hospital, Victoria Street, Darlinghurst, Sydney, New South Wales 2010, Australia
[b] Department of Neurosurgery, St Vincent's Hospital, Sydney, New South Wales, Australia
[c] Professorial Unit, Royal National Throat Nose and Ear Hospital, 330 Grays Inn Road, London WC1X 8DA, UK
* Corresponding author.
E-mail address: richard@richardharvey.com.au

Otolaryngol Clin N Am 44 (2011) 1081–1140
doi:10.1016/j.otc.2011.06.020
0030-6665/11/$ – see front matter © 2011 Elsevier Inc. All rights reserved.

oto.theclinics.com

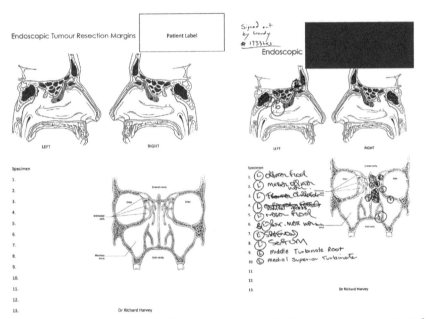

Fig. 1. Surgical margin mapping in the removal of a small adenocystic carcinoma is useful both to ensure orientation, chase follow-up margins that might return unexpected formal positive findings, and aid adjuvant radiotherapy planning.

therapy planning. The access required should be predetermined by the tumor and preoperative imaging (**Table 1**). There should be minimal attempts to be conservative at the expense of gaining adequate access for tumor removal. Functional cavity techniques are a secondary concern. In addition, there should be no hesitancy in removing macroscopically involved tissue, such as dura, periorbital, and other important structures. Although the biology of some tumors may afford an approach of gross removal from dura, carotid, and orbital structures with successful adjuvant therapy, this is not standard care and has yet to be proved as effective therapy for malignancy. This shortcoming should not prevent the surgeon from removing obviously involved anatomic barriers at the time surgery (**Fig. 2**). Much of this is related to surgeon skill and expertise. It differs greatly from managing benign conditions, such as inverted papilloma, in which preserving anatomic barriers to spread is paramount.

Proponents of the traditional craniofacial approach (tCFR) argue that an en bloc resection possible with the tCFR is impossible with endoscopic approaches that, at best, are "piecemeal resection" of the tumor. Proponents of the endoscopic approach are of the opinion that, in resecting tumors involving the anterior skull base an en bloc resection is rarely possible whatever approach is used. Optimum endoscopic visualization enables a wide-field, three-dimensional resection close to an en bloc resection in most cases and a better term is tumor disassembly. Proponents of both approaches agree that the resection is intended to achieve negative margins. An endoscopic approach offers several other advantages.[1] The operation time is shorter, and is associated with less morbidity and shorter hospital stay.[2] Patients do not experience the serious complications that can be associated with the approach in tCFR, nor are they likely to be subject to the reduction in quality of life. Nicolai and colleagues[3] reported a complication rate of 6% following endoscopic resection of malignant tumor

Table 1
Malignant sinonasal tumors: pretreatment imaging

Tasks	CT	Standard MR	Study Planes	Additional MR Sequences
To distinguish tumor from retained mucus	Adequate, but less sensitive than MR (3-mm slice thickness better than 1 mm)	TSE T2-weighted sequences are indicated (slice thickness 3 mm)	Axial and coronal planes	FLAIR sequence to differentiate CSF from the cystic/fluid content of tumors or mucoceles
To assess periorbita invasion	Bone erosion precisely shown by CT. The periorbita is not usually distinguished from tumor signal (slice thickness 1–2 mm)	SE T1-weighted and TSE T2-weighted sequences are indicated. Periorbita can be more easily separated from tumor signal (slice thickness not >3 mm)	Axial and coronal planes	STIR (orbital fat signal suppressed) may be used to increase detection of orbital fat tissue
To assess dura mater invasion	Although skull base erosion is precisely shown by CT, only large dura breakage is detected. Contrast enhancement is required (slice thickness 1–2 mm)	TSE T2-weighted and postcontrast SE T1-weighted sequences are indicated (slice thickness not >3 mm)	Axial, coronal, and sagittal planes	—
To assess perineural spread	Limited to indirect signs (fat effacement or enlargement of foramina, muscular atrophy)	Direct demonstration of the abnormal nerve by enhanced fat-saturated SE T1-weighted sequences (slice thickness not >3 mm)	Axial and coronal planes	GE sequences with submillimetric isotropic slices (FIESTA; VIBE) to image the intraforaminal segment of cranial nerves
To assess relationships of tumor with cisternal cranial nerve segments	Not indicated	TSE T2-weighted sequence (slice thickness <3 mm)	Axial, coronal, and sagittal planes	MR cisternography with submillimetric isotropic slices (3DFT-CISS; DRIVE)
To analyze the intracranial/upper neck internal carotid artery course	CT angiography (requires contrast agent injection, high spatial resolution acquisition). MIP reconstructions	—	Axial, coronal, and sagittal planes	MR angiography (requires contrast agent injection). MIP reconstructions

Abbreviations: CT, computed tomography; DRIVE, driven equilibrium radio frequency reset pulse sequence; FIESTA, fast imaging employing steady state sequence; GE, gradient echo sequence; MIP, maximum intensity projection; MR, magnetic resonance; SE, spin echo sequence; STIR, short tau inversion recovery sequence; TSE, turbo spin echo sequence; VIBE, volume interpolated breath-hold examination sequence; 3DFT-CISS, three-dimensional constructive interference in a steady state sequence.

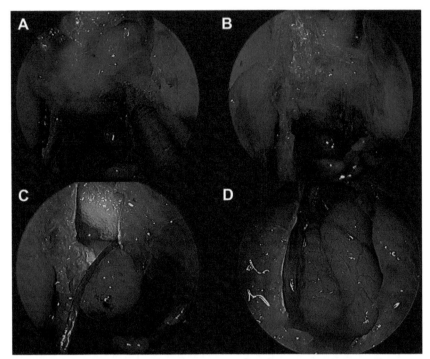

Fig. 2. Small low-grade adenocarcinoma with clear involvement of the olfactory bulb. The bone (*A*) and dura (*B*) look macroscopically normal but there is obvious disease in the olfactory bulb (*C*). There is minimal evidence that removing the tumor to dura then treating with adjuvant therapies replaces formal resection. Intracranial recurrence would have almost been assured if not managed accordingly (*D*).

compared with 16% after craniofacial resection (CFR). The most common complication after endoscopic approach was cerebrospinal fluid (CSF) leak, followed by mucocele formation. Life-threatening complications, such as intracranial bleeding and infection, are a risk regardless of the approach.

The diversity of the malignant disorders seen in the skull base makes reporting of large homogenous cohorts of patient outcomes scarce. The sinonasal tract and skull base is a region with the greatest histologic diversity in the body, and this is reflected in the extensive disorder classification list compiled by the World Health Organization (WHO) (**Box 1**).[4]

INCIDENCE AND EPIDEMIOLOGY
Malignant Tumors

Sinonasal neoplasms are uncommon neoplasms that account only for 1% of all malignancies,[5,6] 3% of all upper respiratory tract malignancies, and only 3% to 5% of all head and neck malignancies.[7,8] Annual incidence is 0.5 to 1 new cases per 100,000 inhabitants in Italy,[9] whereas high rates for sinonasal malignancies (SNM) were found in Asian and African populations, the highest age-adjusted rates, between 2.5 and 2.6 per 100,000 per annum, occurring in Japanese men.[10] Sinonasal malignancies are more common in men. The male/female ratio is reported to be between 1.2 and 2.7/1.[11,12] In the maxillary sinus, the male/female ratio is 2:1, and in the ethmoid sinus the

---

Box 1
WHO Classification of Tumors and associated ICD-O codes

Nasal cavity and paranasal sinuses

1. Malignant epithelial tumors

2. Neuroendocrine tumors

3. Soft tissue tumors

4. Borderline and low malignant potential tumors of soft tissue

5. Malignant tumors of bone and cartilage

6. Hematolymphoid tumors

7. Neuroectodermal tumors

8. Germ cell tumors

9. Secondary tumors

---

male/female ratio is 1.4:1. Overall, 75% of all malignant tumors occur in persons older than 50 years.[13]

The most common sinonasal malignancies are the primary epithelial tumors, followed by the nonepithelial malignant tumors. In the group of epithelial SNMs, the squamous cell carcinoma (SCC) dominated, and, in the nonepithelial SNMs, the most common group was malignant lymphoma. The prevalence of the different malignant tumors in the literature is extremely variable. The incidence of epithelial SNMs ranges between 52.9% and 91%.[13,14] In a series of 115 patients, Svane-Knudsen[15] reported that 64% had well-differentiated SCCs, adenocarcinomas, and adenoid cystic carcinomas. Non-Hodgkin lymphomas and undifferentiated carcinomas represented 9% and 2.6%, respectively. In a German series of 216 cases, Zbaren and colleagues[16] found 56% to be epidermoid carcinomas and 14% to be adenocarcinomas. Similarly, in 60 Japanese patients, Haraguchi and colleagues[17] found a predominance of well-differentiated SCCs (25%) followed by melanomas and NHL (23%) and a small number of undifferentiated carcinomas (5%). However, in areas where there is a high incidence of sinonasal neoplasms, the histopathologic spectrum is different from the spectrum in low-risk areas. Undifferentiated carcinomas in Chinese high-risk areas (eg, Hong Kong) constitute more than 80% of all sinonasal malignancies.[18] Incidence, site, and histologic type can vary in different geographic areas, which may be because of occupational, social, and genetic factors.[19] For all nose and sinus tumors, the nose is the primary site in 25% and the sinuses 75%, and of all sinus neoplasms, 60% to 80% originate from maxillary sinus.[13] However, it is not easy to determine the exact site of origin with large tumors. As a result, the tumor distributions in the literature are variable.[13]

SCC is the most common tumor of the sinonasal malignancies (**Fig. 3**). Approximately 60% to 73% of SCCs originate in the maxillary sinus, 20% to 30% in the nasal cavity, 10% to 15% in the ethmoid sinus, and 1% in the sphenoid and frontal sinuses.[12,13,20] Among the carcinomas of the nose and paranasal sinuses, sinonasal gland carcinomas represent the second most frequent type of malignant epithelial tumor, and the paranasal sinuses are the most common site of minor salivary gland involvement.[21–23] Adenoid cystic carcinoma (ACC) accounts for less than 1% of all head and neck malignancies and 10% of all salivary gland neoplasms.[23,24] Lupinetti and colleagues[25] reported that most patients were white (72.4%), nonsmokers (48.4), and nondrinkers (74.4%) in their ACC series. Sinonasal ACC accounts for

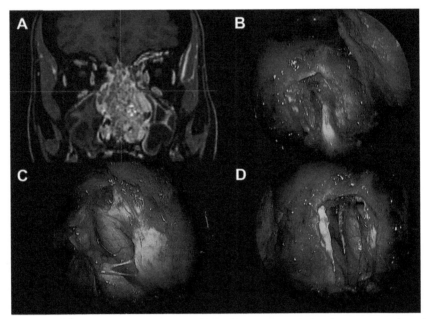

Fig. 3. Squamous cell carcinoma arising from the septum. Magnetic resonance imaging (MRI) shows involvement of the crista galli (*A*), which is removed (*B*) along with the macroscopically involved dura (*C*) for final resection superiorly to include the falx cerebri (*D*).

10% to 25% of all head and neck ACC.[23] The maxillary sinus (47%) and the nasal cavity (30%) were the most common primary tumor sites. ACC has a propensity for perineural spread and bony invasion, which can lead to significant skull base involvement and intracranial extension.[25]

Adenocarcinoma is the third most common mucosal epithelial malignancy found in this area (**Fig. 4**), after SCC and ACC,[26] and represents approximately 8% to 15% of all sinonasal cancers.[27,28] The incidence is less than 1 case per 100,000 inhabitants per year,[29] occurring predominately among men with a mean age of presentation of 60 to 65 years.[30] However, in the northern part of Spain, the incidence is 0.19 cases/100,000 inhabitants per year.[31] The median age of onset lies between 50 and 60 years[30] and even earlier in wood dust–related tumors.[32] Men develop adenocarcinoma 4 times more frequently than women, implying an occupational hazard.[33] It is located most frequently (85%) in the ethmoid sinus and the upper part of the nasal cavity. One study using endoscopic endonasal surgery showed that woodworkers' adenocarcinomas constantly originated in the olfactory cleft, appearing as polyplike neoplasms with well-defined boundaries.[34] They occasionally arise in other sites of the nasal cavity (maxillary sinus in 10%) and these cases are usually not related to wood dust exposure.[35]

Sinonasal mucoepidermoid carcinoma accounts for 0.6% of all salivary tumors and 4.8% of all mucoepidermoid carcinomas. The most common site is maxillary sinus, followed by nasal cavity, nasopharynx, and ethmoid sinuses in order of decreasing frequency.[10,36]

Associated Risk Factors

Wood dust exposure

The association between wood dust exposure and adenocarcinoma of the sinuses is also well established. It is estimated that woodworkers have a 500 times increased risk

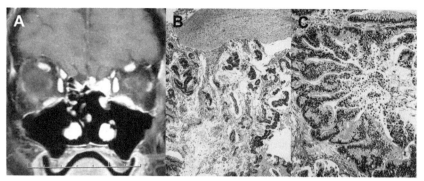

Fig. 4. Left ethmoid adenocarcinoma on computed tomography (*A*) and histology demonstrating invasion into the olfactory bulb (*B*) and typical 'intestinal type' pattern (*C*).

compared with the male population and up to 900 times compared with the population in general.[32] It has been shown that the true risk factor is the exposure to wood dust particles, and not the possible exposure to chemical products used in the industry, such as polish, varnish, or protectors.[32] Hardwood types, such as ebony, oak, and beech, confer the highest risk of developing sinonasal adenocarcinomas,[37] increased further by inhalation of formaldehyde or substances normally used in this type of industry.[38] The strong relation of adenocarcinoma to exposure to wood dust makes it a disease almost exclusive to carpenters and furniture makers. Therefore, in many countries (eg, Australia, Germany, the United Kingdom, Belgium, France), it is considered an industrial disease.[37,39–42] The furniture makers who are likely to be exposed to the fine wood dusts of threshold greater than 5 mg/m^3/d are at greater risk.[14,43,44] Many findings indicate a dose-response relationship,[38,45,46] with a higher incidence of tumors occurring among workers exposed for longer periods of time. Recent studies have shown that even short periods of exposure (<5 years) can lead to an increased risk of carcinoma. In general, the normally long latency period is estimated at 40 years,[47] although it can range between 20 and 70 years.[43] Despite this clear cause, it is still unknown by what molecular mechanism sinonasal adenocarcinomas develop. Because wood dust does not have mutagenic properties, it is hypothesized that prolonged exposure to, and irritation by, wood dust particles stimulate cellular turnover by inflammatory pathways.[33,48]

Smoking
Smoking is associated with an increased risk of nasal cancer, especially SCC of the maxillary sinus.[12,13,49] However, some reports did not find any increased risk for sinonasal tract malignancies associated with tobacco and alcohol.[50] Further research is needed to determine whether smoking is a significant causal factor in sinonasal carcinoma.

Chemical exposure
Thorium dioxide, when used as an imaging agent, may cause antral squamous and mucoepidermoid carcinomas.[13] Although no other definitive risk factors for mucoepidermoid carcinoma have been identified, minor trauma and chronic irritation have been implicated in the cause of sinonasal tract cancers in general.[51] Relative risk rates for sinonasal epithelial malignancies have been determined for several chemical agents (chromates, nickel compounds, isopropylic alcohol, and mustard gas) and for several occupations (ie, nuclear refinery work, leather work in boot and shoe

manufacturing, chrome pigment work, metalwork, textile work, construction work, baking, flour milling, and farming) even in the apparent absence of causal agents.[52] Increased risks to different industries were reported as: the metal industry, relative risk ranging from 3.1 to 5.9; the textile industry, ranging from 2.9 to 17.0; the mining and construction industry, ranging from 2.3 to 5.3; and the agricultural industry, ranging from 1.9 to 3.3.[52] Among women, exposure to textile dust was associated with an increased risk of SCC and adenocarcinoma. For SCC, the risk increased with the duration and the level of exposure. The risks associated with the different types of textile fibers (cotton, wool, and synthetic fibers) were similar and the results did not incriminate a particular type of textile.[53] An association between SCC and nickel exposure has been shown by Pedersen and colleagues[54] who reported that workers at a nickel refinery in Norway developed SCC at 250 times the expected rate, with a latent period varying from 18 to 36 years.

Human papillomavirus infection
The current evidence linking human papillomavirus (HPV) to at least a proportion of benign sinonasal papillomas is convincing. Based on the analysis of more than 1000 such lesions, Syrjaenen[55] reported that HPV-6 and HPV-11 is present in one-third (33.3%) of inverted papillomas and this detection rate is higher than most other reported extragenital papillomas, except those of the larynx and bronchus. Tang and colleagues[56] detected human papilloma virus in up to 86% of inverted papilloma cases. The 2005 International Agency for Research on Cancer evaluation on the carcinogenicity of HPV in humans[57] concluded that there is sufficient evidence for the carcinogenicity of HPV in the oral cavity and oropharynx, limited evidence in the larynx, and inadequate evidence in sinonasal cavities.[58] However, some previous reports have suggested a possible implication of HPV in the development of several carcinomas of the sinonasal region.[55,59,60] In 1993, Kashima and colleagues[61] found that 4% of SCC were HPV positive. Alos and colleagues[58] detected HPV DNA in tumor tissue of 20% of patients with sinonasal SCC. The tumors affected predominantly men, by a ratio of approximately 3:1; no significant differences in sex and age were found between HPV-positive and HPV-negative groups. There were no significant differences in tumor stage at presentation. Despite the similar clinical characteristics and staging at presentation, patients with HPV-positive tumors had a significantly better prognosis than those with HPV-negative neoplasms (**Fig. 5**).[58] Syrjaenen[55] showed that 21.7% of sinonasal carcinomas analyzed were positive for HPV. Low-risk HPV types 6 and 11 are usually confined to benign lesions, whereas the reverse is true for the oncogenic HPV types 16 and 18, and the presence of squamocolumnar junctions and squamous cell metaplasia in the sinonasal system.[55] The discrepancies reported by several studies might result, in part, from technical reasons, but it is also possible that sinonasal lesions have a heterogeneous cause (HPV related and nonrelated) and/or that some novel (as yet unidentified) HPV types exist in these lesions, which are detected by some studies but not by others.

Rare Tumors

Primary sinonasal tract mucosal malignant melanomas are rare, accounting for between 0.3% and 2% of all malignant melanomas and about 4% of head and neck melanomas.[62–66] The head and neck represents the most common site of mucosal malignant melanoma with a suggested incidence of about 0.018/10^5 to 0.051/10^5 per year.[63,67,68] Sinonasal tract mucosal malignant melanomas represent up to 4% of all sinonasal tract neoplasms.[64,67,69] In the National Cancer Database report by the American College of Surgeons Commission on Cancer and the American

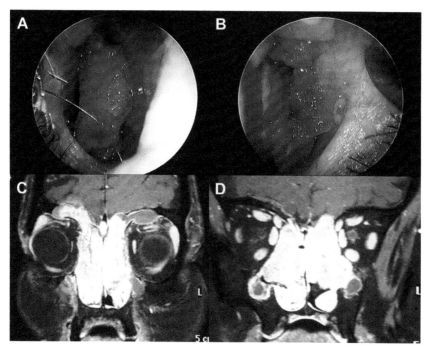

Fig. 5. Massive HPV +ve inverted papilloma of the sinonasal tract on right (*A*) and left (*B*) endoscopy. The coronal post contrast MRI (*C* and *D*) were suspicious for focal SCC change.

Cancer Society of more than 84,000 melanomas seen from 1985 to 1994,[62] only 1.3% were melanomas that arose from mucosal surfaces, of which 55% were of the head and neck. Sinonasal tract mucosal malignant melanomas were found to be equally common in men and women. A higher proportion of melanoma was identified in black patients (10.4%).[70] In general, the mean age for sinonasal tract mucosal malignant melanomas (64.3 years) is later than for cutaneous malignant melanomas. Sinonasal tract mucosal malignant melanoma is a more lethal disease in patients older than 60 years, a finding similar to cutaneous melanoma.[70] Tumors originating in the sinuses are less common than those arising in the nasal cavity, but sinus tumors may grow asymptomatically until late in the disease course.[69,71] One-third of patients had neck metastases, which often preceded distant metastasis, and distant metastasis was always rapidly fatal.[72]

The incidence of olfactory neuroblastoma was 0.4 cases/million inhabitants per year[73] but is difficult to establish, and the tumor is not as rare as is commonly reported and probably represents more than 5% of all nasal malignant tumors.[73–75] Olfactory neuroblastoma occurs in a wide age range (3–90 years), with a bimodal peak in the second and sixth decades of life.[76–78] Occasional cases have also been reported in children younger than 10 years.[15,75] Olfactory neuroblastoma affects male and female patients with similar frequency and can be found in all age groups.[75,79] No known causal factor exists for this tumor,[80] although diethylnitrosamine injections can induce tumors in hamsters at the site of the olfactory epithelium.[81] No hereditary patterns have been described for this neoplasm, and there is no apparent racial predilection.[76]

Extrapulmonary neuroendocrine carcinomas (SNEC) only account for 4% of all SNECs,[82] and few cases of SNECs of head and neck have been reported.[83] Less than 250 cases of head and neck SNEC have been published, including 48 cases of SNEC in the nasal and paranasal cavities.[84,85] Most patients with SNEC of the head and neck are male. Although there seems to be an association with cigarette smoking, the association is not as strong as that with pulmonary SNEC.[86,87] Although the neoplasm has been described at any age between 16 and 77 years, the prevalent distribution is in the fifth and sixth decades.[88,89] No particular risk factors for this tumor have been identified.[85,90,91]

Although tumors of this type occur in a variety of organs and sites, small cell undifferentiated carcinoma (ScCC) of the sinonasal tract is a rare malignancy, with the reported series all having fewer than 10 patients.[86] In the MD Anderson series of neuroendocrine tumors, there were only 7 cases of small cell carcinoma.[92] The paucity of well-documented cases precludes generalization about the clinical features. Within this limitation, the mean age at presentation is approximately 50 years (range 26–77 years), and there is no sex predilection. Anatomic sites include the nasal cavity, ethmoid sinuses, and maxillary sinus.[93]

Sinonasal undifferentiated carcinoma (SNUC) is also a rare tumor, with fewer than 100 reported cases in the world literature.[94] There is a male predominance (2–3:1). The age range is broad, usually ranging from the third to ninth decades; the median age at presentation is in the sixth decade.[95–97] There are no known causal agents. SNUCs are typically negative for Epstein-Barr virus (EBV).[96–98] Some cases have been reported to develop following radiation therapy for nasopharyngeal carcinoma.[96]

The annual incidence of the Ewing's Sarcoma Family of Tumors (ESFT) in the United States is 2.1 cases per million children, and they account for approximately 2% of all cancers in children and young adults.[99] ESFT is more common in male than in female patients and has a greater incidence in white and Hispanic children than in black or Asian children.[100,101] ESFT is not believed to be inherited and is not associated with any cancer syndromes. In 95% of cases, at (11;22)(q24;q12) translocation is detected.[102] Sinonasal tract involvement is rare, with about 50 cases reported in the English literature. Most of them were observed in the maxillary sinus, whereas fewer than 10 cases each involved the ethmoid and nasal fossa (also known as PNET-primitive neuroectodermal tumor).

Hemangiopericytomas are unusual vascular tumors that account for only 1% of all vascular neoplasms and for 3% to 5% of sarcomas.[26] They rarely occur in the paranasal sinuses and nasal cavity. The rate of head and neck involvement ranges between 15% and 25%, with sinonasal tract localization present in 5% of patients.[26] Ethmoid, nasal cavity, and sphenoid sinus are the preferential sites of origin.[103] Although the tumor affects all ages, it occurs most commonly in adults in the sixth and seventh decades of life.[104,105] No gender predominance is reported.[105,106] Trauma, steroid therapy, and altered hormone secretions are proposed as predisposing factors.[107,108]

Sarcomas of the head and neck are rare tumors, accounting for 4% to 10% of all sarcomas[109–112] and fewer than 1% of all malignancies of the head and neck region.[113,114] Sarcomas of the sinonasal tract comprise about 15% of sinonasal tumors.[115] Oral and maxillofacial sarcomas present at any age from 5 months to 77 years (mean 42 years) and there is a male/female ratio of 3:1 with predilection for the mandible.[116,117] The mean age and male/female ratio in Africa is lower than in Western series.[118]

Osteosarcoma is a rare bone tumor that occurs primarily in long bones. Overall incidence is 1:100,000 inhabitants per year. Between 6% and 13% of cases occur in the head and neck region.[119] Osteosarcoma had peak prevalence in the third decade, with equal gender distribution. Occurrence in the pediatric age is rare.[120] In the maxillofacial region, it tends to occur a decade later than in long bones. Osteosarcoma accounts for 0.5% to 1% of all sinonasal tract tumors.[121] In children with osteosarcoma, about 3% carry a germ line mutation in p53, with most of these having a family history suggesting Li-Fraumeni syndrome.[122] The incidence of osteosarcoma has been increasing by about 1.4% per year for the past 25 years.[123] The cause of osteosarcoma remains unknown. Bone abnormalities and diseases such as Paget disease of bone, fibrous dysplasia, myositis ossificans, other hereditary disorders like retinoblastoma, Li-Fraumeni syndrome, and previous chemotherapy and irradiation for other malignancies have been suggested as specific risk factors.[124,125]

Rhabdomyosarcoma is the most frequent soft tissue sarcoma in the pediatric age group, accounting for up to 75% of all child sarcomas and 6% of all pediatric cancers. The embryonal subtype is the most common. Mesenchymal rhabdomyosarcoma is rare. The head and neck region is the most commonly involved site (37%).[126] Occurrence of head and neck rhabdomyosarcoma in adults is rare. Only 10% of all soft tissue tumors and 1% of all neoplasms in the sinonasal tract are rhabdomyosarcomas.[127] Sinonasal tract localization is present in about 8% of all adult-age rhabdomyosarcomas.[128]

Chondrosarcoma make up only 10% to 20% of malignant primary bone tumors, with 5% to 10% located in the head and neck. Maxillary sinus is the most frequently involved site.[129,130] In the skull base, chondrosarcomas typically occur at the petroclival synchondrosis. The lesion is commonly diagnosed in the sixth decade. The pediatric population is rarely affected. There is no gender predominance.[128] However, in some reports it is more frequently seen in men.[118,131] The cause of chondrosarcoma remains unknown. Meanwhile, associated conditions include multiple hereditary exostosis, Ollier disease, Maffucci syndrome, previous intravenous thorium dioxide contrast use, Paget disease of bone, chondromyxoid fibroma, and previous irradiation.[132]

Leiomyosarcoma is unusual in the orofacial region[109] and accounts for approximately 7% of all soft tissue sarcomas. It is the fourth most common sarcoma, mainly in the maxilla, and with a 5:1 male/female ratio.[118] Sinonasal tract localization is rare, with about 40 cases reported in the literature.[133]

Fibrosarcoma with mandibular predominance and equal sex distribution was the fifth most common sarcoma. Liposarcoma, fibromyxosarcoma, neurofibrosarcoma, ameloblastic sarcoma, and synovial sarcoma are rare.[109,118]

Sinonasal lymphomas, either primary or secondary, are mostly non-Hodgkin lymphomas (NHLs) and are the second most common malignant tumors following carcinomas occurring in the sinonasal tract. NHLs are classified into B and T-NK subtypes according to lymphocytic phenotype.[20,134] There is a difference in incidence, epidemiology, and cell type between Western and Asian countries. In Western countries, lymphomas are infrequent and sinonasal tract involvement varies between 0.2% and 2% of all NHLs.[135] They constitute 5.8% to 8% of the extranodal lymphomas arising in the head and neck area.[134,136] B-cell lymphomas are predominant and tend to affect paranasal sinuses in the elderly.[20,134] In Asian and South American countries, the incidence of NHLs of the nasal region is higher than in the United States, they account for 2.6% to 6.7% of all lymphomas, and are the second most frequent group of extranodal lymphomas after gastrointestinal lymphomas. T or NK cell lymphomas are predominant and the nasal cavity is mainly involved in younger people.[137,138]

EBV is considered important in the etiopathogenesis of lymphomas, especially for specific lymphomas such as Burkitt lymphoma and nasal NK-T lymphoma. In Asian countries, the prevalence of EBV-positive T-cell lymphomas is similar to the prevalence of EBV virus infection and differs from the findings of the more common EBV-negative B-cell nasal lymphomas in the United States. These findings suggest that EBV plays a role in the development of nasal T-cell lymphomas and that the incidence of EBV infection may explain the reported East-West difference in the incidence of nasal T-cell lymphomas.[20,134,137]

Most of the malignant tumors of the sinonasal regions are primary in origin. Metastasis of malignant tumors to the sinonasal area occurs infrequently and usually presents at the late stage of primary disease. More than 50% of sinonasal metastases originate from a renal carcinoma.[139] Other most common primary sources, in decreasing order after the kidney, are lung (12%), urogenital ridge (12%), breast (9%), and gastrointestinal tract (GI) tract (6%).[140] The most common metastatic sites are the maxillary sinus (50%), followed by the ethmoid sinus (18%) and nasal cavity (15%).[139–142] However, some reports from east Asia are different from European and North American reports. Different incidences of malignant neoplasms in the primary site may explain the different incidences of sinonasal metastatic tumor.[143] Although the mean age of patients with sinonasal metastases varies in different primary origins, the highest incidence is in the sixth decade in men and the seventh decade in women.[144]

SCC

Results following endoscopic resection of sinonasal SCC Although large series of SCC of the maxillary sinus were found in the literature review,[14,21,145,146] obtaining accurate survival figures was not straightforward. Comparison across studies was often confounded by heterogeneous patient cohorts and treatment modality. Most cases received radiotherapy combined with some form of maxillectomy with or without orbital clearance.[146] In addition, most tumors were T3 or T4 at presentation[14,21] and had frequently extended posteriorly into the pterygoid region, which significantly reduces long-term survival. The overall 5-year survival of maxillary SCC was reported at 25%, although patients with T1 tumors at presentation were higher at 55%.[145]

Few studies reported oncological outcomes of SCC exclusively following endoscopic excision. Some studies reported on endoscopy-assisted surgery combined with conventional open approaches, whereas others compared outcomes between surgery and radiotherapy.[147] Most published data are derived from a heterogeneous patient cohort of varied histologic type, in which the main objective was to compare outcomes between endoscopic and CFR.[2,3,148,149] In studies that did reported outcomes following endoscopic resection of malignant tumors, there were frequently insufficient SCC cases for exclusive analysis.[1,150–154]

One published study was identified from the literature review to have reported outcomes for endoscopic resection of sinonasal SCC.[155] This was a small cohort study of 11 patients with a mean age of 62.5 years. Radiation or chemotherapy was used in 8 patients. Seven patients underwent surgery using a strictly endoscopic approach, whereas 4 required combined endoscopic and neurosurgical resection. Local recurrence and distant metastatic rates were 20% and 0%, respectively. Overall survival and disease-free survival were both calculated at 91%, with mean follow-up of 31.5 (range 6–88) months.

Eighteen studies[2,3,147,149–163] were identified to be potentially relevant and had evaluated oncological results following endoscopic resection, performed as the sole procedure or in combination with CFR. Data related to SCC were scarce. Twelve articles[2,3,147,149–156,158,161] included some reports on SCC (**Table 2**).

A total of 150 patients with SCC were pooled from the data available (see **Table 2**). If a single center had generated more than 1 case series, from overlapping periods, data

Table 2
Publications selected for data related to sinonasal SCC

	First Author, Year	Total Number of Malignant Sinonasal Tumors	Total Number of SCC in the Series
1	Eviatar et al,[156] 2004	6	1
2	Castelnuovo et al,[154] 2006	13	3
3	Poetker et al,[150] 2005	16	5
4	Shipchandler et al,[155] 2005	11	11
5	Buchmann et al,[149] 2006	78	33
6	McKay et al,[147] 2007	73	30
7	Kim et al,[2] 2008	40	7
8	Chen,[161] 2006	7	1
9	Lund et al,[152] 2007	49	3
10	Podboj and Smid,[153] 2007	16	6
11	Nicolai et al,[3] 2008	184	25
12	Eloy et al,[158] 2009	66	25
	Total	559	150

from the most recent series were used. Sixty-four patients underwent the traditional CFR (tCFR), 40 patients underwent endoscopy-assisted surgery with an appropriate open approach, and 39 were managed purely with endoscopic surgery (**Table 3**). Seven patients were deemed unresectable or declined surgery and were treated

Table 3
Number of sinonasal SCC by different approaches

First Author, Year	SCC	tCFR	Combined	Endoscopic	Remarks
Eviatar et al,[156] 2004	1	—	—	1	—
Castelnuovo et al,[154] 2006	3	—	3	—	Endoscopic nasal and anterior craniotomy
Poetker et al,[150] 2005	5	—	—	5	—
Shipchandler et al,[155] 2005	11	—	4	7	—
Buchmann et al,[149] 2006	33	—	33	—	Open approaches complemented with endoscopic
McKay et al,[147] 2007	30	23	—	—	7 underwent radiotherapy with chemotherapy
Kim et al,[2] 2008	7	7	—	—	—
Chen,[161] 2006	1	—	—	1	—
Lund et al,[152] 2007	3	—	—	3	—
Podboj and Smid,[153] 2007	6	—	—	6	—
Nicolai et al,[3] 2008	25	9	—	16	—
Eloy et al,[158] 2009	25	25	—	—	—
Total	150	64	40	39	7 treated with radiotherapy/ chemotherapy

with radiotherapy and chemotherapy. Only 1 study reported exclusively on endoscopic surgery for SCC.[155]

Of the 39 patients who underwent purely endoscopic surgery, data were available only for 23 patients. Individual data were collated from 5 studies,[150,153,155,159,161] and are summarized in **Table 4**. Patient demographics, tumor staging, site of origin, extent of tumor invasion, recurrence, and site of distant metastasis were not consistently reported in all of the 5 studies. Twenty-three patients, with a mean age of 59.8 (range 25–85) years, were analyzed. The male/female ratio was 2:1 (12 male, 6 female, 5 unreported). Contrary to previous studies that reported a preponderance of advanced disease, 65.2% of patients had either T1 or T2 tumors at presentation. This finding may represent selection bias of the investigators to offer endoscopic resection of the tumor. Six patients (26.8%) had local recurrence of SCC, which was higher than the 12% reported by Nicolai and colleagues.[3] One of the 6 patients who had local recurrence also had distant metastasis (patient #5; see **Table 4**). Another patient (patient #16; see **Table 4**), who did not have local recurrence, was found to have distant metastasis to the brain. At latest follow-up, 19 patients (82.6%) were alive with no evidence of disease. Three patients (2 T1 and 1 T2) died of their disease, including the patient who had distant metastasis to the brain. One patient died of other causes.

Other reports of patients who were treated endoscopically lacked data documentation. These include 3 patients with SCC in a cohort of 49 patients reported by Lund and colleagues.[152] One of these patients died at 40-months follow-up, 1 was alive with disease, and the third was disease free. The follow-up of this cohort ranged from 6 to 126 months (mean 36 months). They report overall survival of 88% at 5 years for the entire cohort. There were insufficient data to calculate survival outcome for the patients with SCC. Eviatar and colleagues[156] report 1 case of a 76-year-old patient treated with endoscopic approach in a cohort of 6 patients with malignant sinonasal tumors that were treated in a 7-year period. This patient remains disease free 4 years after the surgery. More recently, Nicolai and colleagues[3] reported their experience of 134 patients with malignant sinonasal tumors managed exclusively with endoscopic approach. This group included 16 patients with SCC. They report a 5-year disease-specific survival of 91.4% (standard deviation [SD] 3.9%) for the entire cohort of 134 patients treated with the endoscopic approach.

Two studies compared endoscopic outcomes with a tCFR cohort,[2,158] whereas another 2 compared endoscopic and combined approaches.[3,149] All studies were retrospective reviews of outcomes, with study cohorts ranging from 2 to 133 patients. When the studies were assessed against the Oxford Center for Evidence-Based Medicine Levels of Evidence criteria,[164] all studies were judged to have level 4 evidence.

Conclusion

- Data on endoscopic surgery for sinonasal SCC are limited, although the accrued data from the pooled patients seems promising. Comparison between the pooled data and previously published outcomes is compounded by the heterogeneous patient population and small cohort of each tumor stage. Nonetheless, the overall disease-free survival rate seems to be comparable with conventional approaches. However, the mean follow-up period is limited to less than 4 years. The overall survival following CFR of sinonasal SCC was 67% at 3 years and decreased to 64% at 5 years' follow-up.[146]
- Whichever surgical technique is used, there is good evidence that the outcome is related to how thoroughly the tumor has been removed. A wide-field three-

Table 4
Summary of data of patients who underwent endoscopic resection for sinonasal SCC

Patient No.	Gender	Age	Extent	Staging	Recurrence	Metastasis	Follow-Up (Mo)	Status
1	M	63	E	T1	N	N	25	DFS
2	F	68	E, CP, LNW, orbital wall	T3	N	N	54	DFS
3	F	66	Septum, M, nasal cavity	T2	N	N	31	DFS
4	M	66	E, M, Mt	T3	N	N	30	DFS
5	M	54	Septum, LNW	T2	Y	N	15	DFS
6	M	85	E, M, S, CP, PMF, LNW	T4a	Y	N	6	DFS
7	M	54	Ant and LNW	T1	N	N	9	DFS
8	Unknown	70	M, E	T1N0	N	N	89	DFS
9	Unknown	40	St	T1N2b	Y	Y	10	DOD
10	Unknown	61	Mt	T1N0	N	N	21	DFS
11	Unknown	63	E, M	T2N0	Y	N	92	DFS
12	Unknown	65	Septum	T2N0	Y	Y	7	DOD
13	M	49	Not stated	Stage IVB	Y	N	57	DFS
14	M	69	E, NF	T2	N	N	63	DFS
15	F	47	NF	T1	N	N	62	DFS
16	F	80	NF	T1	N	Y	28	DOD
17	M	50	E	T3	N	N	34	DFS
18	M	35	E	T2	N	N	89	DFS
19	M	40	E	T4	N	N	78	DFS
20	F	71	IT, NF, septum, and torus	T4b	N	N	77	DFS
21	M	25	E, PE, St, Mt, ant wall SS	T4	N	N	58	DFS
22	F	77	E and MT	T2	N	N	19	DOC
23	M	77	NC	T1	N	N	3	DFS
Summary	12 men 6 women 5 unknown	59.78 (mean) 25–85 (range)	—	T1 = 8 T2 = 7 T3 = 3 T4 = 4	Yes = 6 No = 17	Yes = 3 No = 20	41.6 (mean) 3–92 (range)	DFS = 21 DOD = 3 DOC = 1 AWD = 1

Abbreviations: AWD, alive with disease; CP, cribriform plate; DFS, disease-free survival; DOC, died of other causes; DOD, died of disease; E, ethmoids; LNW, lateral nasal wall; M, maxillary sinus; Mt, middle turbinate; NC, nasal cavity; NF, nasal fossa; PE, posterior ethmoids; PMF, pterygomaxillary fossa; SS, sphenoid sinus; St, superior turbinate.

Data from Refs. [150,153,155,159,161]

dimensional resection undertaken with optimum endoscopic visualization, achieving negative margins, offers resection of the tumor that is close to an en bloc resection, which is rarely possible in practice (**Fig. 6**). The overall morbidity and mortality associated with endoscopic resection of sinonasal SCC seems to be less than with traditional approaches.

Adenocarcinoma

Adenocarcinoma is a glandular malignancy of the sinonasal tract. It is divided into 2 main groups: (1) intestinal-type adenocarcinoma (ITAC), and (2) nonintestinal-type adenocarcinoma. Nonintestinal-type adenocarcinoma is further divided into low-grade and high-grade subtypes.[165]

ITAC

This carcinoma resembles adenocarcinoma of the intestinal tract.

Epidemiology and causes This tumor has a male predominance, probably caused by occupational exposure, and usually presents in the fifth and sixth decades (mean age at presentation 58 years).[166] Wood dust and leather dust have been shown to be associated with the development of this tumor in several different countries, with a considerable delay between exposure and presentation (up to 40 years).[167] It is believed that the larger dust particles may be involved because they are preferentially accumulated in the nose. The carcinogens involved are still unknown but may include alkaloids, saponins, stilbenes, aldehydes, quinones, flavonoids, terpenes, fungal proteins, and tannins.[52,168]

Histology There are 2 published classifications of these tumors, those of Barnes[166] and Kleinsasser and Schroeder.[30] The Barnes classification[166] is preferred because it is simpler, and is the classification presented in **Table 5**. The Kleinsasser and Shroeder[30] classification divides the mucinous type of tumor into alveolar and signet ring tumors.[30] Franchi and colleagues[165] showed that such a division had no prognostic significance.

ITAC are generally locally aggressive with a local recurrence rate of around 50%, local lymph node spread of about 10%, and distant metastasis rate of 20%.[30,165,166,169] The cumulative, disease-specific, 5-year survival rate is between 40% and 60%, with most deaths occurring in the first 3 years. Because the average presentation of these tumors is generally late, with most being T3 and T4 tumors,

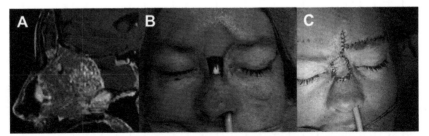

Fig. 6. (*A*) SCC extended to nasal dorsum (CT) and requires resection to clear the margins (*B*) the remaining part was performed endoscopically. Local glabella flap was used for reconstruction (*C*). The goal of surgery is near-field 3 dimensional resection controlled by histological assessment - not an open or endoscopic debate.

Table 5
The Barnes[166] classification of adenocarcinoma

Types	Approximate Prevalence Varies from Author to Author (%)	Differentiation	3-y Cumulative Survival (%)[a]
Papillary	18	Well differentiated	82
Colonic	40	Moderately differentiated	54
Solid	20	Poorly differentiated	36
Mucinous	14	Mucinous	48
Mixed	8	Mixed differentiation	71

[a] Derived from Kleinsasser and Schroeder.[30]
Data from Barnes L. Intestinal-type adenocarcinoma of the nasal cavity and paranasal sinuses. Am J Surg Pathol 1986;10(3):192–202.

staging tumors according to the tumor-node-metastasis (TNM) staging system has little prognostic significance.[165]

Sinonasal nonintestinal-type adenocarcinomas

The tumors are divided into low-grade and high-grade subtypes, with low-grade presenting mostly in the ethmoid cells and the high-grade in the maxillary sinus.[170] These tumors may present in the nasal cavity or in any combination of the locations discussed earlier. Low-grade tumors have a more indolent course, presenting with unilateral nasal obstruction and epistaxis, whereas high-grade tumors may present with additional symptoms associated with extension of the tumor into the orbit (double vision, proptosis), infratemporal fossa (infraorbital nerve sensory changes), or intracranial cavity (frontal lobe symptoms and headache).[170]

Low-grade tumors have an excellent prognosis, with 5-year survival of up to 85%,[171] whereas high-grade tumors have a poor prognosis, with 3-year survival of around 20%.[170]

Salivary Gland–type Carcinomas

Salivary gland–type adenocarcinomas are uncommon, occurring in 5% to 10% of sinonasal adenocarcinomas.[172] They are believed to originate from the seromucinous glands of the nasal and sinus epithelium. **Table 6** lists the types and occurrence of all sinonasal salivary tumors (both malignant and benign).

Table 6
Types and occurrence of all sinonasal salivary tumors

Tumor Type	Percentage Occurrence
High-grade adenocarcinoma not otherwise specified	30
ACC	17
Mucoepidermoid carcinoma	5
Low-grade salivary-type adenocarcinoma (various types including mucoepidermoid and acinic cell carcinoma	21
Pleomorphic adenoma[a]	23

This nomenclature predates the most recent WHO classification.
[a] Benign.
Data from Refs.[51,170,172,353]

Adenocarcinoma not otherwise specified may be considered a diagnostic entity on its own and is often poorly differentiated with a poor prognosis, in keeping with other poorly differentiated adenocarcinomas.[166,170,172] ACC is the most common salivary gland malignant tumor, originating most commonly in the maxillary sinus (60%) and nasal cavity (25%). The extent of tumor spread is often underestimated by radiology as perineural spread, which is common in this tumor and often remains undetected, and the long-term survival is poor with 7% 10-year survival[173] with most patients dying of local recurrence rather than distant metastasis.[174] Long-term follow-up is thus mandatory to detect late recurrences. The other salivary gland malignancies are all very rare and not individually presented.

Treatment

Most studies on the treatment of sinonasal malignancies do not separate the histologic types of tumors and present series in which the treatment of these tumors are grouped together (**Table 7**).[1,148–154,157,161,163,175–177] There are only a few published studies[48,168,171,172,178–180] in which the adenocarcinomas have been separately reported. A great deal of the evidence for the treatment of nonepidermoid malignancies comes from separating these tumors from other tumors in the published studies.

The central issue in the treatment of adenocarcinomas is to prevent locoregional recurrence, because most patients die as consequence of a local recurrence rather than as a result of either local or systemic metastasis.[152,172,181] Treatment is focused on removing the tumor, where possible with a clear margin, and this depends on the site of the tumor. Pedunculated or isolated tumors attaching to turbinates or the septum can be easily removed with a good margin of normal tissue either by endoscopic or open approach. The treatment controversy is around tumors that abut or transgress the skull base or orbit. The current gold standard for the treatment of these tumors remains a CFR (tCFR),[48,148,157,175,178,180] which involves a craniotomy to expose the anterior skull base from above and, traditionally, an open approach to

Table 7
Numbers of adenocarcinomas reported in the literature

First Author, Year	Total Number of Malignant Sinonasal Tumors	Total Number of Adenocarcinomas
Lund et al,[157] 1998	167	42
Stammberger et al,[177] 1999	43	7
Thaler et al,[163] 1999	4	1
Goffart et al,[1] 2000	78	40
Roh et al,[151] 2004	47	2
Poetker et al,[150] 2005	16	2
Ganly et al,[176] 2005	334	107
Batra et al,[148] 2005	25	3
Buchmann et al,[149] 2006	78	2
Castelnuovo et al,[154] 2006	18	10
Chen,[161] 2006	7	4
Howard et al,[175] 2006	259	62
Lund et al,[152] 2007	49	15
Podboj and Smid,[153] 2007	16	5
Total	1141	302

the nasal and sinus cavity allowing resection of the cribiform plate, ethmoids, fovea ethmodalis, anterior face of sphenoid, and septum. Orbital involvement is determined by whether or not the orbital periostium is breached. If not breached, this structure is preserved. Postoperative irradiation is advocated by most investigators, although the evidence for its usefulness is lacking.[48,178,179,182,183] Adjuvant chemotherapy is rarely given.[48] The 3-year disease-specific survival rate is around 72%, and the 5-year survival rate for this procedure is around 60%.[48] However, it is well recognized that CFR resection is not a benign procedure and has a significant morbidity, with 33% of patients suffering complications, and a mortality of 4.5%.[176] With the increased usage of the endoscope in the 1990s, the nasal component of the CFR was more commonly performed endoscopically and this procedure was termed a combined endoscopic CFR (CECFR). In 2008, Nicolai and colleagues[3] compared their results for CECFR with wholly endoscopic resection and found that, for adenocarcinoma, the 5-year disease-free survival was 60% compared with 80% for the wholly endoscopic approach. However, the indication for performing a combined approach was in patients who had more extensive tumor, usually with dura and brain invasion, so it is not possible to compare these outcomes.

In the 1990s, reports began to detail wholly endoscopic resection of adenocarcinomas of the sinonasal cavity.[181] Again, most of these publications combined adenocarcinoma with other histologic groups, making true outcome assessment of this new technique difficult (**Table 8**).

The initial limitations of the wholly endoscopic approach were the ability of the surgeon to access extension of the tumor onto and through the dura and into brain.[1,3]

Table 8
Adenocarcinoma resected by an entirely endoscopic approach

First Author, Year	Total Cases (n)	Adenocarcinoma (n)	DXT (n)	Recurrence Rate for Entirely Endoscopic Resection (Follow-up is Mean Time for All Patients)
Stammberger et al,[177] 1999	36	7	—	5 clear of disease at 30 mo
Shah et al,[181] 1999	1	1	—	1 clear of disease at 12 mo
Goffart et al,[1] 2000	66	40[a]	87.9%	5-y disease-specific survival 57.6%
Roh et al,[151] 2004	19	2	78.9%	1 recurrence at 40 mo
Poetker et al,[150] 2005	16	2	0%	No recurrences at 19 mo
Batra et al,[148] 2005	9	2	78%	1 recurrence at 24 mo
Lund et al,[152] 2007	47	14	76%	1 recurrence at 36 mo
Podboj and Smid,[153] 2007	16	5	60%	No recurrence at 84 mo
Nicolai et al,[3] 2008	134	44	35%	5-y disease-specific survival 94.4%
Bogaerts et al,[178] 2008	44	44	100%	5-y disease-specific survival 83%
Jardeleza et al,[180] 2009	12	12	75%	91.6% disease-specific survival at 30 mo

[a] Some of these patients may have had an additional craniotomy as part of the procedure.

The stated principles of a wholly endoscopic resection remain the same as those for CFR in that the aim is to achieve a complete local resection to prevent local recurrence.[178,180] The wholly endoscopic approach is different from the standard CFR approach in that the tumor in the nose is debulked until the tumor attachment is clearly identified. Once this is clear, the surgical approach to resect the entire tumor, including a margin of normal tissue, is planned.[3,177,180,184] New endoscopic techniques for accessing previously difficult regions such as the frontal sinus, areas of the maxillary sinus, and infratemporal fossa are now available.[148,160,178,180] Techniques such as frontal drillout or Draf III procedure allow full access to tumor extension into the frontal sinus or onto the posterior wall of the frontal sinus.[185] Endoscopic medial maxillectomy gives access to the entire maxillary sinus and the infratemporal fossa.[186] The current major controversy is whether the wholly endoscopic resection compromises the outcome by the resection being performed in most instances in a piecemeal fashion.[160,181,186,187] The other area of debate is whether it is necessary to achieve clear margins and whether it is worthwhile documenting such margins during both the endoscopic and CFR approaches. The margins of an anterior skull base resection (either including or excluding the lamina papyracea) are usually bony or cartilaginous and this can make it difficult for the surgeon to obtain a representative sample to send for frozen section.[178] In addition, it has been found that the incidence of recurrence after surgery in patients with positive and negative margins is similar.[178] Because most patients receive postoperative radiotherapy, the positive margins (and normal resection margins) are all included in the postoperative treatment fields. Additional advantages of an endoscopic resection are the improved visualization of the tumor borders provided by the magnification achieved with the use of endoscopes, lack of skin incisions, and lack of resection of normal tissue (maxilla, nasal bones, sinuses) to be able to visualize the extent of the tumor.[148,160,178,180,184,187] However, it is well recognized that wholly endoscopic resection of tumors abutting or breaching the normal confines of the sinonasal cavity is technically demanding, that the learning curve for such techniques is significant and takes considerable time to achieve, and that these procedures should not be adopted until such a level of expertise has been developed within the skull base team (see **Fig. 2**).[180]

Conclusion

- Endoscopic resection is possible for many tumors
- Adjuvant radiotherapy is used for all but very small tumors
- Stripping of the tumor from involved structures is not considered standard of care, and involved structures such as the dura should be resected as they would be in tCFR.

MALIGNANT NEUROECTODERMAL TUMORS
Olfactory Neuroblastoma/Esthesioneuroblastoma

Incidence and cause
The incidence of olfactory neuroblastoma is difficult to establish, but the tumor is not as rare as is commonly reported, and probably represents more than 5% of all nasal malignant tumors. Olfactory neuroblastoma occurs in a wide age range (3–90 years) with a bimodal peak in the second and sixth decades of life (**Fig. 7**).[78,188] Sporadic cases have also been reported in children less than 10 years of age.[76]

The exact cell of origin of olfactory neuroblastoma is believed to be the basal reserve cell, the olfactory stem cell that gives rise to both the neuronal and the epithelial sustentacular cells. Proposed sources have included Jacobson vomeronasal

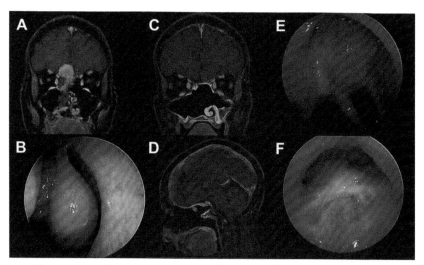

Fig. 7. Olfactory neuroblastoma in a 60 year old female. There is a significant intracranial portion on MRI (*A*) and it extends through the septum superiorly to the contralateral olfactory cleft on the left on endoscopy (*B*). The resection encompasses dura, falx cerebri and margins over the orbital roof (*C*) and low left septal flap and nasal floor was used for reconstruction (*D* and *E*). A endoscopic Lothrop is critical for access during endoscopic resection of these tumors (*F*) and should be considered standard for neoplasms where the resection extends beyond the anterior ethmoid artery.

organ, the sphenopalatine ganglion, the ectodermal olfactory placode, Loci ganglion, autonomic ganglia in the nasal mucosa, and the olfactory epithelium.[75] Although a neuronal or neural crest origin is supported by the presence of neurofilaments in olfactory neuroblastoma, until recently[189] little evidence has linked olfactory neuroblastoma directly to the olfactory epithelium despite the clinical association (**Fig. 8**).

No known causal factor exists for this tumor,[80] although diethylnitrosamine injections can induce tumors in hamsters at the site of the olfactory epithelium.[81] No hereditary patterns have been described for this neoplasm and there is no apparent racial predilection.

Staging

Kadish and colleagues[190] were the first to propose a staging classification, using 3 categories, group A, B, and C (**Table 9**). A further system was proposed with the advent of advances in imaging,[79] based on the TNM system (**Table 10**). Although a system of classification has been proposed, various attempts have been made to modify the Kadish system.[78,191] Other investigators suggest that, by using the Kadish staging system and the Hyams grading system independently, they can predict patients' outcome with more accuracy.[192] The Hyams grading system is based on histology and is referred to later.

Treatment and Results

The primary site

A combination of surgery and radiotherapy is the most frequently used approach, and the one that achieved the highest cure rates.[193,194] Despite the lack of support for single-modality treatment regimes,[195] a substantial number of patients are treated by surgery or radiotherapy alone. The difference in survival between the combined

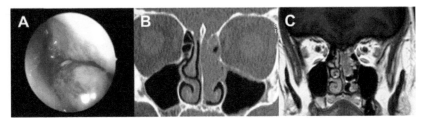

Fig. 8. Olfactory neuroblastoma with origin visible in the olfactory cleft. Endoscopic view with attachment high in the olfactory cleft (*A*), CT showing a mass medial to the middle turbinate (*B*), MRI of the contrast enhancement on T1 (*C*).

treatments and radiotherapy alone is significant (**Table 11**). The 5-year disease-specific survival in the literature is between 52% and 90%.[79] Surgery alone was associated with lower survival combined with a combination of radiotherapy and chemotherapy, or triple modality treatment (surgery, radiotherapy, and chemotherapy). Although the results were 15% to 20% better, the differences from the best combination were not statistically significant, probably because of the limited number of patients.[193] These results were complied from the MEDLINE database from the period 1990 to 2000, without language tags. There were 26 treatment studies that formed the basis for the tabulations described earlier, and data extracted from these studies comprised the total number of patients, the staging system used, the patients' distributions by stage and the histologic grade, and the treatment used. Outcome data consisted of recurrence-free survival at 3 and 5 years; overall survival at 5 and 10 years; and the results by stage, grade, and treatment modality.

In 5 studies, olfactory neuroblastoma were histopathologically graded and, according to Hyams and colleagues, the mean 5-year survival was 56% (SD 20) in patients with grade I or II tumors and 25% (95% confidence interval [CI] SD 20) in those with grade III or IV tumors. This difference was significant (odds ratio 6.18; 1.30–29.3). In 25 studies that used the Kadish classification, the mean 5-year survival for group A was 72% (SD 41), group B 59% (SD 44), and group C 47% (SD 16). On average, 5% (SD 7) of patients presented with cervical lymph node metastases. In the studies of survival data according to N stage, only 29% of N+ patients were treated successfully, compared with 64% of N0, a significant difference (odds ratio 5.1; 95% CI 1.6–17.0).

Table 9
Olfactory neuroblastoma staging according to Kadish and colleagues[190] and modified by Morita and colleagues[78]

Type	Extension
A	Tumor limited to the nasal cavity
B	Tumor involving the nasal and paranasal sinuses
C	Tumor extending beyond the nasal and paranasal sinuses, including involvement of the cribriform plate, base of the skull, orbit cavity, or intracranial cavity
D	Tumor with metastasis to cervical nodes or distant sites

Data from Kadish S, Goodman M, Wang CC. Olfactory neuroblastoma. A clinical analysis of 17 cases. Cancer 1976;37(3):1571–6; and Morita A, Ebersold MJ, Olsen KD, et al. Esthesioneuroblastoma: prognosis and management. Neurosurgery 32(5):706–14 [discussion: 714–5].

Table 10 Olfactory neuroblastoma: staging system after Dulguerov and Calcaterra[79]	
Stage	**Characteristics**
T1	Tumor involving the nasal cavity and/or paranasal sinuses (excluding the sphenoid sinus), sparing the most superior ethmoidal cells
T2	Tumor involving the nasal cavity and/or paranasal sinuses (including the sphenoid sinus) with extension to, or erosion of, the cribriform plate
T3	Tumor extending into the orbit or protruding into the anterior cranial fossa, without dural invasion
T4	Tumor involving the brain
N0	No cervical lymph node metastases
N1	Any form of cervical lymph node metastases
M0	No metastases
M1	Any distant metastases

Data from Dulguerov P, Calcaterra T. Esthesioneuroblastoma: the UCLA experience 1970–1990. Laryngoscope 1992;102(8):843–9.

Surgery

Most institutions favor surgery as the first treatment modality, followed by radiotherapy.[78,157,191,196–201]

Endocranial extension and a close relation to the ethmoid roof and cribriform plate have conventionally led to a combined transfacial and neurosurgical approach. CFR allows for an en bloc resection of the tumor with better assessment of any intracranial extension and protection of the brain and optic nerve. The resection should include the entire cribriform plate and crista galli. It is said that the olfactory bulb and overlying dura should be removed with the specimen, although there is no clear evidence to support the assertion that the whole of the bulb should be removed.[202] Open surgery has long been regarded as the gold standard, with results available for decades. A craniotomy is probably not justified for T1 tumors if there is clear radiological evidence of a normal cribriform plate and no involvement of the upper ethmoidal cells, although this clinical picture is seldom seen. The evolution of surgical techniques has created another surgical option in the form of endonasal endoscopic surgery. The use of

Table 11 Olfactory neuroblastoma: distribution of patients and survival by treatment modality (1992–2008) according to the meta-analysis by Devaiah and Andreoli[205]					
Modality	**No. of Patients**	**Frequency (%)**	**Survival (%)**	**Odds Ratio**	**Confidence Interval**
Surgery alone	87	20 ± 22	48 ± 40	1.9	0.7–4.9
Surgery plus radiotherapy	169	44 ± 20	65 ± 25	1	—
Radiation alone	49	13 ± 19	37 ± 33	2.5	1.02–6.0
Surgery plus radiotherapy plus chemotherapy	48	7 ± 16	47 ± 37	2.1	0.68–16.5
Radiation plus chemotherapy	26	0 ± 1	0	—	—
Chemotherapy	6	2 ± 4	40 ± 55	—	—

Data from Devaiah AK, Andreoli MT. Treatment of esthesioneuroblastoma: a 16-year meta-analysis of 361 patients. Laryngoscope 2009;119(7):1412–6.

endoscopic surgery for olfactory neuroblastoma followed by the use of the stereo-tactic radiosurgical γ knife therapy has recently been used.[77,203] One report of 10 cases with a mean follow-up of 38 months used endoscopic resection alone without any recurrence, although only 2 had Kadish stage C.[204] In the last decade, numerous articles with small numbers have been published on the endoscopic resection of olfactory neuroblastoma. Devaiah and Andreoli[205] reviewed the literature with a meta-analysis and showed that an endoscopic approach gave a better survival rate. The aim of this study was to compare results of open, endoscopic, endos-copy-assisted, and nonsurgical treatments since the first publication in the literature that mentioned an endoscopic removal. This analysis extracted sufficient data in 361 subjects and the statistically significant results for the full cohort are summarized in **Table 12**.[150,160,194,206–215]

Endoscopic surgery produced overall better survival rates than open surgery, with no significant difference between follow-up times in the endoscopic and open surgery groups. Because the gold standard open procedure considerably predated endo-scopic treatment, they also grouped the data according to the publication year. The endoscopic surgery group maintained better survival rates (**Table 13**). These data show evidence for the efficacy of endoscopic surgery in olfactory neuroblastoma. There are more cases of long-term follow-up in the open surgery group than the endo-scopic treatment group and most of the open surgery tumors belonged to the Kadish C and D stages, whereas the endoscopic techniques were used more commonly for Kadish A and B tumors. This finding reflects how endoscopic surgery has mainly been used for less extensive lesions, which might not only be a reflection of the size of the tumor but their symptoms, because more extensive lesions might be expected to be more invasive and less differentiated, although this cannot be ascertained from the data available.[205] The most recent publication on endoscopic endonasal resection for all Kadish groups has recently been published by Folbe and colleagues[216] This is a retrospective, multicenter study with 23 patients operated endoscopically, with postoperative radiotherapy in 16 patients. The mean follow-up was 45.2 months with 1 recurrence. The investigators conclude that endoscopic surgery is replacing CFR and that oncological control is not sacrificed when good endoscopic resection techniques are used.

Radiotherapy

Standard radiotherapy techniques include external megavoltage beam and a 3-field technique; an anterior port is later combined with wedge fields to provide a homoge-neous dose distribution. The doses range from 55 Gy to 65 Gy, with most receiving more than 60 Gy. Currently, it is considered that radiotherapy should play a role in the management of olfactory neuroblastoma, particularly in patients who have had incomplete surgical resection or who present with residual disease.[210,213,217] In a small

Table 12				
Olfactory neuroblastoma: comparison of survival results (1992–2008) according to the meta-analysis by Devaiah and Andreoli[205]				
Treatment A	**Number**	**Treatment B**	**Number**	**P**
Surgery	279	No surgery	52	<.001
Open surgery	214	Endoscopic surgery	40	.0019 (endoscopic better)
Open surgery	214	Endoscopy assisted	57	.0123 (endoscopic better)

Data from Devaiah AK, Andreoli MT. Treatment of esthesioneuroblastoma: a 16-year meta-analysis of 361 patients. Laryngoscope 2009;119(7):1412–6.

Table 13
Olfactory neuroblastoma: comparison of survival results (2002–2008) according to the meta-analysis by Devaiah and Andreoli[205]

Treatment A	Number	Treatment B	Number	P
Open surgery	145	Endoscopic surgery	40	.0018 (endoscopic better)
Open surgery	145	Endoscopy assisted	57	.0133 (endoscopic better)

Data from Devaiah AK, Andreoli MT. Treatment of esthesioneuroblastoma: a 16-year meta-analysis of 361 patients. Laryngoscope 2009;119(7):1412–6.

retrospective series, a comparison was made between conventional radiotherapy and stereotactically guided conformal radiotherapy (SCRT). It was concluded that SCRT improved target coverage and sparing of organs at risk.[218]

Chemotherapy

Olfactory neuroblastoma is regarded as a chemosensitive tumor based on multiple reported responses to treatment.[207,219–221] Neoadjuvant therapy is seldom curative on its own and it may be of no benefit in some patients. Individuals who respond to preoperative chemotherapy have a greater chance of long-term disease-free survival.[219] It has been proposed that Hyams' grading is an important predictor of response to chemotherapy,[222] and it has been suggested that cisplatin-based chemotherapy is helpful in advanced, high-grade olfactory neuroblastoma and should be considered the treatment of choice in the systemic treatment of these patients.

Neoadjuvant chemotherapy has been advocated for patients with advanced disease at the University of Virginia in a 20-year period.[197] In 34 consecutive patients, two-thirds showed a significant reduction of tumor burden with adjuvant therapy and patients who showed a response to neoadjuvant therapy showed a significantly greater disease-free mortality. Preoperative chemotherapy consisted of cyclophosphamide (650 mg/m^2) and vincristine (1.5 mg/m^2; maximal dose, 2 mg), administered every 3 weeks for 6 cycles. Adriamycin was used in combination with cyclosphosphamide in 2 patients. Most patients also received a total dose of 50 Gy of preoperative fractionated radiation therapy.

CNS Metastases

CNS metastases (as opposed to direct intracranial extension) can occur in olfactory neuroblastoma. These lesions are believed to arise when tumor cells violate the ependymal epithelium of the ventricles to gain free access to the ventricular fluid. Tumor cells then disseminate through the CSF pathways to distant sites.[223] More than 17 patients identified from the literature had CNS metastases from olfactory neuroblastoma.[223,224] The trends were found in these patients (1) most patients in whom CNS metastases developed had Kadish stage C disease at diagnosis; (2) there was a highly variable time to onset of CNS metastases, ranging from 1 to 228 months after initial diagnosis of olfactory neuroblastoma; (3) survival after CNS metastases was generally less than 2 years; and (4) the treatment regimen that appeared to result in the longest survival after CNS metastases included surgical resection of the metastatic lesion followed by radiation and/or chemotherapy.

Neck Metastases

Neck metastases are found at presentation in 5% of patients. Such patients should be treated by neck dissection or radiotherapy. It has been estimated from a review of the literature[76] that up to 23.4% may develop cervical lymph node metastases. Thus, treatment of the clinically negative neck may be warranted. In general, an elective neck dissection is not considered because these cervical nodes metastases may not develop for 2 years or more. It is pragmatic to treat them when they are clinically apparent. However, nodal metastases are associated with the development of distant metastases; hence, should these patients undergo an elective neck dissection in advance of the development of metastatic neck disease? The high frequency of occurrence of lymph node metastases is sufficient to refute the claim that olfactory neuroblastoma is a low-grade malignant tumor. Distant metastases synchronous at presentation have been reported in 6.6% (3/45).[191]

Primary Tumor Recurrence

The assessment of recurrent olfactory neuroblastoma at the primary site is usually undertaken with magnetic resonance imaging (MRI). The appearance of the recurrent tumor does not differ from that imaged at initial presentation.[224] Enhanced computed tomography (CT) and MRI images in the coronal plane are helpful in identifying small recurrences and/or intracranial extensions. The meta-analysis by Dulguerov and colleagues[193] found that the 5-year survival of 45% was associated with recurrent disease. Local recurrence in olfactory neuroblastoma occurs in approximately 30%. CFR followed by radiotherapy is associated with fewer recurrences (around 10%). Salvage after local recurrence is possible in 33% to 50% of cases.[74]

Regional and Distant Recurrence

Regional recurrence in the cervical lymph nodes, where the primary site is disease free, occurs in 15% to 20% of cases and is salvageable by treating these in one-third.

Distant metastases with locoregional control are common (8%) and carry a poor prognosis. The time to metastases in varies from 1 to 20 months.[191] Sites involved include the lung, liver, eye, parotid, CNS, bone, vertebrae, and epidural space.

Assessment of Recurrence and Further Treatment

Median survival after recurrence is 12 months, so it is imperative to deal with the primary site initially to minimize the risk of metastatic disease.[214]

There is a delayed neck metastatic rate of 16%, and some consider that this is an indication for elective neck dissection in all cases of olfactory neuroblastoma. Patients with advanced local disease should undergo radiological examination of the neck and may be candidates for regional treatment[212] that may include either treating the neck with radiotherapy or performing an elective neck dissection followed by radiotherapy.

The principle site for distant metastases in one series[191] was bone, with vertebrae being the most common location (86%). Asymptomatic bone metastases were found in 3 patients at presentation coincidentally with a bone scan that was performed after bone marrow biopsies showed aplasia. Hence, a bone scan and bone marrow biopsy should be considered if the likelihood of distant metastases is raised. The significant risk factor for developing distant metastases is the presence of cervical metastases at initial presentation.

There is a single case report of a woman with an olfactory neuroblastoma with epithelial and endocrine differentiation that transformed into a mature ganglioneuroma after chemoradiotherapy.[225]

Recommended Follow-up

Olfactory neuroblastoma is a neoplastic disease with a long natural history characterized by frequent local and regional recurrences after conventional treatment,[212] and so extended follow-up of patients is warranted. The mean time for recurrence is 5 years for evaluating most other cancers of the head and neck, but this is not valid for olfactory neuroblastoma; there the survival data at 10, 15, and even 20 years is important in evaluating the result of treatment.[226]

Girod and colleagues[200] have suggested that MRI with gadolinium should be done 2 to 4 months after completion of all therapy, and should be repeated 4 to 6 monthly for 5 years and then annually for the patient's lifetime.[224,227] Continued clinical follow-up is indicated annually thereafter and any symptoms should be investigated. An annual chest radiograph should be performed to exclude the presence of metastases.

Conclusion

- The current recommended treatment strategy is:
  - ○ Kadish A: –surgery, in selected cases combined with radiotherapy.
  - ○ Kadish B: radiotherapy before or after surgery, to the primary tumor site and subclinical lymph nodes. Adjunctive chemotherapy may be added to this treatment depending on the degree of differentiation of the tumor.
  - ○ Kadish C/D: preoperative chemotherapy and/or radiotherapy followed by surgery. The use of adjuvant chemotherapy has yet to be further elucidated, as well as the timing of the surgery and the radiotherapy. Surgery may be followed by chemoradiotherapy at centers with extensive skull base experience.

MALIGNANT MELANOMA
Introduction

Malignant melanoma of the sinonasal mucosa is an uncommon disease, and survival is poor. Diagnosis is often delayed because the onset of symptoms is insidious and patients present with advanced disease. The rarity and long natural history of malignant tumors make it difficult to accrue cohorts to compare endoscopic resection with the established gold standard of CFR.[152]

Incidence and Cause

Malignant melanoma (MM) is a rare disorder of the nasal cavity and paranasal sinus mucosa. Primary sinonasal tract mucosal MMs are rare, accounting for between 0.3% and 2% of all malignant melanomas and about 4% of head and neck melanomas.[62–67,69] In the National Cancer Database report by the American College of Surgeons Commission on Cancer and the American Cancer Society of more than 84,000 melanomas seen from 1985 to 1994, only 1.3% were melanomas that arose from mucosal surfaces, of which 55% were of the head and neck. Sinonasal tract mucosal MMs were equally common in men and women. A higher proportion of melanoma was identified in black patients (10.4%).[66] In general, the mean age for sinonasal tract mucosal MMs is 64.3 years, being later in life than cutaneous malignant melanomas. Sinonasal tract mucosal MMs have a worse prognosis over 60 years.[66] Tumors originating in the sinuses are less common than those arising in the nasal cavity, and they tend to grow asymptomatically until late in the disease course.[19,69] One-third of patients present with neck metastases, which often preceded more distant metastasis, and distant metastasis, the latter usually being rapidly fatal.[72]

Approximately 80% of MM are found within the nasal vault and 20% in the sinuses (**Fig. 9**).[63,67,68] The incidence is not increasing, unlike that of cutaneous melanoma, which has increased significantly in the past few years.

Preexisting melanosis in the nasal mucosa is uncommon, and is believed to be a risk factor for developing MM, and this is supported by a higher incidence in the black

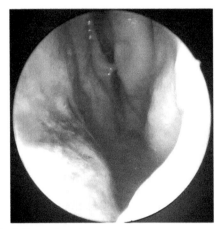

Fig. 9. Melanoma of the left nasal septum.

population. The cause is unclear, although several series have found that occupational exposure to formaldehyde may be a factor.[70,228,229]

Staging

Staging the disease before treatment is essential for documentation and comparing the results of treatment.

Thompson and colleagues[70] suggested using the TNM classification as a predictor of biologic behavior.

Ballantyne[230] described a simple system that has been used by many because of its simplicity:

Stage I: disease confined to the primary site
Stage II: primary lesion with regional lymph node metastasis
Stage III: presence of systemic metastasis

Treatment and Results

The primary therapeutic modality is surgical resection with wide local margins. Incomplete local control is a predictor of poor survival in mucosal melanomas.[231] Although no formal randomized trials have shown benefit from radiation therapy in sinonasal melanoma, some studies suggest that radiotherapy may provide some improved local control but none show an increase in life expectancy. Postoperative radiation is often recommended for advanced disease, but with little evidence to support its use with any improvement in survival rates. Chemotherapy is currently only used for disseminated disease and palliation and its benefit is uncertain.

Local recurrence is a major problem and Huang and colleagues[232] had an average time from surgery to local recurrence of 5 months. Regional recurrence is similarly a problem, being 7.45 months in the same series.[232]

Prophylactic neck dissection in an N0 neck is not done because the incidence of node metastases is low.[233]

Distant metastases have been reported between 10.3 months[232] and 23.2 months.[70] Dauer and colleagues[72] reported a median time between diagnosis and death of 19 months in their series of 61 patients, with a cancer-specific survival rate of 22.1% at 5 years. In a series of 115 patients reported by Thompson and colleagues,[70] 55% died of disseminated disease after a mean of 2.3 years, although

Bridger and colleagues,[234] who propose initial radical surgery and postoperative radiotherapy, reported a mean survival time of 4.3 years in their series of 27 patients. The completeness of resection seems to be important.

Nicolai and colleagues[3] retrospectively analyzed 17 patients with MM in a series of 184 skull base tumors. Fourteen sinonasal MM were removed endoscopically and 3 using a craniofacial endoscopic approach. The staging of these patients was not described. Nine of the endoscopic group recurred (64%) and 2 of the craniofacial endoscopic approach (67%) after a mean follow-up of 34.1 months. It is not possible to determine the survival rates for MM from the data in the large mixed group of skull base tumors that they reported.

In MM of all mucosal sites in the head and neck, positive margins are associated with a greatly increased mortality.[235]

Whatever the therapy, median survival is poor. Beyond the negative risk factors of size, deep thickness, and invasion, a review from the Mayo Clinic found statistically significant survival benefit from the primary lesion being located on the nasal septum, as opposed to the sinuses or lateral nasal wall.[72]

Mucosal melanomas of the sinonasal tract tend to be more aggressive and have a poorer prognosis than their cutaneous counterparts, having 22% to 46% 5-year survival rate.[70,232,234] The poor prognosis with MM is attributable to both local recurrence and distant metastasis. Several new biologic and immune modulator treatments are currently being investigated for use in patients with mucosal melanoma, and the results of these treatments is eagerly awaited.

Surgery and/or Radiotherapy

A retrospective review by Lund and colleagues[236] examined whether surgery combined with radiotherapy confers any survival benefit compared with radical local excision alone. From a cohort of 72 patients treated between 1963 and 1996 within a single unit, complete data were available for 58 individuals who were examined. The investigators came to the conclusion that overall survival was poor and did not seem to be improved by the addition of radiotherapy. Thompson and colleagues,[70] who advocated surgery and radiotherapy in a series of 115 patients, concluded that the specific type of therapy did not seem to influence the overall patient outcome, because there was no significant difference between patients managed by surgery, surgery with chemotherapy, surgery with radiotherapy, or all 3.

A minority of workers have been proponents of radiotherapy, although MM has historically been regarded as not being radiosensitive. Owens and colleagues[237] treated 11 patients with adjuvant radiotherapy and found that it decreased local recurrence but did not significantly improve survival, although the sample size was small. Wada and colleagues[238] retrospectively studied 21 patients who received radiotherapy alone and 10 for gross residual disease after surgery. They reported a 29% complete response rate and a 58% partial response rate, but their disease-specific survival rates were in line with other studies. Other studies of mucosal MM of the head and neck suggest that radiotherapy increases the local and neck disease-free period but does not increase survival.[239] Temam and colleagues[240] treated 46 patients with paranasal sinus MM as well as 23 with MM of the oral cavity or pharynx. Patients with small tumors who received postoperative radiotherapy had better local disease-free survival than patients with larger tumors who did not receive radiotherapy. Their conclusion that postoperative radiotherapy increases local control is open to criticism given the bias in the staging of disease between those who did and did not receive radiotherapy. Both Nandapalan and colleagues[241] and Patel and colleagues[233] found that radiotherapy did not provide any local control.

Bridger and colleagues[234] reported favorable survival rates compared with most other series advocating wide local excision followed by radiotherapy (**Table 14**).

Brandwein and colleagues[228] from Mount Sinai Medical University did a retrospective study as well as a meta-analysis of the English-language literature for cases of documented sinonasal melanoma from 1977 to 1995. The population in this study included 10 men and 15 women aged 23 to 83 years (mean 65 years). Tumor sites included the inferior turbinate, superior nasal cavity, nasal cavity floor/palate, ethmoid sinuses, and maxillary sinus. They reported that, in spite of advances in imaging, surgical techniques, and adjuvant therapeutics, the mean survival for patients with sinonasal melanoma remains poor. They identified a total of 163 cases from the literature: the 5-year median survival for all patients was 36 months.

In another large cohort of patients, the Mayo Clinic retrospectively reviewed 61 cases from the period between 1955 and 2003.[72] The most common treatment was surgical excision alone (48%). The cancer-specific survival rate (ie, rate of death caused by disease) was 48.9% and 22.1% at 3 and 5 years respectively. Median time between diagnosis and death caused by disease was 19 months. They concluded that wide local excision is the treatment of choice, and some patients may benefit from postoperative radiotherapy. Local recurrence and distant metastasis are common and any improvement in survival is likely to depend on the development of better systemic therapies.[242] In a more recent prospective study by Lund and colleagues,[152] all 11 MM tumors were removed endoscopically with the intention to cure the patient. Three patients had previously had a lateral rhinotomy. Following endoscopic resection, 1 patient had a further endoscopic resection, another had a lateral rhinotomy, and 2 patients had neck dissections (6 and 16 months). The overall survival at 5 years for this specific group was 80%, of whom 36% were disease-free patients. Lund and colleagues[152] found that the endoscopic removal of MM is as effective as by other means but emphasized that CFR remains the gold standard for tumors that contact or traverse the skull base.

Discussion

In general the prognosis of paranasal sinus MM is poor,[70] although lesions that affect the septum do better.[72] The 5-year survival rate is worse than for cutaneous malignant melanoma. This difference may relate to a delay in diagnosis because of its hidden site and the nonspecific nature of its presenting symptoms.

The place of radiotherapy remains uncertain. The small size of most series and lack of randomization and the variation in treatment modalities used makes it difficult to extract any meaningful data from the literature. The disorder and its propensity to recur locally and metastasize remain the primary problem. Whether the primary lesion is removed endoscopically via an external incision or midfacial degloving seems to make little difference to the prognosis. There are some data to favor wide local excision rather than local removal.[234] Lund and colleagues[152] concluded that the intention with endoscopic surgery is not limited but it should always be done with the intention to cure the patient by removing the tumor with the same margin as might be achieved by an open procedure. Long-term follow-up is mandatory (up to 15 or 20 years to help compare different treatment modalities.

Conclusion

- Patients with sinonasal MM often present late because it often has an insidious onset.
- The initial resection should be wide with intention to cure.

Table 14
Results of treatment of sinonasal malignant melanoma in the literature

Authors	Number of Patients	Primary Treatment to Local Recurrence	Primary Treatment to Regional Recurrence	Primary Treatment to Distant Metastases	Survival and Disease-free Interval
Thompson et al,[70] 2003 (ethos: wide local excision plus some radiotherapy/chemotherapy)	115	Unable to extract data	Unable to extract data	Unable to extract data	45% alive at a mean of 2.3 y, 22% alive at 5 y
Bridger et al,[234] 2005 (ethos: radical surgery and radiotherapy)	27	14.7 mo (mean)	Unable to extract data	23.2 mo (mean)	46% alive at 5 y, mean survival 52 mo
Huang et al,[232] 2007 (ethos: surgery plus some with radiotherapy/chemotherapy)	15	5 mo (mean)	7.45 mo (mean)	10.3 mo (mean)	49.5% alive at 2 y, 33% at 5 y
Lund et al,[152] 2007 (all endoscopic resection, intention to cure, prospective)	11	Unable to extract data	Unable to extract data	Unable to extract data	80% alive at 5 y, 36% disease free
Dauer et al,[72] 2008 (ethos: wide local excision plus some radiotherapy)	61	9 mo (mean)	Unable to extract data	13 mo (mean)	48.9% alive at 3 y, 22.1% at 5 y Median survival 19 mo
Brandwein et al,[228] 1997	25	Unable to extract data	Unable to extract data	Unable to extract data	60% survival at a mean of 21 mo 44% disease free at 5 y
Nicolai et al,[3] 2008 (endoscopic resection, probable radiotherapy but not detailed)	14	Unable to extract data	Unable to extract data	Unable to extract data	18% disease free, mean follow-up of 34.1 mo

- The limited evidence at present suggests that the endoscopic removal of MM is as effective as by other means.
- Radiotherapy may help local control but does not affect survival.
- Local recurrence is a problem.
- Sinonasal MM is associated with poor survival rates.
- MM of the septum is associated with a better prognosis than elsewhere in the nose and paranasal sinuses.

BONE AND CARTILAGE
Chondrosarcoma

Introduction and incidence
Chondrosarcomas are rare, slow-growing malignancies of cartilage that mainly affect the pelvis and long bones. In general, chondrosarcomas affect older adults, and show a male predilection (**Fig. 10**).[4] Skull base chondrosarcomas often arise from remnants of cartilage after ossification and constitute 0.15% of all intracranial tumors and 6% of all skull base tumors.[243] Chondrosarcomas are even more rare in the facial skeleton and the sinonasal tract, accounting for less than 16% of all sarcomas of the nasal cavity, paranasal sinuses, and nasopharynx.

Histology
Histologically, chondrosarcomas are divided into 3 grades (grade 1, well differentiated (**Fig. 11**); grade 2, intermediate differentiated; grade 3, poorly differentiated), according to the degree of cellularity, nuclear size and atypia, and mitotic activity.[244] Analyzed in a multivariate fashion, histologic grade is the single most important predictor of local recurrence and metastasis, along with surgical stage (margins).[245–247]

Treatment
En bloc excision is the preferred surgical treatment of intermediate-grade and high-grade chondrosarcoma; however, this option is rarely possible in the skull base areas. For low-grade chondrosarcoma, extensive curettage may provide satisfactory local control[4] but is not ideal. However, status of the surgical margins and grading are the most important predictive factors.[245–247] Management of skull base chondrosarcomas is difficult because of their challenging location along the median and paramedian ventral skull base, often extending along the petroclival fissures. By virtue of their location, critical arteries, cranial nerves, and cavernous sinuses surround chondrosarcomas. En bloc resection is not possible for these lesions.

Chondrosarcomas are radioresistant, so doses greater than 60 Gy are needed to achieve local control after incomplete resection. Compared with other forms of radiation therapy, proton beam therapy has been used to increase the dose delivered to the

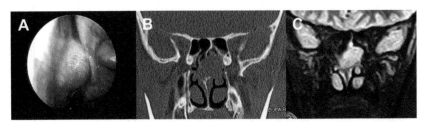

Fig. 10. Chondrosarcoma of the septum/clivus. Endoscopic view (*A*), CT (*B*), and typical enhancing T2 MRI appearance (*C*).

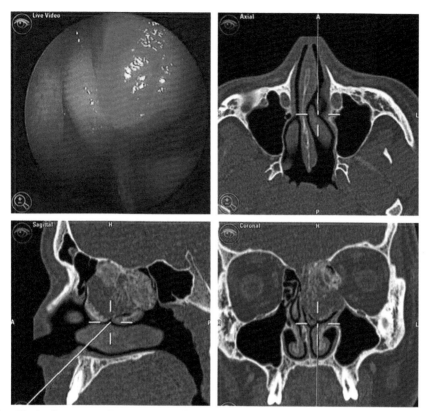

Fig. 11. An intraoperative image guidance screenshot of a chondrosarcoma of the left ethmoid.

tumor while elegantly sparing dosing to adjacent critical normal structures.[248] An extensive review of the literature led some investigators to conclude that the use of proton therapy following maximal surgical resection shows a high probability of medium-term and long-term cure with a low risk of significant complications, although there are no available prospective studies.[249] Others, reporting the use of a 68-Gy dose for chondrosarcomas (n = 22), reported an actuarial 5-year local control rate of 94% for chondrosarcomas. Brainstem compression at the time of proton therapy (P = .007) and gross tumor volume greater than 25 mL (P = .03) were associated with lower local control rates.[250] Chemotherapy is possibly effective only for mesenchymal chondrosarcoma, and is of uncertain value for undifferentiated chondrosarcoma.[251]

Various external and endoscopic approaches have been described for the surgical resection of chondrosarcomas of the skull base. Despite extensive external approaches, total resection is difficult and subtotal resection is the most common scenario. Similarly, others have noted that complications are to be expected with the management of these lesions.[246] Conventional transcranial/transfacial skull base approaches are often associated with postoperative cranial neuropathies because of the need to obtain an adequate surgical exposure.[246] Gay and colleagues[252] reported a series of 60 patients with either chordomas or chondrosarcomas, in which only 28 patients (47%) had total resection based on postoperative imaging. However, 48 patients (80%) suffered new cranial neuropathies. They noted a significant difference in recurrence and survival rates between total or near-total resection with patients who underwent subtotal or partial resection.[252]

In a review of 64 patients by Sekhar and colleagues,[253] only 50% of patients had total resection but 41% of patients incurred additional neurologic deficits. Oghalai and colleagues[246] reported a series of 33 patients in whom only 8 patients (28%) had total resection and 6 patients (18%) suffered surgical complications.

Tzortzidis and colleagues[254] reviewed 47 patients who underwent microsurgical resection in a 20-year period. A gross total resection was obtained in 61.7% of patients and subtotal resection was obtained in 38.3% of patients. A postoperative complication rate, including CSF leaks and new cranial nerve palsies, of 18% was reported. Patients who underwent a gross total resection, especially as a primary procedure, showed better local control and quality of life.[254]

Results

Chondrosarcomas, especially low-grade tumors, are associated with an excellent prognosis if the lesions are completely resected (**Table 15**). Their tendency to present in well-differentiated form (grade 1) explains why chondrosarcoma is the head and neck soft tissue malignancy with initially the best prognosis. However, overall 5-year survival, combined for the different grades, varies from 56% to 87%, and this deteriorates markedly with time.[175] Conversely, mesenchymal chondrosarcoma is a high-grade tumor with an unpredictable and generally poor prognosis.

Discussion

Endoscopy may be used for sampling. Its role for the surgical resection is not well defined. A literature search reveals a lack of randomized trials comparing open and endoscopic approaches regarding completeness of surgical excision and outcome for either skull base or sinonasal lesions. There are various case reports of endoscopic removal of chondrosarcomas affecting the septum[131,244,255–258] and the posterior septum and sphenoid rostrum.[259] These reports suggest that small lesions without skull base or orbital involvement, especially if located at the level of the nasal septum, are amenable to an endoscopic resection. Others have described the techniques for the endoscopic removal of deep-seated lesions, including chondrosarcomas with other disorders arising in the sphenoid sinus,[153,259,260] clivus,[261–263] petrous apex,[264] and pterygopalatine fossa.[265] However, long-term follow-up is lacking.

In a recent report by Frank and colleagues,[261] the endoscopic transnasal approach for chordomas and chondrosarcomas was reviewed. Using this technique, the mean hospital stay was 5 days and no perioperative complications, including CSF leaks or neurologic deficits, were noted. However, only 2 of the 9 patients had skull base chondrosarcomas.

Conclusion

- Surgical resection (and occasionally, for high-grade tumors or positive margins, postoperative radiotherapy) provides the best long-term results.
- Tumor recurrence has been associated with advanced histologic grading and adequacy of treatment. Therefore, the recurrence rate is directly proportional to the degree of resection as well as the histologic grade.
- A total resection can be achieved with endoscopic endonasal approaches for most tumors in the median sinonasal tract.
- Skull base lesions are often adjacent to critical neurovascular structures; therefore, their removal is achieved in a piecemeal fashion regardless of the approach.

Table 15
Chondrosarcomas removed via an endonasal endoscopic approach in the literature

Location	Series	Study Design	Total No. of Patients	Chondrosarcomas (N)	Extent of Resection	Mean Follow-Up Range (Mo)	Morbidity	Recurrence
Septum	Matthews[257]	Case series	1	1	Complete	—	None	—
Septum	Giger[258]	Case series	1	1	Complete	36	None	—
Septum	Coppit[246]	Case series	2	2	Complete	—	None	—
Septum	Betz[259]	Case series	2	1	Incomplete	12	None	Early recurrence removed
Septum	Jenny[260]	Case series	1	1	Complete	—	None	—
Sphenoid	Carrau[261]	Case series	1	1	Complete	—	None	—
Sphenoid	Castelnuovo[262]	Case series	41	1	—	—	—	—
Sphenoid	Tami[354]	Case series	8	1	—	—	—	—
Clivus and sphenopetrous	Frank[263]	Case series	11	2	—	—	—	—
Clivus	Zhang[264]	Case series	9	2	Complete/ subtotal	3–39	—	—
Pterygopalatine area	Hu[267]	Case series	1	1	—	—	—	—

First author only given for each series.

- An endonasal corridor offers the advantage of avoiding the manipulation of cranial nerves that is required by the external lateral approaches.

POSTOPERATIVE SURVEILLANCE

Postoperative surveillance, mainly based on magnetic resonance (MR) studies, is intended to detect residual/recurrent lesions and possible complications (eg, mucocele). Understanding the radiologic features of the healing process in a large surgical cavity created at the interface between the sinonasal tract and the adjacent skull base is of paramount importance for correct interpretation of the MR images obtained during follow-up.[266] Furthermore, preoperative examination should be available for comparison and the radiologist should obtain information about the exact extent of the resection, the residual presence of microscopic or macroscopic disease, possible interposition of flaps, results of pathologic analysis of the specimen, and the postoperative use of adjuvant treatment. Because many vascular flaps have been recently introduced to close large dural defects with the intent of preventing CSF leak and to promote faster and more complete healing, understanding their appearance with few variables at MR can allow the radiologist to avoid mistakes in differential diagnosis between findings related to a regular or impaired (flap displacement or necrosis) healing process and presence of a persistent/recurrent lesion.[266,267]

Another key issue in posttreatment MR follow-up is distinguishing between the lesion and inflammatory tissues, such as granulation tissue, which may escape detection even by expert clinicians and radiologists.[268] In such cases, positron emission tomography (PET)/CT examination may give additional information. However, most of the experience acquired with PET/CT has relied on fluorodeoxyglucose (FDG) uptake. However, FDG accumulates in both cancer and inflammatory cells because of an increased glycolytic activity, making it uncertain whether an area of increased FDG uptake necessarily represents tumor.[266] The introduction of new agents, such fluorodeoxythymidine, which accumulate only in actively replicating cells, might help in differentiating tumor and inflammatory lesions.

Postoperative imaging is mandatory in all malignancies involving the sinonasal tract and the skull base, as well as in some benign lesions such as osteoma, juvenile angiofibroma, pituitary adenomas, epidermoid cysts, craniopharyngiomas, and meningiomas that, because of their deep location or submucosal pattern of growth, are not easily picked up by endoscopic evaluation.

Recurrent malignant lesions, if diagnosed at an early stage, may be still amenable to salvage treatment. Therefore, it is necessary that patients are followed with periodic MR. Commonly accepted schedules include examination at 4-month or 6-month intervals for the first 2 years after treatment, and subsequently every 6 to 12 months[3,269] in conjunction with 3-monthly clinical assessments in the first 2 years with 6-monthly reviews following. In tumors that are prone to develop late recurrences, such as chondrosarcoma, ACC, and olfactory neuroblastoma, imaging surveillance should be extended for life, rather than the usual 5-year date from treatment.

PROGNOSTIC FACTORS
General Considerations

The prognosis varies according to the diversity of pathohistologic and individual features (type of tumor, size, location, grade and growth pattern, regional and distant spread, general health status of the patient) and also to differing treatment strategies. Some of these factors are constitutive elements of the TNM classification system.[160,236,270,271]

In malignant disease, involvement of the orbita, dura, retromaxillary fossa, intra-dural extension, or brain infiltration has a significant negative impact on survival.[149,175,193,272–277] One of the most important negatively prognostic signs is a positive surgical margin at the first extirpative procedure.[145,278] Size of the tumor (bulk), sphenoid sinus involvement, limited invasion of the dura and brain tissue, site of orbit invasion (anterior vs posterior), age, and sex have been a matter of debate.[178,274,275,279–281] In general, a higher rate of recurrence is observed for more advanced disease, regardless of the surgical technique.[282]

Concerning endoscopic surgery, the analysis of these data indicates that the strategy should be to perform a complete removal, and this strategy has to be based on the staging of the tumor. However, en bloc versus piecemeal resection does not make a prognostic difference.[283]

Some tumors have special prognostic features. MM generally has a poor overall survival.[236] In olfactory neuroblastomas, histopathologic grading according to Hyams can predict the outcome.[192,211,284] However, in inverted papillomas, for example, no prognostic factor of local control has been defined,[285] whereas younger patients and smokers show a trend to recurrence of these tumors.[286] In chordomas, tumor bulk matters: tumor volume of more than 70 mL is associated with a worse prog-nosis.[261] Eligibility for the endonasal approach and T staging do not parallel each other.[178]

ADJUNCTIVE THERAPY FOR SINONASAL AND SKULL BASE TUMORS
Radiotherapy

External radiotherapy
Interpretation of results of treatment in general, and radiotherapy in particular, for sino-nasal cancers is complicated by the high variety of histology, biologic behavior, the site, and the extent of the disease. Moreover, because of the low incidence of these tumors, large series of homogenous patients are rare to nonexistent. Comparison and analysis of the role of individual treatments is therefore difficult.

It is generally accepted that most sinonasal cancers are radiosensitive and that radiotherapy results in a success rate of about 35% as single-modality treatment.[21,287] The radiosensitivity largely depends on the histology and growth rate of the tumor.

However, there is a consensus that the primary treatment of choice for most sino-nasal cancers is, whenever possible, complete surgical resection followed by postop-erative radiotherapy, with or without chemotherapy.[21,288] The added value of radiotherapy to the surgical resection can be estimated at 10% on local control rates as well as improvement in survival (ranging from 5% to 50%) after 5 years.[287–294]

To list specific data on treatment techniques is difficult because the treatment itself is also determined by variables such as the histology and the extension, both of which also determine the outcome. Specifically in the large stage III/IV carcinomas, multi-modal treatment improves the outcome[290] and this is irrespective of the surgical margin status. In inoperable/unresectable cases, the results with radiotherapy as single-treatment modality are poor, as expected, but may still reach 15% to 20%.[295]

The classic radiotherapy regimen consists of repeated doses of 1.8 to 2.0 Gy, 5 days per week, during 6 to 7 weeks, resulting in a total dose of 60 to 70 Gy.

Radiotherapy has side effects including acute and late toxicity and long-term complications.[22,289,292,296–300] The most important and most relevant traditional side effects for sinonasal cancers can be loss of smell, which is present in almost 100% of patients, possibly because of a combination of causes; mucositis with dryness and crust formation of the nasal mucosa; orbital complications including conjunctivitis, keratitis, retinopathy; optic neuropathy with vision loss; and brain necrosis. Hypopituitarism may rarely occur, resulting in clinical hormonal disturbances.[301] A secondary concern related to the toxicity of radiotherapy is underdosage in regions of risk, compromising the long-term local control and survival rates.

To reduce these complications, improvements in radiotherapy have been developed and now are already integrated in the treatment regimens in most Western countries. Three-dimensional radiotherapy (3D-CRT)[302–304] was the first major improvement and intensity-modulated radiotherapy (IMRT) has become the gold standard for radiotherapy. Using intensity-modulated radiotherapy (IMRT), the high-dose areas that can be sculpted around the target volumes, with steep dose decrease immediately outside these regions. IMRT significantly reduces the risk for acute and chronic ocular toxicity and therefore prevents irreversible late optic nerve damage[302,305–311] **(Table 16)**. However, these new developments in radiotherapy have not been shown to offer an improved oncological outcome.[296,304–308,311]

Chemotherapy

Systemic chemotherapy
There is evidence that adjuvant chemotherapy concurrent with radiotherapy (concurrent chemoradiotherapy) can be beneficial for the patient in specific indications. Survival is improved by 4%.[312–316]

In the palliative treatment of metastases, both radiotherapy and chemotherapy may be indicated depending on the tumor histology, the location and number of metastases, and the related symptoms.

Local chemotherapy
Local application of 5-fluorouracil (5-FU) in the treatment of adenocarcinoma of the sinuses was introduced by Sato and colleagues[317]: minimally invasive transantral clearance followed by topical chemotherapy with 5-FU has also been used in the Netherlands by Knegt and colleagues[171,318] with excellent success. After an extended ethmoidectomy through a Caldwell-Luc approach, the cavity was packed with ribbon gauze impregnated with 5% 5-FU cream. On a regular weekly or twice-weekly basis,

Table 16
Acute and chronic toxicity and optic neuropathy associated with IMRT

References	N	Acute Toxicity (Grade 3/4) (%)[a]		Chronic Toxicity (Grade 3/4) (%)[b]		Optic Neuropathy (%)[c]	
Duthoy et al,[305] 2005	39	8	(21)	6	(15)	3	(8)
Combs et al,[306] 2006	46	2	(4)	0	(0)	0	(0)
Dirix (2) et al,[308] 2007	21	0	(0)	0	(0)	0	(0)
Daly et al,[307] 2007	36	6	(17)	2	(6)	0	(0)
Hoppe et al,[309] 2008	37	3	(8)	0	(0)	0	(0)
Madani et al,[310] 2008	84	4	(5)	6	(7)	1	(1)
Total	263	23	(9)	14	(5)	4	(2)

[a] Acute toxicity according to the Common Toxicity Criteria (CTC version 3.0) published august 2006, available on the Internet at http://ctep.info.nih.gov/protocolDevelopment/electronic_applications/docs/ctcaev3.pdf. Grade3/4 indicates at least severe toxicity affecting active daily life.
[b] Chronic toxicity indicating adverse events occurring greater than 90 days after radiation therapy, according to the RTOG/EORTC morbidity scoring scheme available on the Internet at http://www.rtog.org/members/toxicity/late.html.
[c] Visual acuity impairment not caused by other ocular toxicity.

the gauze was removed and debriding of necrotic tissue was performed under general anesthesia or under local anesthesia with analgesia and sedation. The cavity was then packed again with gauze impregnated with 5-FU. Five-year disease-specific survival rates and local control rates of 78% and 87% have been reported.[171] However, this treatment is not always well tolerated by the patients and has a high morbidity rate: orbital inflammation (40%) and CSF leakage (8%).These results have not been reproduced by many investigators[319] and should not be considered as standard of care in most centers.

All patients with head and neck malignancies should be seen in a multidisciplinary clinic before deciding on treatment protocols.

ARE ONCOLOGICAL OUTCOMES THE SAME WITH EXPANDED ENDOSCOPIC SURGERY AS WITH OPEN CRANIOFACIAL SURGERY?

Although the introduction of endoscopic technology has had a profound impact on the management of sinonasal tumors, it is of utmost importance to realize that the endoscope is simply an enabling technology that may be used in any surgical corridor. The primary benefit of the endoscope is enhanced visualization. Because of the optical properties of the endoscope, there is no loss of light and line-of-sight problems are avoided. The use of the endoscope for the removal of benign tumors such as inverting papillomas and angiofibromas was introduced in the early 1990s[320–326] and is now readily accepted by most sinus surgeons.[327–333] Published series have showed that endoscopic excision of properly selected tumors is associated with improved local tumor control and decreased morbidity compared with standard open approaches.[282,285,334–337] The application of endonasal endoscopic techniques to the management of malignant sinonasal tumors has been more controversial.[3,152,272,338,339] The primary concern is adherence to oncological principles: complete en bloc excision with adequate margins of the neoplasm. Secondary concerns include visualization, the ability to achieve hemostasis and deal with vascular complications, and reconstruction.

In contrast, the role of endoscopic endonasal techniques in malignant tumors of the sinuses and skull base is mostly defined by retrospective chart analysis presenting data primarily on survival (eg, 5-years and 10-year disease-free survival rate/overall survival rate; patient being alive with disease, dead of disease, dead of intercurrent disease, or lost to follow-up), control of disease (local/regional control, distant metastases; need for additional treatment modalities), and surgical complications. Sometimes additional data, such as for operative time, estimated blood loss, postoperative discomfort (morbidity), as well as length of hospitalization and follow-up time, are provided referring to 1 or more cohorts of patients (exclusively endoscopic, endoscopy-assisted, or nonendoscopic resections) suffering from comparable types and sizes of tumors according to established staging systems.[3,77,148–152,158–161,236,339,340]

According to the literature, endoscopic surgery is usually performed on well-selected, localized cases. Improved cosmetic outcome following endonasal interventions is sometimes mentioned,[158] but it is rarely evaluated. The same is true for postoperative development of atrophic rhinitis, which may be potentiated by adjunctive radiotherapy.[160,216,341,342]

For the moment, the levels of evidence in endoscopic tumor surgery are mainly level 3 (case series) (**Table 17**) and level 4 (expert opinion). In the next decade, higher levels of evidence will be needed. Because of the paucity of patient numbers, joint efforts will be crucial. Questions remain on the use of staging to decide on the management, behavior, or treatment based on histology or new molecular biology, whether the accuracy of

Table 17
Case series of endoscopic surgery for sinonasal malignancy

Author	Histology	N	Mean Follow-up (mo)	Survival
Stammberger et al,[177] 2000	Olfactory neuroblastoma	6	57	100% 1 CFR
Goffart et al,[1] 2000	Mixed	66	26	66%
Roh et al,[151] 2004	Mixed	13	26	86% DFS
Shipchandler et al,[155] 2005	SCC	7	31	91%
Poetker et al,[150] 2005	Mixed	16	17	Recurrence rate 31%
Bockmuhl et al,[351] 2005	Adenocarcinoma, SCC, olfactory neuroblastoma	29	65	78% 5-y survival
Castelnuovo et al,[204] 2006	Mixed	18	25	61% 19.8 mo
Bogaerts et al,[178] 2008	Adenocarcinoma	44	36	81% overall 73% local control
Dave et al,[160] 2007	Mixed	17	?	94% local control
Lund et al,[152] 2007	Mixed	49	36	88% overall 68% DFS
Nicolai et al,[159] 2007	Mixed	16	47	87% DFS
Podboj and Smid,[153] 2007	Mixed	16	67	87% DFS
Gardner et al,[352] 2008	Meningioma	34	—	—
Nicolai et al,[3] 2009	Mixed	184 134 EEA	34	91% for EEA

Abbreviation: EEA, exclusive endoscopic approach.

tumor-free margins achieved endoscopically equate or exceed open surgery, and the impact of endoscopic resection on quality of life compared with open procedures.

SUMMARY

In the published literature, outcomes in endonasal tumor surgery are favorable. However, there exists a publication bias in favor of reports on successful surgery that has been noted in other disciplines.[343] In endonasal skull base surgery, the mandatory learning curve of the surgeon calls for specific training programs addressing technical demands and also crisis management.[344–349] In addition, advanced skull base techniques should be undertaken only in centers where all other surgical approaches can be performed if required.[177] Constant training of the multidisciplinary skull base team should help to keep the rate of complications minimal.[345,350] The possibilities of grading tumors based on new molecular biology techniques and the tailoring of the treatment based on the behavior of the tumor will further refine decision making in the future.

ACKNOWLEDGMENTS

The data presented are extracted from Lund V, Stammberger H, Nicolai P, et al. European position paper on endoscopic management of tumors of the nose, paranasal sinuses and skull base tumors. Rhinology 2010;Suppl 22:1–144, with permission.

EBM Question	Author's Reply
Are oncological outcomes the same with EES compared to open craniofacial surgery?	For some tumors, such as olfactory neuroblastoma, there is good evidence that endoscopic resection is as good or better than open (Level 3a Grade C). However, for all others, the paucity of cases and heterogeneity of published reports suggest similar outcomes in specially selected cases (Grade D).

REFERENCES

1. Goffart Y, Jorissen M, Daele J, et al. Minimally invasive endoscopic management of malignant sinonasal tumours. Acta Otorhinolaryngol Belg 2000;54(2): 221–32.
2. Kim B, Kim D, Kim S, et al. Endoscopic versus traditional craniofacial resection for patients with sinonasal tumors involving the anterior skull base. Clin Exp Otorhinolaryngol 2008;1(13):148–53.
3. Nicolai P, Battaglia P, Bignami M, et al. Endoscopic surgery for malignant tumors of the sinonasal tract and adjacent skull base: a 10-year experience. Am J Rhinol 2008;22(3):308–16.
4. Barnes L, Eveson JW, Reichart P, et al. Pathology and genetics of head and neck tumours. Lyon (France): IARC Press; 2005.
5. Tufano RP, Mokadam NA, Montone KT, et al. Malignant tumors of the nose and paranasal sinuses: hospital of the University of Pennsylvania experience 1990-1997. Am J Rhinol 1999;13(2):117–23.
6. Rinaldo A, Ferlito A, Shaha AR, et al. Is elective neck treatment indicated in patients with squamous cell carcinoma of the maxillary sinus? Acta Otolaryngol 2002;122(4):443–7.
7. Le QT, Fu KK, Kaplan M, et al. Treatment of maxillary sinus carcinoma: a comparison of the 1997 and 1977 American Joint Committee on cancer staging systems. Cancer 1999;86(9):1700–11.
8. Tiwari R, Hardillo JA, Mehta D, et al. Squamous cell carcinoma of maxillary sinus. Head Neck 2000;22(2):164–9.
9. Magnani C, Ciambellotti E, Salvi U, et al. The incidence of tumors of the nasal cavity and the paranasal sinuses in the district of Biella, 1970-1986. Acta Otorhinolaryngol Ital 1989;9(5):511–9 [in Italian].
10. Muir CS, Nectoux J. Descriptive epidemiology of malignant neoplasms of nose, nasal cavities, middle ear and accessory sinuses. Clin Otolaryngol Allied Sci 1980;5(3):195–211.
11. Zylka S, Bien S, Kaminski B, et al. Epidemiology and clinical characteristics of the sinonasal malignancies. Otolaryngol Pol 2008;62(4):436–41 [in Polish].
12. Barbieri PG, Lombardi S, Candela A, et al. Nasal sinus cancer registry of the province of Brescia. Epidemiol Prev 2003;27(4):215–20 [in Italian].
13. Olsen KD. Nose and sinus tumors. In: McCaffrey T, editor. Rhinologic diagnosis and treatment. New York: Thieme; 1997. p. 334–59.
14. Fasunla AJ, Lasisi AO. Sinonasal malignancies: a 10-year review in a tertiary health institution. J Natl Med Assoc 2007;99(12):1407–10.
15. Svane-Knudsen V, Jorgensen KE, Hansen O, et al. Cancer of the nasal cavity and paranasal sinuses: a series of 115 patients. Rhinology 1998;36(1):12–4.
16. Zbaren P, Richard JM, Schwaab G, et al. Malignant neoplasms of the nasal cavity and paranasal sinuses. Analysis of 216 cases of malignant neoplasms of nasal cavity and paranasal sinuses. HNO 1987;35(6):246–9 [in German].

17. Haraguchi H, Ebihara S, Saikawa M, et al. Malignant tumors of the nasal cavity: review of a 60-case series. Jpn J Clin Oncol 1995;25(5):188–94.

18. Van Hasselt CA, Skinner DW. Nasopharyngeal carcinoma. An analysis of 100 Chinese patients. S Afr J Surg 1990;28(3):92–4.

19. Lund VJ. Malignancy of the nose and sinuses. Epidemiological and aetiological considerations. Rhinology 1991;29(1):57–68.

20. Maroldi R, Lombardi D, Farina D, et al. Malignant neoplasms. In: Maroldi R, Nicolai P, editors. Imaging in treatment planning for sinonasal diseases. Berlin: Springer; 2005. p. 159–220.

21. Dulguerov P, Jacobsen MS, Allal AS, et al. Nasal and paranasal sinus carcinoma: are we making progress? A series of 220 patients and a systematic review. Cancer 2001;92(12):3012–29.

22. Katz TS, Mendenhall WM, Morris CG, et al. Malignant tumors of the nasal cavity and paranasal sinuses. Head Neck 2002;24(9):821–9.

23. Rhee CS, Won TB, Lee CH, et al. Adenoid cystic carcinoma of the sinonasal tract: treatment results. Laryngoscope 2006;116(6):982–6.

24. da Cruz Perez DE, Pires FR, Lopes MA, et al. Adenoid cystic carcinoma and mucoepidermoid carcinoma of the maxillary sinus: report of a 44-year experience of 25 cases from a single institution. J Oral Maxillofac Surg 2006;64(11): 1592–7.

25. Lupinetti AD, Roberts DB, Williams MD, et al. Sinonasal adenoid cystic carcinoma: the M. D. Anderson Cancer Center experience. Cancer 2007;110(12): 2726–31.

26. Batsakis J. Tumors of the head and neck: clinical and pathological considerations. Baltimore (MD): Williams & Wilkins; 1979.

27. Orvidas LJ, Lewis JE, Weaver AL, et al. Adenocarcinoma of the nose and paranasal sinuses: a retrospective study of diagnosis, histologic characteristics, and outcomes in 24 patients. Head Neck 2005;27(5):370–5.

28. Roush GC. Epidemiology of cancer of the nose and paranasal sinuses: current concepts. Head Neck Surg 1979;2(1):3–11.

29. Alessi DM, Trapp TK, Fu YS, et al. Nonsalivary sinonasal adenocarcinoma. Arch Otolaryngol Head Neck Surg 1988;114(9):996–9.

30. Kleinsasser O, Schroeder HG. Adenocarcinomas of the inner nose after exposure to wood dust. Morphological findings and relationships between histopathology and clinical behavior in 79 cases. Arch Otorhinolaryngol 1988;245(1):1–15.

31. Nunez F, Suarez C, Alvarez I, et al. Sino-nasal adenocarcinoma: epidemiological and clinico-pathological study of 34 cases. J Otolaryngol 1993;22(2): 86–90.

32. Acheson ED, Cowdell RH, Hadfield E, et al. Nasal cancer in woodworkers in the furniture industry. Br Med J 1968;2(5605):587–96.

33. Llorente JL, Perez-Escuredo J, Alvarez-Marcos C, et al. Genetic and clinical aspects of wood dust related intestinal-type sinonasal adenocarcinoma: a review. Eur Arch Otorhinolaryngol 2009;266(1):1–7.

34. Georgel T, Jankowski R, Henrot P, et al. CT assessment of woodworkers' nasal adenocarcinomas confirms the origin in the olfactory cleft. AJNR Am J Neuroradiol 2009;30(7):1440–4.

35. Hermsen MA, Llorente JL, Perez-Escuredo J, et al. Genome-wide analysis of genetic changes in intestinal-type sinonasal adenocarcinoma. Head Neck 2009;31(3):290–7.

36. Spiro RH, Huvos AG, Berk R, et al. Mucoepidermoid carcinoma of salivary gland origin. A clinicopathologic study of 367 cases. Am J Surg 1978;136(4):461–8.

37. Wolf J, Schmezer P, Fengel D, et al. The role of combination effects on the etiology of malignant nasal tumours in the wood-working industry. Acta Otolaryngol Suppl 1998;535:1–16.

38. Luce D, Gerin M, Leclerc A, et al. Sinonasal cancer and occupational exposure to formaldehyde and other substances. Int J Cancer 1993;53(2):224–31.

39. Bussi M, Gervasio CF, Riontino E, et al. Study of ethmoidal mucosa in a population at occupational high risk of sinonasal adenocarcinoma. Acta Otolaryngol 2002;122(2):197–201.

40. Holt GR. Sinonasal neoplasms and inhaled air toxics. Otolaryngol Head Neck Surg 1994;111(1):12–4.

41. Van den Oever R. Occupational exposure to dust and sinonasal cancer. An analysis of 386 cases reported to the N.C.C.S.F. Cancer Registry. Acta Otorhinolaryngol Belg 1996;50(1):19–24.

42. Wilhelmsson B, Lundh B. Nasal epithelium in woodworkers in the furniture industry. A histological and cytological study. Acta Otolaryngol 1984;98(3–4): 321–34.

43. Engzell U. Occupational etiology and nasal cancer. An internordic project. Acta Otolaryngol Suppl 1979;360:126–8.

44. Jinadu M. Review of occupational health problems of wood industrial workers. Nigerian Medical Practitioner 1983;5:25–8.

45. Magnani C, Comba P, Ferraris F, et al. A case-control study of carcinomas of the nose and paranasal sinuses in the woolen textile manufacturing industry. Arch Environ Health 1993;48(2):94–7.

46. Bolm-Audorff U, Vogel C, Woitowitz H. Occupation and smoking as risk factors of nasal and nasopharyngeal cancer. In: Sakurai H, Okazaki I, Omae K, editors. Occupational epidemiology: proceedings of the seventh International Symposium on Epidemiology in Occupational Health, Tokyo, Japan. Amsterdam: Excerpta Medica; 1990. p. 71–4.

47. Nylander LA, Dement JM. Carcinogenic effects of wood dust: review and discussion. Am J Ind Med 1993;24(5):619–47.

48. Choussy O, Ferron C, Vedrine PO, et al. Adenocarcinoma of Ethmoid: a GETTEC retrospective multicenter study of 418 cases. Laryngoscope 2008;118(3):437–43.

49. Zhu K, Levine RS, Brann EA, et al. Case-control study evaluating the homogeneity and heterogeneity of risk factors between sinonasal and nasopharyngeal cancers. Int J Cancer 2002;99(1):119–23.

50. Goldenberg D, Golz A, Fradis M, et al. Malignant tumors of the nose and paranasal sinuses: a retrospective review of 291 cases. Ear Nose Throat J 2001; 80(4):272–7.

51. Thomas GR, Regalado JJ, McClinton M. A rare case of mucoepidermoid carcinoma of the nasal cavity. Ear Nose Throat J 2002;81(8):519–22.

52. Comba P, Belli S. Etiological epidemiology of tumors of the nasal cavities and the paranasal sinuses. Ann Ist Super Sanita 1992;28(1):121–32 [in Italian].

53. Luce D, Leclerc A, Morcet JF, et al. Occupational risk factors for sinonasal cancer: a case-control study in France. Am J Ind Med 1992;21(2):163–75.

54. Pedersen E, Hogetveit AC, Andersen A. Cancer of respiratory organs among workers at a nickel refinery in Norway. Int J Cancer 1973;12(1):32–41.

55. Syrjanen KJ. HPV infections in benign and malignant sinonasal lesions. J Clin Pathol 2003;56(3):174–81.

56. Tang AC, Grignon DJ, MacRae DL. The association of human papillomavirus with Schneiderian papillomas: a DNA in situ hybridization study. J Otolaryngol 1994;23(4):292–7.

57. International Agency for Research on Cancer. Natural history and epidemiology of HPV infection. Lyon (France): International Agency for Research on Cancer; 2007. p. 112–35.

58. Alos L, Moyano S, Nadal A, et al. Human papillomaviruses are identified in a subgroup of sinonasal squamous cell carcinomas with favorable outcome. Cancer 2009;115(12):2701–9.

59. Hoffmann M, Klose N, Gottschlich S, et al. Detection of human papillomavirus DNA in benign and malignant sinonasal neoplasms. Cancer Lett 2006;239(1): 64–70.

60. El Mofty SK, Lu DW. Prevalence of high-risk human papillomavirus DNA in non-keratinizing (cylindrical cell) carcinoma of the sinonasal tract: a distinct clinico-pathologic and molecular disease entity. Am J Surg Pathol 2005;29(10):1367–72.

61. Kashima HK, Kessis T, Hruban RH, et al. Human papillomavirus in sinonasal papillomas and squamous cell carcinoma. Laryngoscope 1992;102(9):973–6.

62. Chang AE, Karnell LH, Menck HR. The National Cancer Data Base report on cutaneous and noncutaneous melanoma: a summary of 84,836 cases from the past decade. The American College of Surgeons Commission on Cancer and the American Cancer Society. Cancer 1998;83(8):1664–78.

63. Chiu NT, Weinstock MA. Melanoma of oronasal mucosa. Population-based analysis of occurrence and mortality. Arch Otolaryngol Head Neck Surg 1996; 122(9):985–8.

64. Freedman HM, DeSanto LW, Devine KD, et al. Malignant melanoma of the nasal cavity and paranasal sinuses. Arch Otolaryngol 1973;97(4):322–5.

65. Kingdom TT, Kaplan MJ. Mucosal melanoma of the nasal cavity and paranasal sinuses. Head Neck 1995;17(3):184–9.

66. Thompson AC, Morgan DA, Bradley PJ. Malignant melanoma of the nasal cavity and paranasal sinuses. Clin Otolaryngol Allied Sci 1993;18(1):34–6.

67. Iversen K, Robins RE. Mucosal malignant melanomas. Am J Surg 1980;139(5): 660–4.

68. Lentsch EJ, Myers JN. Melanoma of the head and neck: current concepts in diagnosis and management. Laryngoscope 1980;111(7):1209–22.

69. Manolidis S, Donald PJ. Malignant mucosal melanoma of the head and neck: review of the literature and report of 14 patients. Cancer 1980;80(8):1373–86.

70. Thompson LD, Wieneke JA, Miettinen M, et al. Sinonasal tract and nasopharyngeal melanomas: a clinicopathologic study of 115 cases with a proposed staging system. Am J Surg Pathol 1980;27(5):594–611.

71. Lund VJ. Malignant melanoma of the nasal cavity and paranasal sinuses. Ear Nose Throat J 1980;72(4):285–90.

72. Dauer EH, Lewis JE, Rohlinger AL, et al. Sinonasal melanoma: a clinicopathologic review of 61 cases. Otolaryngol Head Neck Surg 1980;138(3):347–52.

73. Theilgaard SA, Buchwald C, Ingeholm P, et al. Esthesioneuroblastoma: a Danish demographic study of 40 patients registered between 1978 and 2000. Acta Otolaryngol 1980;123(3):433–9.

74. Bradley PJ, Jones NS, Robertson I, et al. Diagnosis and management of esthesioneuroblastoma. Curr Opin Otolaryngol Head Neck Surg 1980;11(2):112–8.

75. Broich G, Pagliari A, Ottaviani F, et al. Esthesioneuroblastoma: a general review of the cases published since the discovery of the tumour in 1924. Anticancer Res 1980;17(4A):2683–706.

76. Rinaldo A, Ferlito A, Shaha AR, et al. Esthesioneuroblastoma and cervical lymph node metastases: clinical and therapeutic implications. Acta Otolaryngol 1980; 122(2):215–21.

77. Walch C, Stammberger H, Anderhuber W, et al. The minimally invasive approach to olfactory neuroblastoma: combined endoscopic and stereotactic treatment. Laryngoscope 1980;110(4):635–40.
78. Morita A, Ebersold MJ, Olsen KD, et al. Esthesioneuroblastoma: prognosis and management. Neurosurgery 1980;32(5):706–14 [discussion: 714–5].
79. Dulguerov P, Calcaterra T. Esthesioneuroblastoma: the UCLA experience 1970–1990. Laryngoscope 1980;102(8):843–9.
80. Mills S, Gaffey M, Frierson H Jr, et al. Tumors of the upper aerodigestive tract and ear. Washington, DC: Armed Forces Institute of Pathology under the auspices of Universities Associated for Research and Education in Pathology; 2000.
81. Kairemo KJ, Jekunen AP, Kestila MS, et al. Imaging of olfactory neuroblastoma–an analysis of 17 cases. Auris, Nasus, Larynx 1980;25(2):173–9.
82. Ibrahim NB, Briggs JC, Corbishley CM, et al. Extrapulmonary oat cell carcinoma. Cancer 1980;54(8):1645–61.
83. Raychowdhuri RN. Oat-cell carcinoma and paranasal sinuses. J Laryngol Otol 1980;79:253–5.
84. Mineta H, Miura K, Takebayashi S, et al. Immunohistochemical analysis of small cell carcinoma of the head and neck: a report of four patients and a review of sixteen patients in the literature with ectopic hormone production. Ann Otol Rhinol Laryngol 1980;110(1):76–82.
85. Babin E, Rouleau V, Vedrine PO, et al. Small cell neuroendocrine carcinoma of the nasal cavity and paranasal sinuses. J Laryngol Otol 1980;120(4):289–97.
86. Renner G. Small cell carcinoma of the head and neck: a review. Semin Oncol 1980;34(1):3–14.
87. Lin CH, Chiang TP, Shum WY, et al. Primary small cell neuroendocrine carcinoma of the nasal cavity after successful curative therapy of nasopharyngeal carcinoma: a case report. Kaohsiung J Med Sci 1980;25(3):145–50.
88. Perez-Ordonez B, Caruana SM, Huvos AG, et al. Small cell neuroendocrine carcinoma of the nasal cavity and paranasal sinuses. Human Pathol 1980;29(8):826–32.
89. Smith SR, Som P, Fahmy A, et al. A clinicopathological study of sinonasal neuroendocrine carcinoma and sinonasal undifferentiated carcinoma. Laryngoscope 1980;110(10 pt 1):1617–22.
90. Silva EG, Butler JJ, Mackay B, et al. Neuroblastomas and neuroendocrine carcinomas of the nasal cavity: a proposed new classification. Cancer 1980;50(11):2388–405.
91. Rischin D, Coleman A. Sinonasal malignancies of neuroendocrine origin. Hematol Oncol Clin North Am 1980;22(6):1297–316, xi.
92. Rosenthal DI, Barker JL Jr, El-Naggar AK, et al. Sinonasal malignancies with neuroendocrine differentiation: patterns of failure according to histologic phenotype. Cancer 1980;101(11):2567–73.
93. Iezzoni JC, Mills SE. "Undifferentiated" small round cell tumors of the sinonasal tract: differential diagnosis update. Am J Clin Pathol 1980;124(Suppl):s110–121.
94. Frierson H Jr. Sinonasal undifferentiated carcinoma. In: Barnes L, editor. Pathology and genetics of head and neck tumours. Lyon (France): IARC Press; 2005. p. 19.
95. Musy PY, Reibel JF, Levine PA. Sinonasal undifferentiated carcinoma: the search for a better outcome. Laryngoscope 2002;112(8 Pt 1):1450–5.
96. Cerilli LA, Holst VA, Brandwein MS, et al. Sinonasal undifferentiated carcinoma: immunohistochemical profile and lack of EBV association. Am J Surg Pathol 2001;25(2):156–63.

97. Jeng YM, Sung MT, Fang CL, et al. Sinonasal undifferentiated carcinoma and nasopharyngeal-type undifferentiated carcinoma: two clinically, biologically, and histopathologically distinct entities. Am J Surg Pathol 2002;26(3):371–6.

98. Wenig BM. Undifferentiated malignant neoplasms of the sinonasal tract. Arch Pathol Lab Med 2009;133(5):699–712.

99. Grier HE. The Ewing family of tumors. Ewing's sarcoma and primitive neuroectodermal tumors. Pediatr Clin North Am 1997;44(4):991–1004.

100. Obata H, Ueda T, Kawai A, et al. Clinical outcome of patients with Ewing sarcoma family of tumors of bone in Japan: the Japanese Musculoskeletal Oncology Group cooperative study. Cancer 2007;109(4):767–75.

101. Damron TA, Ward WG, Stewart A. Osteosarcoma, chondrosarcoma, and Ewing's sarcoma: National Cancer Data Base report. Clin Orthop Relat Res 2007;459:40–7.

102. Vaccani JP, Forte V, de Jong AL, et al. Ewing's sarcoma of the head and neck in children. Int J Pediatr Otorhinolaryngol 1999;48(3):209–16.

103. Serrano E, Coste A, Percodani J, et al. Endoscopic sinus surgery for sinonasal haemangiopericytomas. J Laryngol Otol 2002;116(11):951–4.

104. Compagno J. Hemangiopericytoma-like tumors of the nasal cavity: a comparison with hemangiopericytoma of soft tissues. Laryngoscope 1978;88(3):460–9.

105. Weber W, Henkes H, Metz KA, et al. Haemangiopericytoma of the nasal cavity. Neuroradiology 2001;43(2):183–6.

106. Herve S, Abd Alsamad I, Beautru R, et al. Management of sinonasal hemangiopericytomas. Rhinology 1999;37(4):153–8.

107. Reiner SA, Siegel GJ, Clark KF, et al. Hemangiopericytoma of the nasal cavity. Rhinology 1990;28(2):129–36.

108. Castelnuovo P, Pagella F, Delu G, et al. Endoscopic resection of nasal haemangiopericytoma. Eur Arch Otorhinolaryngol 2003;260(5):244–7.

109. Yamaguchi S, Nagasawa H, Suzuki T, et al. Sarcomas of the oral and maxillofacial region: a review of 32 cases in 25 years. Clin Oral Investig 2004;8(2):52–5.

110. Chindia ML. Osteosarcoma of the jaw bones. Oral Oncol 2001;37(7):545–7.

111. Ajagbe HA, Junaid TA, Daramola JO. Osteogenic sarcoma of the jaw in an African community: report of twenty-one cases. J Oral Maxillofac Surg 1986; 44(2):104–6.

112. Regezi J, Scuibba J, Jordan R. Oral pathology: clinical pathologic correlations. 4th edition. St Louis (MO): Saunders; 2003.

113. Gorsky M, Epstein JB. Head and neck and intra-oral soft tissue sarcomas. Oral Oncol 1998;34(4):292–6.

114. Figueiredo MT, Marques LA, Campos-Filho N. Soft-tissue sarcomas of the head and neck in adults and children: experience at a single institution with a review of literature. Int J Cancer 1988;41(2):198–200.

115. Sercarz JA, Mark RJ, Nasri S, et al. Pediatric rhabdomyosarcoma of the head and neck. Int J Pediatr Otorhinolaryngol 1995;31(1):15–22.

116. Fokkens W, Lund V, Mullol J, European Position Paper on Rhinosinusitis and Nasal Polyps group. European position paper on rhinosinusitis and nasal polyps 2007. Rhinol Suppl 2007;(20):1–136.

117. Shekelle PG, Woolf SH, Eccles M, et al. Clinical guidelines: developing guidelines. BMJ 1999;318(7183):593–6.

118. Chidzonga MM, Mahomva L. Sarcomas of the oral and maxillofacial region: a review of 88 cases in Zimbabwe. Br J Oral Maxillofac Surg 2007;45(4):317–8.

119. Ha PK, Eisele DW, Frassica FJ, et al. Osteosarcoma of the head and neck: a review of the Johns Hopkins experience. Laryngoscope 1999;109(6):964–9.

120. Gadwal SR, Gannon FH, Fanburg-Smith JC, et al. Primary osteosarcoma of the head and neck in pediatric patients: a clinicopathologic study of 22 cases with a review of the literature. Cancer 2001;91(3):598–605.
121. Park YK, Ryu KN, Park HR, et al. Low-grade osteosarcoma of the maxillary sinus. Skeletal Radiol 2003;32(3):161–4.
122. Picci P. Osteosarcoma (osteogenic sarcoma). Orphanet J Rare Dis 2007;2:6.
123. Caudill JS, Arndt CA. Diagnosis and management of bone malignancy in adolescence. Adolesc Med 2007;18(1):62–78, ix.
124. Oda D, Bavisotto LM, Schmidt RA, et al. Head and neck osteosarcoma at the University of Washington. Head Neck 1997;19(6):513–23.
125. Galera-Ruiz H, Sanchez-Calzado JA, Rios-Martin JJ, et al. Sinonasal radiation-associated osteosarcoma after combined therapy for rhabdomyosarcoma of the nose. Auris Nasus Larynx 2001;28(3):261–4.
126. Callender TA, Weber RS, Janjan N, et al. Rhabdomyosarcoma of the nose and paranasal sinuses in adults and children. Otolaryngol Head Neck Surg 1995;112(2):252–7.
127. Hicks J, Flaitz C. Rhabdomyosarcoma of the head and neck in children. Oral Oncol 2002;38(5):450–9.
128. Carrau RL, Segas J, Nuss DW, et al. Role of skull base surgery for local control of sarcoma of the nasal cavity and paranasal sinuses. Eur Arch Otorhinolaryngol 1994;251(6):350–6.
129. Gadwal SR, Fanburg-Smith JC, Gannon FH, et al. Primary chondrosarcoma of the head and neck in pediatric patients: a clinicopathologic study of 14 cases with a review of the literature. Cancer 2000;88(9):2181–8.
130. Downey TJ, Clark SK, Moore DW. Chondrosarcoma of the nasal septum. Otolaryngol Head Neck Surg 2001;125(1):98–100.
131. Kainuma K, Netsu K, Asamura K, et al. Chondrosarcoma of the nasal septum: a case report. Auris Nasus Larynx 2009;36(5):601–5.
132. Burkey BB, Hoffman HT, Baker SR, et al. Chondrosarcoma of the head and neck. Laryngoscope 1990;100(12):1301–5.
133. Lippert BM, Godbersen GS, Luttges J, et al. Leiomyosarcoma of the nasal cavity. Case report and literature review. ORL J Otorhinolaryngol Relat Spec 1996;58(2):115–20.
134. Vidal RW, Devaney K, Ferlito A, et al. Sinonasal malignant lymphomas: a distinct clinicopathological category. Ann Otol Rhinol Laryngol 1999;108(4):411–9.
135. Quraishi MS, Bessell EM, Clark D, et al. Non-Hodgkin's lymphoma of the sinonasal tract. Laryngoscope 2000;110(9):1489–92.
136. Campo E, Cardesa A, Alos L, et al. Non-Hodgkin's lymphomas of nasal cavity and paranasal sinuses. An immunohistochemical study. Am J Clin Pathol 1991;96(2):184–90.
137. Arber DA, Weiss LM, Albujar PF, et al. Nasal lymphomas in Peru. High incidence of T-cell immunophenotype and Epstein-Barr virus infection. Am J Surg Pathol 1993;17(4):392–9.
138. Nakamura K, Uehara S, Omagari J, et al. Primary non-Hodgkin lymphoma of the sinonasal cavities: correlation of CT evaluation with clinical outcome. Radiology 1997;204(2):431–5.
139. Simo R, Sykes AJ, Hargreaves SP, et al. Metastatic renal cell carcinoma to the nose and paranasal sinuses. Head Neck 2000;22(7):722–7.
140. Bernstein JM, Montgomery WW, Balogh K Jr. Metastatic tumors to the maxilla, nose, and paranasal sinuses. Laryngoscope 1966;76(4):621–50.

141. Pignataro L, Peri A, Ottaviani F. Breast carcinoma metastatic to the ethmoid sinus: a case report. Tumori 2001;87(6):455–7.

142. Friedmann I, Osborn DA. Metastatic tumours in the ear, nose and throat region. J Laryngol Otol 1965;79:576–91.

143. Huang HH, Fang TJ, Chang PH, et al. Sinonasal metastatic tumors in Taiwan. Chang Gung Med J 2008;31(5):457–62.

144. Izquierdo J, Armengot M, Cors R, et al. Hepatocarcinoma: metastasis to the nose and paranasal sinuses. Otolaryngol Head Neck Surg 2000;122(6): 932–3.

145. Bhattacharyya N. Factors predicting survival for cancer of the ethmoid sinus. Am J Rhinol 2002;16(5):281–6.

146. Kermer C, Poeschl PW, Wutzl A, et al. Surgical treatment of squamous cell carcinoma of the maxilla and nasal sinuses. J Oral Maxillofac Surg 2008;66(12): 2449–53.

147. McKay SP, Shibuya TY, Armstrong WB, et al. Cell carcinoma of the paranasal sinuses and skull base. Am J Otol 2007;28(5):294–301.

148. Batra PS, Citardi MJ, Worley S, et al. Resection of anterior skull base tumors: comparison of combined traditional and endoscopic techniques. Am J Rhinol 2005;19(5):521–8.

149. Buchmann L, Larsen C, Pollack A, et al. Endoscopic techniques in resection of anterior skull base/paranasal sinus malignancies. Laryngoscope 2006;116(10): 1749–54.

150. Poetker DM, Toohill RJ, Loehrl TA, et al. Endoscopic management of sinonasal tumors: a preliminary report. Am J Rhinol 2005;19(3):307–15.

151. Roh HJ, Batra PS, Citardi MJ, et al. Endoscopic resection of sinonasal malignancies: a preliminary report. Am J Rhinol 2004;18(4):239–46.

152. Lund V, Howard DJ, Wei WI. Endoscopic resection of malignant tumors of the nose and sinuses. Am J Rhinol 2007;21(1):89–94.

153. Podboj J, Smid L. Endoscopic surgery with curative intent for malignant tumors of the nose and paranasal sinuses. Eur J Surg Oncol 2007;33(9):1081–6.

154. Castelnuovo P, Belli E, Bignami M, et al. Endoscopic nasal and anterior craniotomy resection for malignant nasoethmoid tumors involving the anterior skull base. Skull Base 2006;16(1):15–8.

155. Shipchandler TZ, Batra PS, Citardi MJ, et al. Outcomes for endoscopic resection of sinonasal squamous cell carcinoma. Laryngoscope 2005;115(11):1983–7.

156. Eviatar E, Vaiman M, Shlamkovitch N, et al. Removal of sinonasal tumors by the endonasal endoscopic approach. Isr Med Assoc J 2004;6(6):346–9.

157. Lund VJ, Howard DJ, Wei WI, et al. Craniofacial resection for tumors of the nasal cavity and paranasal sinuses–a 17-year experience. Head Neck 1998;20(2): 97–105.

158. Eloy JA, Vivero RJ, Hoang K, et al. Comparison of transnasal endoscopic and open craniofacial resection for malignant tumors of the anterior skull base. Laryngoscope 2009;119(5):834–40.

159. Nicolai P, Castelnuovo P, Lombardi D, et al. Role of endoscopic surgery in the management of selected malignant epithelial neoplasms of the nasoethmoidal complex. Head Neck 2007;29(12):1075–82.

160. Dave SP, Bared A, Casiano RR. Surgical outcomes and safety of transnasal endoscopic resection for anterior skull tumors. Otolaryngol Head Neck Surg 2007;136(6):920–7.

161. Chen MK. Minimally invasive endoscopic resection of sinonasal malignancies and skull base surgery. Acta Otolaryngol 2006;126(9):981–6.

162. Solares CA, Fakhri S, Batra PS, et al. Transnasal endoscopic resection of lesions of the clivus: a preliminary report. Laryngoscope 2005;115(11):1917–22.
163. Thaler ER, Kotapka M, Lanza DC, et al. Endoscopically assisted anterior cranial skull base resection of sinonasal tumors. Am J Rhinol 1999;13(4):303–10.
164. Phillips B, Ball C, Sackett D, et al. Oxford centre for evidence-based medicine - levels of evidence. Available at: http://www.cebm.net/index.aspx?o=1025. Accessed March 28, 2011.
165. Franchi A, Gallo O, Santucci M. Clinical relevance of the histological classification of sinonasal intestinal-type adenocarcinomas. Hum Pathol 1999;30(10):1140–5.
166. Barnes L. Intestinal-type adenocarcinoma of the nasal cavity and paranasal sinuses. Am J Surg Pathol 1986;10(3):192–202.
167. Macbeth R. Malignant disease of the paranasal sinuses. J Laryngol Otol 1965; 79:592–612.
168. Klintenberg C, Olofsson J, Hellquist H, et al. Adenocarcinoma of the ethmoid sinuses. A review of 28 cases with special reference to wood dust exposure. Cancer 1984;54(3):482–8.
169. Franquemont DW, Fechner RE, Mills SE. Histologic classification of sinonasal intestinal-type adenocarcinoma. Am J Surg Pathol 1991;15(4):368–75.
170. Heffner DK, Hyams VJ, Hauck KW, et al. Low-grade adenocarcinoma of the nasal cavity and paranasal sinuses. Cancer 1982;50(2):312–22.
171. Knegt PP, Ah-See KW, vd Velden LA, et al. Adenocarcinoma of the ethmoidal sinus complex: surgical debulking and topical fluorouracil may be the optimal treatment. Arch Otolaryngol Head Neck Surg 2001;127(2):141–6.
172. Leivo I. Update on sinonasal adenocarcinoma: classification and advances in immunophenotype and molecular genetic make-up. Head Neck Pathol 2007; 1(1):38–43.
173. Spiro RH, Huvos AG, Strong EW. Adenoid cystic carcinoma of salivary origin. A clinicopathologic study of 242 cases. Am J Surg 1974;128(4):512–20.
174. Wiseman SM, Popat SR, Rigual NR, et al. Adenoid cystic carcinoma of the paranasal sinuses or nasal cavity: a 40-year review of 35 cases. Ear Nose Throat J 2002;81(8):510–4, 516–7.
175. Howard DJ, Lund VJ, Wei WI. Craniofacial resection for tumors of the nasal cavity and paranasal sinuses: a 25-year experience. Head Neck 2006;28(10):867–73.
176. Ganly I, Patel SG, Singh B, et al. Craniofacial resection for malignant paranasal sinus tumors: report of an International Collaborative Study. Head Neck 2005; 27(7):575–84.
177. Stammberger H, Anderhuber W, Walch C, et al. Possibilities and limitations of endoscopic management of nasal and paranasal sinus malignancies. Acta Oto-rhinolaryngol Belg 1999;53(3):199–205.
178. Bogaerts S, Vander Poorten V, Nuyts S, et al. Results of endoscopic resection followed by radiotherapy for primarily diagnosed adenocarcinomas of the paranasal sinuses. Head Neck 2008;30(6):728–36.
179. Claus F, Boterberg T, Ost P, et al. Postoperative radiotherapy for adenocarcinoma of the ethmoid sinuses: treatment results for 47 patients. Int J Radiat Oncol Biol Phys 2002;54(4):1089–94.
180. Jardeleza C, Seiberling K, Floreani S, et al. Surgical outcomes of endoscopic management of adenocarcinoma of the sinonasal cavity. Rhinology 2009;47(4): 354–61.
181. Shah UK, Hybels RL, Dugan J. Endoscopic management of low-grade papillary adenocarcinoma of the ethmoid sinus: case report and review of the literature. Am J Otol 1999;20(3):190–4.

182. Shidnia H, Hornback NB, Saghafi N, et al. The role of radiation therapy in the treatment of malignant tumors of the paranasal sinuses. Laryngoscope 1984; 94(1):102–6.

183. Housset M, Huart J. Role of radiotherapy in the treatment of epitheliomas of the anterior skull base. Neurochirurgie 1997;43(2):85–7 [in French].

184. Jorissen M. The role of endoscopy in the management of paranasal sinus tumours. Acta Otorhinolaryngol Belg 1995;49(3):225–8.

185. Wormald PJ. Salvage frontal sinus surgery: the endoscopic modified Lothrop procedure. Laryngoscope 2003;113(2):276–83.

186. Robinson S, Patel N, Wormald PJ. Endoscopic management of benign tumors extending into the infratemporal fossa: a two-surgeon transnasal approach. Laryngoscope 2005;115(10):1818–22.

187. Singh H, Sethi D, Jern-Lin L. Minimally invasive endoscopic management (MIEM) of malignant sino-nasal tumours - is there a future? SGH Proceedings 2008;17(1):26–30.

188. Spiro JD, Soo KC, Spiro RH. Nonsquamous cell malignant neoplasms of the nasal cavities and paranasal sinuses. Head Neck 1995;17(2):114–8.

189. Carney ME, O'Reilly RC, Sholevar B, et al. Expression of the human Achaete-scute 1 gene in olfactory neuroblastoma (esthesioneuroblastoma). J Neurooncol 1995;26(1):35–43.

190. Kadish S, Goodman M, Wang CC. Olfactory neuroblastoma. A clinical analysis of 17 cases. Cancer 1976;37(3):1571–6.

191. Koka VN, Julieron M, Bourhis J, et al. Aesthesioneuroblastoma. J Laryngol Otol 1998;112(7):628–33.

192. Miyamoto RC, Gleich LL, Biddinger PW, et al. Esthesioneuroblastoma and sino-nasal undifferentiated carcinoma: impact of histological grading and clinical staging on survival and prognosis. Laryngoscope 2000;110(8):1262–5.

193. Dulguerov P, Allal AS, Calcaterra TC. Esthesioneuroblastoma: a meta-analysis and review. Lancet Oncol 2001;2(11):683–90.

194. Rastogi M, Bhatt M, Chufal K, et al. Esthesioneuroblastoma treated with non-craniofacial resection surgery followed by combined chemotherapy and radio-therapy: an alternative approach in limited resources. Jpn J Clin Oncol 2006; 36(10):613–9.

195. Biller HF, Lawson W, Sachdev VP, et al. Esthesioneuroblastoma: surgical treat-ment without radiation. Laryngoscope 1990;100(11):1199–201.

196. Resto VA, Eisele DW, Forastiere A, et al. Esthesioneuroblastoma: the Johns Hop-kins experience. Head Neck 2000;22(6):550–8.

197. Polin RS, Sheehan JP, Chenelle AG, et al. The role of preoperative adjuvant treatment in the management of esthesioneuroblastoma: the University of Virginia experience. Neurosurgery 1998;42(5):1029–37.

198. Chao KS, Kaplan C, Simpson JR, et al. Esthesioneuroblastoma: the impact of treatment modality. Head Neck 2001;23(9):749–57.

199. Shah JP. Surgery of the anterior skull base for malignant tumors. Acta Otorhino-laryngol Belg 1999;53(3):191–4.

200. Girod D, Hanna E, Marentette L. Esthesioneuroblastoma. Head Neck 2001; 23(6):500–5.

201. Boyle JO, Shah KC, Shah JP. Craniofacial resection for malignant neoplasms of the skull base: an overview. J Surg Oncol 1998;69(4):275–84.

202. Carta F, Kania R, Sauvaget E, et al. Endoscopic skull base resection for adeno-carcinoma and olfactory neuroblastoma. Rhinology 2011;49(1):74–9.

203. Unger F, Walch C, Stammberger H, et al. Olfactory neuroblastoma (esthesio-neuroblastoma): report of six cases treated by a novel combination of endo-scopic surgery and radiosurgery. Minim Invasive Neurosurg 2001;44(2): 79–84.

204. Castelnuovo P, Delu G, Sberze F, et al. Esthesioneuroblastoma: endonasal endoscopic treatment. Skull Base 2006;16(1):25–30.

205. Devaiah AK, Andreoli MT. Treatment of esthesioneuroblastoma: a 16-year meta-analysis of 361 patients. Laryngoscope 2009;119(7):1412–6.

206. Zafereo ME, Fakhri S, Prayson R, et al. Esthesioneuroblastoma: 25-year experi-ence at a single institution. Otolaryngol Head Neck Surg 2008;138(4):452–8.

207. Kiyota N, Tahara M, Fujii S, et al. Nonplatinum-based chemotherapy with irino-tecan plus docetaxel for advanced or metastatic olfactory neuroblastoma: a retrospective analysis of 12 cases. Cancer 2008;112(4):885–91.

208. Unger F, Haselsberger K, Walch C, et al. Combined endoscopic surgery and radiosurgery as treatment modality for olfactory neuroblastoma (esthesioneuro-blastoma). Acta Neurochir (Wien) 2005;147(6):595–601 [discussion: 601–2].

209. Yuen AP, Fan YW, Fung CF, et al. Endoscopic-assisted cranionasal resection of olfactory neuroblastoma. Head Neck 2005;27(6):488–93.

210. Eich HT, Hero B, Staar S, et al. Multimodality therapy including radiotherapy and chemotherapy improves event-free survival in stage C esthesioneuroblastoma. Strahlenther Onkol 2003;179(4):233–40.

211. Hwang SK, Paek SH, Kim DG, et al. Olfactory neuroblastomas: survival rate and prognostic factor. J Neurooncol 2002;59(3):217–26.

212. Simon JH, Zhen W, McCulloch TM, et al. Esthesioneuroblastoma: the University of Iowa experience 1978-1998. Laryngoscope 2001;111(3):488–93.

213. Slevin NJ, Irwin CJ, Banerjee SS, et al. Olfactory neural tumours–the role of external beam radiotherapy. J Laryngol Otol 1996;110(11):1012–6.

214. Eriksen JG, Bastholt L, Krogdahl AS, et al. Esthesioneuroblastoma–what is the optimal treatment? Acta Oncol 2000;39(2):231–5.

215. Wang C, Chen Y, Hsu Y, et al. Transcranial resection of olfactory neuroblastoma. Skull Base 2005;15(3):163–71.

216. Folbe A, Herzallah I, Duvvuri U, et al. Endoscopic endonasal resection of esthe-sioneuroblastoma: a multicenter study [Erratum appears in Am J Rhinol Allergy; 23(2):238]. Am J Rhinol Allergy 2009;23(1):91–4.

217. Eich HT, Staar S, Micke O, et al. Radiotherapy of esthesioneuroblastoma. Int J Radiat Oncol Biol Phys 2001;49(1):155–60.

218. Zabel A, Thilmann C, Milker-Zabel S, et al. The role of stereotactically guided conformal radiotherapy for local tumor control of esthesioneuroblastoma. Strah-lenther Onkol 2002;178(4):187–91.

219. Sheehan JM, Sheehan JP, Jane JA Sr, et al. Chemotherapy for esthesioneuro-blastomas. Neurosurg Clin N Am 2000;11(4):693–701.

220. Mishima Y, Nagasaki E, Terui Y, et al. Combination chemotherapy (cyclophos-phamide, doxorubicin, and vincristine with continuous-infusion cisplatin and etoposide) and radiotherapy with stem cell support can be beneficial for adolescents and adults with estheisoneuroblastoma. Cancer 2004;101(6): 1437–44.

221. Bhattacharyya N, Thornton AF, Joseph MP, et al. Successful treatment of esthe-sioneuroblastoma and neuroendocrine carcinoma with combined chemo-therapy and proton radiation. Results in 9 cases. Arch Otolaryngol Head Neck Surg 1997;123(1):34–40.

222. McElroy EA Jr, Buckner JC, Lewis JE. Chemotherapy for advanced esthesio-neuroblastoma: the Mayo Clinic experience. Neurosurgery 1998;42(5):1023–7 [discussion: 1027–8].

223. Shaari CM, Catalano PJ, Sen C, et al. Central nervous system metastases from esthesioneuroblastoma. Otolaryngol Head Neck Surg 1996;114(6):808–12.

224. Chamberlain MC. Treatment of intracranial metastatic esthesioneuroblastoma. J Clin Oncol 2002;20(1):357–8.

225. Miura K, Mineta H, Yokota N, et al. Olfactory neuroblastoma with epithelial and endocrine differentiation transformed into ganglioneuroma after chemoradiotherapy. Pathol Int 2001;51(12):942–7.

226. Levine PA. Would Dr. Ogura approve of endoscopic resection of esthesioneuroblastomas? An analysis of endoscopic resection data versus that of craniofacial resection. Laryngoscope 2009;119(1):3–7.

227. Olsen KD, DeSanto LW. Olfactory neuroblastoma. Biologic and clinical behavior. Arch Otolaryngol 1983;109(12):797–802.

228. Brandwein MS, Rothstein A, Lawson W, et al. Sinonasal melanoma. A clinicopathologic study of 25 cases and literature meta-analysis. Arch Otolaryngol Head Neck Surg 1997;123(3):290–6.

229. Holmstrom M, Lund VJ. Malignant melanomas of the nasal cavity after occupational exposure to formaldehyde. Br J Ind Med 1991;48(1):9–11.

230. Ballantyne AJ. Malignant melanoma of the skin of the head and neck. An analysis of 405 cases. Am J Surg 1970;120(4):425–31.

231. Lee SP, Shimizu KT, Tran LM, et al. Mucosal melanoma of the head and neck: the impact of local control on survival. Laryngoscope 1994;104(2):121–6.

232. Huang SF, Liao CT, Kan CR, et al. Primary mucosal melanoma of the nasal cavity and paranasal sinuses: 12 years of experience. J Otolaryngol 2007;36(2):124–9.

233. Patel SG, Prasad ML, Escrig M, et al. Primary mucosal malignant melanoma of the head and neck. Head Neck 2002;24(3):247–57.

234. Bridger AG, Smee D, Baldwin MA, et al. Experience with mucosal melanoma of the nose and paranasal sinuses. ANZ J Surg 2005;75(4):192–7.

235. Penel N, Mallet Y, Mirabel X, et al. Primary mucosal melanoma of head and neck: prognostic value of clear margins. Laryngoscope 2006;116(6):993–5.

236. Lund VJ, Howard DJ, Harding L, et al. Management options and survival in malignant melanoma of the sinonasal mucosa. Laryngoscope 1999;109(2 Pt 1):208–11.

237. Owens JM, Roberts DB, Myers JN. The role of postoperative adjuvant radiation therapy in the treatment of mucosal melanomas of the head and neck region. Arch Otolaryngol Head Neck Surg 2003;129(8):864–8.

238. Wada H, Nemoto K, Ogawa Y, et al. A multi-institutional retrospective analysis of external radiotherapy for mucosal melanoma of the head and neck in Northern Japan. Int J Radiat Oncol Biol Phys 2004;59(2):495–500.

239. Krengli M, Masini L, Kaanders JH, et al. Radiotherapy in the treatment of mucosal melanoma of the upper aerodigestive tract: analysis of 74 cases. A Rare Cancer Network study. Int J Radiat Oncol Biol Phys 2006;65(3):751–9.

240. Temam S, Mamelle G, Marandas P, et al. Postoperative radiotherapy for primary mucosal melanoma of the head and neck. Cancer 2005;103(2):313–9.

241. Nandapalan V, Roland NJ, Helliwell TR, et al. Mucosal melanoma of the head and neck. Clin Otolaryngol Allied Sci 1998;23(2):107–16.

242. Dwivedi R, Dwivedi R, Kazi R, et al. Mucosal melanoma of nasal cavity and paranasal sinus. J Cancer Res Ther 2008;4(4):200–2.

243. Berkmen YM, Blatt ES. Cranial and intracranial cartilaginous tumours. Clin Radiol 1968;19(3):327–33.

244. Coppit GL, Eusterman VD, Bartels J, et al. Endoscopic resection of chondrosarcomas of the nasal septum: a report of 2 cases. Otolaryngol Head Neck Surg 2002;127(6):569–71.

245. Giuffrida AY, Burgueno JE, Koniaris LG, et al. Chondrosarcoma in the United States (1973 to 2003): an analysis of 2890 cases from the SEER database. J Bone Joint Surg Am 2009;91(5):1063–72.

246. Oghalai JS, Buxbaum JL, Jackler RK, et al. Skull base chondrosarcoma originating from the petroclival junction. Otol Neurotol 2005;26(5):1052–60.

247. Bloch OG, Jian BJ, Yang I, et al. A systematic review of intracranial chondrosarcoma and survival. J Clin Neurosci 2009;16(12):1547–51.

248. Nguyen QN, Chang EL. Emerging role of proton beam radiation therapy for chordoma and chondrosarcoma of the skull base. Curr Oncol Rep 2008; 10(4):338–43.

249. Amichetti M, Amelio D, Cianchetti M, et al. A systematic review of proton therapy in the treatment of chondrosarcoma of the skull base. Neurosurg Rev 2010; 33(2):155–65.

250. Ares C, Hug EB, Lomax AJ, et al. Effectiveness and safety of spot scanning proton radiation therapy for chordomas and chondrosarcomas of the skull base: first long-term report. Int J Radiat Oncol Biol Phys 2009;75(4):1111–8.

251. Gelderblom H, Hogendoorn PC, Dijkstra SD, et al. The clinical approach towards chondrosarcoma. Oncologist 2008;13(3):320–9.

252. Gay E, Sekhar LN, Rubinstein E, et al. Chordomas and chondrosarcomas of the cranial base: results and follow-up of 60 patients. Neurosurgery 1995;36(5): 887–96 [discussion: 896–7].

253. Sekhar LN, Pranatartiharan R, Chanda A, et al. Chordomas and chondrosarcomas of the skull base: results and complications of surgical management. Neurosurg Focus 2001;10(3):E2.

254. Tzortzidis F, Elahi F, Wright DC, et al. Patient outcome at long-term follow-up after aggressive microsurgical resection of cranial base chondrosarcomas. Neurosurgery 2006;58(6):1090–8 [discussion: 1090–8].

255. Matthews B, Whang C, Smith S. Endoscopic resection of a nasal septal chondrosarcoma: first report of a case. Ear Nose Throat J 2002;81(5):327–9.

256. Giger R, Kurt AM, Lacroix JS. Endoscopic removal of a nasal septum chondrosarcoma. Rhinology 2002;40(2):96–9.

257. Betz CS, Janda P, Arbogast S, et al. Myxoma and myxoid chondrosarcoma of the nasal septum: two case reports. HNO 2007;55(1):51–5 [in German].

258. Jenny L, Harvinder S, Gurdeep S. Endoscopic resection of primary nasoseptal chondrosarcoma. Med J Malaysia 2008;63(4):335–6.

259. Carrau RL, Aydogan B, Hunt JL. Chondrosarcoma of the sphenoid sinus resected by an endoscopic approach. Am J Otol 2004;25(4):274–7.

260. Castelnuovo P, Pagella F, Semino L, et al. Endoscopic treatment of the isolated sphenoid sinus lesions. Eur Arch Otorhinolaryngol 2005;262(2):142–7.

261. Frank G, Sciarretta V, Calbucci F, et al. The endoscopic transnasal transsphenoidal approach for the treatment of cranial base chordomas and chondrosarcomas. Neurosurgery 2006;59(1 Suppl 1):ONS50–7 [discussion: ONS50–7].

262. Zhang Q, Kong F, Yan B, et al. Endoscopic endonasal surgery for clival chordoma and chondrosarcoma. ORL J Otorhinolaryngol Relat Spec 2008;70(2):124–9.

263. Ceylan S, Koc K, Anik I. Extended endoscopic approaches for midline skull-base lesions. Neurosurg Rev 2009;32(3):309–19 [discussion: 318–9].

264. Zanation AM, Snyderman CH, Carrau RL, et al. Endoscopic endonasal surgery for petrous apex lesions. Laryngoscope 2009;119(1):19–25.

265. Hu A, Thomas P, Franklin J, et al. Endoscopic resection of pterygopalatine chondrosarcoma. J Otolaryngol Head Neck Surg 2009;38(3):E100–3.

266. Harvey RJ, Pitzer G, Nissman DB, et al. PET/CT in the assessment of previously treated skull base malignancies. Head Neck 2010;32(1):76–84.

267. Kang MD, Escott E, Thomas AJ, et al. The MR imaging appearance of the vascular pedicle nasoseptal flap [Erratum appears in AJNR Am J Neuroradiol 2009;30(7):E113]. AJNR Am J Neuroradiol 2009;30(4):781–6.

268. Fatterpekar GM, Delman BN, Som PM. Imaging the paranasal sinuses: where we are and where we are going. Anat Rec (Hoboken) 2008;291(11):1564–72.

269. Madani G, Beale TJ, Lund VJ. Imaging of sinonasal tumors. Semin Ultrasound CT MR 2009;30(1):25–38.

270. Bhattacharyya N. Cancer of the nasal cavity: survival and factors influencing prognosis. Arch Otolaryngol Head Neck Surg 2002;128(9):1079–83.

271. Blanch JL, Ruiz AM, Alos L, et al. Treatment of 125 sinonasal tumors: prognostic factors, outcome, and follow-up. Otolaryngol Head Neck Surg 2004;131(6): 973–6.

272. Snyderman CH, Carrau RL, Kassam AB, et al. Endoscopic skull base surgery: principles of endonasal oncological surgery. J Surg Oncol 2008;97(8):658–64.

273. Alvarez I, Suarez C, Rodrigo JP, et al. Prognostic factors in paranasal sinus cancer. Am J Otol 1995;16(2):109–14.

274. Cantu G, Solero CL, Mariani L, et al. A new classification for malignant tumors involving the anterior skull base. Arch Otolaryngol Head Neck Surg 1999; 125(11):1252–7.

275. Carrillo JF, Guemes A, Ramirez-Ortega MC, et al. Prognostic factors in maxillary sinus and nasal cavity carcinoma. Eur J Surg Oncol 2005;31(10):1206–12.

276. Dulguerov P, Allal AS. Nasal and paranasal sinus carcinoma: how can we continue to make progress? Curr Opin Otolaryngol Head Neck Surg 2006; 14(2):67–72.

277. Nazar G, Rodrigo JP, Llorente JL, et al. Prognostic factors of maxillary sinus malignancies. Am J Rhinol 2004;18(4):233–8.

278. Har-El G, Casiano RR. Endoscopic management of anterior skull base tumors. Otolaryngol Clin North Am 2005;38(1):133–44, ix.

279. Bachar G, Goldstein DP, Shah M, et al. Esthesioneuroblastoma: the Princess Margaret Hospital experience. Head Neck 2008;30(12):1607–14.

280. McCaffrey TV, Olsen KD, Yohanan JM, et al. Factors affecting survival of patients with tumors of the anterior skull base. Laryngoscope 1994;104(8 Pt 1): 940–5.

281. Van Tuyl R, Gussack GS. Prognostic factors in craniofacial surgery. Laryngoscope 1991;101(3):240–4.

282. Sautter NB, Cannady SB, Citardi MJ, et al. Comparison of open versus endoscopic resection of inverted papilloma. Am J Rhinol 2007;21(3):320–3.

283. Wellman B, Traynelis V, McCulloch T, et al. Midline anterior craniofacial approach for malignancy: results of en bloc versus piecemeal resections. Skull Base Surg 1999;9(1):41–6.

284. Dias FL, Sa GM, Lima RA, et al. Patterns of failure and outcome in esthesioneuroblastoma. Arch Otolaryngol Head Neck Surg 2003;129(11):1186–92.

285. Mortuaire G, Arzul E, Darras JA, et al. Surgical management of sinonasal inverted papillomas through endoscopic approach. Eur Arch Otorhinolaryngol 2007;264(12):1419–24.

286. Jardine AH, Davies GR, Birchall MA. Recurrence and malignant degeneration of 89 cases of inverted papilloma diagnosed in a non-tertiary referral population

between 1975 and 1995: clinical predictors and p53 studies. Clin Otolaryngol Allied Sci 2000;25(5):363–9.

287. Amendola BE, Eisert D, Hazra TA, et al. Carcinoma of the maxillary antrum: surgery of radiation therapy? Int J Radiat Oncol Biol Phys 1981;7(6):743–6.

288. Jansen EP, Keus RB, Hilgers FJ, et al. Does the combination of radiotherapy and debulking surgery favor survival in paranasal sinus carcinoma? Int J Radiat Oncol Biol Phys 2000;48(1):27–35.

289. Blanco AI, Chao KS, Ozyigit G, et al. Carcinoma of paranasal sinuses: long-term outcomes with radiotherapy. Int J Radiat Oncol Biol Phys 2004;59(1):51–8.

290. Guntinas-Lichius O, Kreppel MP, Stuetzer H, et al. Single modality and multimodality treatment of nasal and paranasal sinuses cancer: a single institution experience of 229 patients. Eur J Surg Oncol 2007;33(2):222–8.

291. Jiang GL, Morrison WH, Garden AS, et al. Ethmoid sinus carcinomas: natural history and treatment results. Radiother Oncol 1998;49(1):21–7.

292. Mendenhall WM, Amdur RJ, Morris CG, et al. Carcinoma of the nasal cavity and paranasal sinuses. Laryngoscope 2009;119(5):899–906.

293. Paulino AC, Marks JE, Bricker P, et al. Results of treatment of patients with maxillary sinus carcinoma. Cancer 1998;83(3):457–65.

294. St-Pierre S, Baker SR. Squamous cell carcinoma of the maxillary sinus: analysis of 66 cases. Head Neck Surg 1983;5(6):508–13.

295. Hoppe BS, Nelson CJ, Gomez DR, et al. Unresectable carcinoma of the paranasal sinuses: outcomes and toxicities. Int J Radiat Oncol Biol Phys 2008;72(3):763–9.

296. Chen AM, Daly ME, Bucci MK, et al. Carcinomas of the paranasal sinuses and nasal cavity treated with radiotherapy at a single institution over five decades: are we making improvement? Int J Radiat Oncol Biol Phys 2007;69(1):141–7.

297. Ellingwood KE, Million RR. Cancer of the nasal cavity and ethmoid/sphenoid sinuses. Cancer 1979;43(4):1517–26.

298. Karim AB, Kralendonk JH, Njo KH, et al. Ethmoid and upper nasal cavity carcinoma: treatment, results and complications. Radiother Oncol 1990;19(2):109–20.

299. Shukovsky LJ, Fletcher GH. Retinal and optic nerve complications in a high dose irradiation technique of ethmoid sinus and nasal cavity. Radiology 1972;104(3):629–34.

300. Takeda A, Shigematsu N, Suzuki S, et al. Late retinal complications of radiation therapy for nasal and paranasal malignancies: relationship between irradiated-dose area and severity. Int J Radiat Oncol Biol Phys 1999;44(3):599–605.

301. Snyers A, Janssens GORJ, Twickler MB, et al. Malignant tumors of the nasal cavity and paranasal sinuses: long-term outcome and morbidity with emphasis on hypothalamic-pituitary deficiency. Int J Radiat Oncol Biol Phys 2009;73(5):1343–51.

302. Hoppe BS, Stegman LD, Zelefsky MJ, et al. Treatment of nasal cavity and paranasal sinus cancer with modern radiotherapy techniques in the postoperative setting–the MSKCC experience. Int J Radiat Oncol Biol Phys 2007;67(3):691–702.

303. Padovani L, Pommier P, Clippe SS, et al. Three-dimensional conformal radiotherapy for paranasal sinus carcinoma: clinical results for 25 patients. Int J Radiat Oncol Biol Phys 2003;56(1):169–76.

304. Dirix P, Nuyts S, Geussens Y, et al. Malignancies of the nasal cavity and paranasal sinuses: long-term outcome with conventional or three-dimensional conformal radiotherapy. Int J Radiat Oncol Biol Phys 2007;69(4):1042–50.

305. Duthoy W, Boterberg T, Claus F, et al. Postoperative intensity-modulated radiotherapy in sinonasal carcinoma: clinical results in 39 patients. Cancer 2005; 104(1):71–82.

306. Combs SE, Konkel S, Schulz-Ertner D, et al. Intensity modulated radiotherapy (IMRT) in patients with carcinomas of the paranasal sinuses: clinical benefit for complex shaped target volumes. Radiat Oncol 2006;1:23.

307. Daly ME, Chen AM, Bucci MK, et al. Intensity-modulated radiation therapy for malignancies of the nasal cavity and paranasal sinuses. Int J Radiat Oncol Biol Phys 2007;67(1):151–7.

308. Dirix P, Nuyts S, Vanstraelen B, et al. Post-operative intensity-modulated radiotherapy for malignancies of the nasal cavity and paranasal sinuses. Radiother Oncol 2007;85(3):385–91.

309. Hoppe BS, Wolden SL, Zelefsky MJ, et al. Postoperative intensity-modulated radiation therapy for cancers of the paranasal sinuses, nasal cavity, and lacrimal glands: technique, early outcomes, and toxicity. Head Neck 2008;30(7):925–32.

310. Madani I, Bonte K, Vakaet L, et al. Intensity-modulated radiotherapy for sinonasal tumors: Ghent University Hospital update. Int J Radiat Oncol Biol Phys 2009;73(2):424–32.

311. Veldeman L, Madani I, Hulstaert F, et al. Evidence behind use of intensity-modulated radiotherapy: a systematic review of comparative clinical studies [Erratum appears in Lancet Oncol 2008;9(6):513]. Lancet Oncol 2008;9(4): 367–75.

312. Homma A, Oridate N, Suzuki F, et al. Superselective high-dose cisplatin infusion with concomitant radiotherapy in patients with advanced cancer of the nasal cavity and paranasal sinuses: a single institution experience. Cancer 2009; 115(20):4705–14.

313. Lee MM, Vokes EE, Rosen A, et al. Multimodality therapy in advanced paranasal sinus carcinoma: superior long-term results. Cancer J Sci Am 1999; 5(4):219–23.

314. Licitra L, Locati LD, Cavina R, et al. Primary chemotherapy followed by anterior craniofacial resection and radiotherapy for paranasal cancer. Ann Oncol 2003; 14(3):367–72.

315. Nishimura G, Tsukuda M, Mikami Y, et al. The efficacy and safety of concurrent chemoradiotherapy for maxillary sinus squamous cell carcinoma patients. Auris Nasus Larynx 2009;36(5):547–54.

316. Enepekides DJ. Sinonasal undifferentiated carcinoma: an update. Curr Opin Otolaryngol Head Neck Surg 2005;13(4):222–5.

317. Sato Y, Morita M, Takahashi HO, et al. Combined surgery, radiotherapy, and regional chemotherapy in carcinoma of the paranasal sinuses. Cancer 1970; 25(3):571–9.

318. Knegt PP, de Jong PC, van Andel JG, et al. Carcinoma of the paranasal sinuses. Results of a prospective pilot study. Cancer 1985;56(1):57–62.

319. Almeyda R, Capper J. Is surgical debridement and topical 5 fluorouracil the optimum treatment for woodworkers' adenocarcinoma of the ethmoid sinuses? A case-controlled study of a 20-year experience. Clin Otolaryngol 2008;33(5): 435–41.

320. Waitz G, Wigand ME. Results of endoscopic sinus surgery for the treatment of inverted papillomas. Laryngoscope 1992;102(8):917–22.

321. McCary WS, Gross CW, Reibel JF, et al. Preliminary report: endoscopic versus external surgery in the management of inverting papilloma. Laryngoscope 1994; 104(4):415–9.

322. Stankiewicz JA, Girgis SJ. Endoscopic surgical treatment of nasal and paranasal sinus inverted papilloma. Otolaryngol Head Neck Surg 1993;109(6): 988–95.

323. Kamel RH. Transnasal endoscopic surgery in juvenile nasopharyngeal angiofibroma. J Laryngol Otol 1996;110(10):962–8.

324. Tseng HZ, Chao WY. Transnasal endoscopic approach for juvenile nasopharyngeal angiofibroma. Am J Otol 1997;18(2):151–4.

325. Fagan JJ, Snyderman CH, Carrau RL, et al. Nasopharyngeal angiofibromas: selecting a surgical approach. Head Neck 1997;19(5):391–9.

326. Zicot AF, Daele J. Endoscopic surgery for nasal and sinusal vascular tumours: about two cases of nasopharyngeal angiofibromas and one case of turbinate angioma. Acta Otorhinolaryngol Belg 1996;50(3):177–82.

327. Midilli R, Karci B, Akyildiz S. Juvenile nasopharyngeal angiofibroma: analysis of 42 cases and important aspects of endoscopic approach. Int J Pediatr Otorhinolaryngol 2009;73(3):401–8.

328. Sham CL, Woo JK, van Hasselt CA, et al. Treatment results of sinonasal inverted papilloma: an 18-year study. Am J Rhinol Allergy 2009;23(2):203–11.

329. Reh DD, Lane AP. The role of endoscopic sinus surgery in the management of sinonasal inverted papilloma. Curr Opin Otolaryngol Head Neck Surg 2009; 17(1):6–10.

330. Gupta AK, Rajiniganth MG. Endoscopic approach to juvenile nasopharyngeal angiofibroma: our experience at a tertiary care centre. J Laryngol Otol 2008; 122(11):1185–9.

331. Bleier BS, Kennedy DW, Palmer JN, et al. Current management of juvenile nasopharyngeal angiofibroma: a tertiary center experience 1999-2007. Am J Rhinol Allergy 2009;23(3):328–30.

332. Seiberling K, Floreani S, Robinson S, et al. Endoscopic management of frontal sinus osteomas revisited. Am J Rhinol Allergy 2009;23(3):331–6.

333. Lawson W, Patel ZM. The evolution of management for inverted papilloma: an analysis of 200 cases. Otolaryngol Head Neck Surg 2009;140(3):330–5.

334. Woodworth BA, Bhargave GA, Palmer JN, et al. Clinical outcomes of endoscopic and endoscopic-assisted resection of inverted papillomas: a 15-year experience [Erratum appears in Am J Rhinol 2008;22(1):97]. Am J Rhinol 2007;21(5):591–600.

335. Busquets JM, Hwang PH. Endoscopic resection of sinonasal inverted papilloma: a meta-analysis. Otolaryngol Head Neck Surg 2006;134(3):476–82.

336. Yiotakis I, Eleftheriadou A, Davilis D, et al. Juvenile nasopharyngeal angiofibroma stages I and II: a comparative study of surgical approaches. Int J Pediatr Otorhinolaryngol 2008;72(6):793–800.

337. Karkos PD, Fyrmpas G, Carrie SC, et al. Endoscopic versus open surgical interventions for inverted nasal papilloma: a systematic review. Clin Otolaryngol 2006;31(6):499–503.

338. Samant S, Kruger E. Cancer of the paranasal sinuses. Curr Oncol Rep 2007; 9(2):147–51.

339. Cohen MA, Liang J, Cohen IJ, et al. Endoscopic resection of advanced anterior skull base lesions: oncologically safe? ORL J Otorhinolaryngol Relat Spec 2009; 71(3):123–8.

340. Kuhn UM, Mann WJ, Amedee RG. Endonasal approach for nasal and paranasal sinus tumor removal. ORL J Otorhinolaryngol Relat Spec 2001;63(6):366–71.

341. Casiano RR, Numa WA, Falquez AM. Endoscopic resection of esthesioneuroblastoma. Am J Rhinol 2001;15(4):271–9.

342. Suriano M, De Vincentiis M, Colli A, et al. Endoscopic treatment of esthesioneuroblastoma: a minimally invasive approach combined with radiation therapy. Otolaryngol Head Neck Surg 2007;136(1):104–7.

343. Yoshimoto Y. Publication bias in neurosurgery: lessons from series of unruptured aneurysms. Acta Neurochir (Wien) 2003;145(1):45–8.

344. Russell PT, Weaver KD. Anterior endoscopic skull-base surgery getting started: an otolaryngologist's perspective. Curr Opin Otolaryngol Head Neck Surg 2007; 15(1):1–5.

345. Snyderman C, Kassam A, Carrau R, et al. Acquisition of surgical skills for endonasal skull base surgery: a training program. Laryngoscope 2007;117(4): 699–705.

346. Castelnuovo P, Pistochini A, Locatelli D. Different surgical approaches to the sellar region: focusing on the "two nostrils four hands technique". Rhinology 2006;44(1):2–7.

347. Castelnuovo P, Valentini V, Giovannetti F, et al. Osteomas of the maxillofacial district: endoscopic surgery versus open surgery. J Craniofac Surg 2008; 19(6):1446–52.

348. Carrabba G, Dehdashti AR, Gentili F. Surgery for clival lesions: open resection versus the expanded endoscopic endonasal approach. Neurosurg Focus 2008;25(6):E7.

349. Cappabianca P, Cavallo LM, Colao A, et al. Surgical complications associated with the endoscopic endonasal transsphenoidal approach for pituitary adenomas. J Neurosurg 2002;97(2):293–8.

350. Stamm AM. Transnasal endoscopy-assisted skull base surgery. Ann Otol Rhinol Laryngol Suppl 2006;196:45–53.

351. Bockmuhl U, Minovi A, Kratzsch B, et al. Endonasal micro-endoscopic tumor surgery: state of the art. Laryngorhinootologie Dec 2005;84(12):884–91 [in German].

352. Gardner PA, Kassam AB, Thomas A, et al. Endoscopic endonasal resection of anterior cranial base meningiomas. Neurosurgery 2008;63(1):36–52 [discussion: 52–4].

353. Eveson J. Salivary gland-type carcinomas. In: Barnes L, Eveson J, Reichart P, et al, editors. Pathology and genetics of head and neck tumours. Lyon: IARC Press; 2005. p. 24–6.

354. Tami TA. Surgical management of lesions of the sphenoid lateral recess. American Journal of Rhinology 2006;20(4):412–6.

355. Hyams VJ, Batsakis JG, Michaels L. Tumors of the upper respiratory tract and ear. Washington, DC: Armed Forces Institute of Pathology; 1988.

APPENDIX

Histopathology and International Classification of Diseases Oncology ICD-O codes[a] according to WHO classification of tumors

1. Malignant epithelial tumors
   a. Lymphoepithelial carcinoma ICD-O 8082/3
   b. Sinonasal undifferentiated carcinoma ICD-O 8020/3
   c. Squamous cell carcinoma
      1. Keratinizing squamous cell carcinoma ICD-O 8070/3
      2. Nonkeratinizing (cylindrical cell, transitional) carcinoma, currently no separate ICD-O
      3. Verrucous carcinoma ICD-O 8051/3
      4. Papillary squamous cell carcinoma ICD-O 8052/3
      5. Basaloid squamous cell carcinoma ICD-O 8083/3
      6. Spindle cell carcinoma ICD-O 8074/3
      7. Adenosquamous carcinoma ICD-O 8560/3
      8. Acantholytic squamous cell carcinoma ICD-O 8075/3
   d. Keratinizing squamous cell carcinoma ICD-O 8070/3
   e. Nonkeratinizing (cylindrical cell, transitional) carcinoma (currently no separate ICD O)
   f. Verrucous carcinoma ICD-O 8051/3
   g. Papillary squamous cell carcinoma ICD-O 8052/3
   h. Basaloid squamous cell carcinoma ICD-O 8083/3
   i. Spindle cell carcinoma ICD-O 8074/3
   j. Adenosquamous carcinoma ICD-O 8560/3
   k. Acantholytic squamous cell carcinoma ICD-O 8075/3
   l. Adenocarcinoma
      i. Intestinal-type adenocarcinomas ICD-O 8144/3 (Subclassification according to Barnes166 1986)
         1. Papillary type
         2. Colonic type
         3. Solid type
         4. Mucinous type
         5. Mixed
      ii. Sinonasal nonintestinal-type adenocarcinomas ICD-0 8140/3
         1. Low-grade adenocarcinoma
         2. High-grade adenocarcinoma
   m. Salivary gland–type carcinoma
      i. Adenoid cystic carcinoma ICD-O 8200/3
      ii. Acinic cell carcinoma ICD-O 8550/3
      iii. Mucoepidermoid carcinoma ICD-O 8430/3
      iv. Epithelial-myoepithelial carcinoma ICD-O 8562/3
      v. Clear cell carcinoma ICD-O 8310/3

2. Neuroendocrine tumors
   a. Typical carcinoid ICD-O 8240/3
   b. Atypical carcinoid ICD-O 8249/3
   c. Small cell carcinoma, neuroendocrine type ICD-O 8041/3

3. Malignant soft tissue tumors
   a. Fibrosarcoma ICD-O 8810/3
   b. Undifferentiated high-grade pleomorphic Sarcoma (MFH) ICD-O 8830/3
   c. Leiomyosarcoma ICD-O 8890/3
   d. Embryonal rhabdomyosarcoma ICD-O 8910/3
   e. Alveolar rhabdomyosarcoma ICD-O 8920/3
   f. Angiosarcoma ICD-O 9120/3
   g. Malignant peripheral nerve sheath tumor ICD-O 9540/3

4. Borderline and low malignant potential tumors of soft tissue
   a. Desmoid-type fibromatosis ICD-O 8821/1
   b. Inflammatory myofibroblastic tumor ICD-O 8825/1
   c. Glomangiopericytoma (sinonasal-type hemangiopericytoma) ICD-O 9150/1
   d. Extrapleural solitary fibrous tumor IDC-O 8815/1

5. Malignant tumors of bone and cartilage
   a. Chondrosarcoma ICD-O 9220/3
   b. Mesenchymal chondrosarcoma ICD-O 9240/3
   c. Osteosarcoma ICD-O 9180/3
   d. Chordoma ICD-O 9370/3

6. Hematolymphoid tumors
   a. Extranodal natural killer (NK)/T-cell lymphoma ICD-O 9719/3
   b. Diffuse large B-cell lymphoma ICD-O 9680/3
   c. Extramedullary plasmacytoma ICD-O 9734/3
   d. Extramedullary myeloid sarcoma ICD-O 9930/3
   e. Histiocytic sarcoma ICD-O 9755/3
   f. Langerhans cell histiocytosis ICD-O 9751/1
   g. Juvenile xanthogranuloma; no ICD-O Code
   h. Rosai-Dorfman disease (sinus histiocytosis with massive lymphadenopathy); no ICD-O code

7. Neuroectodermal tumors
   a. Ewing sarcoma ICD-O 9260/3
   b. Primitive neuroectodermal tumor (PNET) ICD-O 9364/3
   c. Olfactory neuroblastoma (esthesioneuroblastoma) ICD-O 9522/3
      Grading (grade 1–4) according to Hyams 1988[355] based on:
      • Architecture
      • Pleomorphism
      • Neurofibrillary matrix
      • Rosettes
      • Mitosis
      • Necrosis
      • Glands
      • Calcification
   d. Melanotic neuroectodermal tumor of infancy ICD-O 9363/0
   e. Mucosal malignant melanoma ICD-O 8720/3
   f. Heterotopic central nervous system (CNS) tissue(nasal glioma) ICD-O none

8. Germ cell tumors
   a. Immature teratoma ICD-O 9080/3
   b. Teratoma with malignant transformation ICD-O 9084/3
   c. Sinonasal yolk sac tumor (endodermal sinus tumor) ICD-O 9071/3
   d. Sinonasal teratocarcinosarcoma ICD-O none
   e. Mature teratoma ICD-O 9080/0
   f. Dermoid cyst ICD-O 9084/0

9. Secondary tumors (mainly metastases from primary tumors of:
   a. Kidney
   b. Lung
   c. Breast
   d. Thyroid
   e. Prostate
   f. Others

[a] Whenever available.

Endoscopic Nasopharyngectomy and its Role in Managing Locally Recurrent Nasopharyngeal Carcinoma

Yew Kwang Ong, MD[a],*, C. Arturo Solares, MD[b],
Steve Lee, MD, PhD[c], Carl H. Snyderman, MD[d,e],
Juan Fernandez-Miranda, MD[e], Paul A. Gardner, MD[e]

KEYWORDS

- Nasopharynx • Endoscope • Nasopharyngeal carcinoma
- Nasopharyngectomy

EBM Question	Level of Evidence	Grade of Recommendation
What is role of endoscopic surgery for recurrent nasopharyngeal carcinoma?	4	C

EPIDEMIOLOGY OF NASOPHARYNGEAL CARCINOMA

Nasopharyngeal carcinoma (NPC) is an epithelial malignancy that arises within the nasopharynx. It has a distinct racial and geographic distribution, with high prevalence in Southern China and Southeast Asia.[1] The highest rates are registered among Cantonese in the Guangdong province of Southern China (of which Hong

The authors have nothing to disclose.

[a] Department of Otolaryngology-Head & Neck Surgery, National University Hospital, 1E Kent Ridge Road, Singapore 119228
[b] Department of Otolaryngology-Head & Neck Surgery, Medical College of Georgia, 1120 15th Street Augusta, GA 30912, USA
[c] Department of Otolaryngology-Head & Neck Surgery, Loma Linda University Medical Center, 11234 Anderson Street, #2586A Loma Linda, CA 92354, USA
[d] Department of Otolaryngology-Head & Neck Surgery, University of Pittsburgh School of Medicine, 200 Lothrop Street, Pittsburgh, PA 15213, USA
[e] Department of Neurological Surgery, University of Pittsburgh School of Medicine, 200 Lothrop Street, Pittsburgh, PA 15213, USA
* Corresponding author.
E-mail address: entv2@nus.edu.sg

Otolaryngol Clin N Am 44 (2011) 1141–1154
doi:10.1016/j.otc.2011.07.002
0030-6665/11/$ – see front matter © 2011 Published by Elsevier Inc.

Kong is a part). The age-standardized incidence for Hong Kong males is 21.5 per 100,000 persons year.[1] The male/female ratio is 2 to 3:1. NPC can be divided into keratinizing and nonkeratinizing, which is further subdivided into differentiated or undifferentiated (**Fig. 1**).[2] Most NPC in high-incidence areas is of the nonkeratinizing type and has an etiologic association with Epstein-Barr virus.[2] Most of the literature deals with the nonkeratinizing type, and this type is implied when no distinction is made.

TREATMENT OF PRIMARY NASOPHARYNGEAL CARCINOMA

NPC is highly radiosensitive and thus the primary treatment of NPC is radiation therapy. Early disease (stage I and II) NPC is treated with radiation alone whereas advanced disease (stage III and IV) is treated with concomitant chemoradiation. With advances in radiotherapy planning and delivery techniques such as intensity-modulated radiotherapy (IMRT) and the use of chemoradiation, a 5-year local control rate of 76% to 91% can be achieved.[3–6] Nevertheless, local recurrence remains a common sign of treatment failure and a major cause of morbidity and mortality.

INVESTIGATIONS

The diagnosis of a recurrence is based on endoscopic or radiological detection of a suspicious mass in the nasopharynx followed by histologic confirmation. Detection of recurrence using traditional computed tomography (CT) or magnetic resonance imaging (MRI) can be challenging. Changes to nasopharyngeal tissue after radiotherapy such as edema, loss of tissue planes, fibrosis, and scarring can obscure the detection of tumor recurrence.[7] Both CT and MRI scans have been reported to have a low sensitivity and moderate specificity in differentiating tumor recurrence from posttherapy changes.[7,8] Positron emission tomography (PET) using fluorodeoxyglucose, apart from its use in the detection of distant metastases, has been shown to be more sensitive than both MRI and CT scan in detecting residual or recurrent tumor. In addition, combined PET/CT imaging can give accurate localization of focal uptake, allowing distinction of disease from normal physiology and better treatment planning.[7]

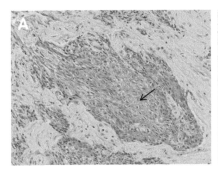 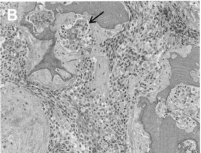

Fig. 1. Photomicrographs of tumor specimens (hematoxylin-eosin, original magnification ×20). (*A*) NPC, keratinizing type. Observe the presence of keratin (*pink material, black arrow*) between the cancer cells. (*B*) Undifferentiated carcinoma. Observe the bony invasion (*black arrow*) and the absence of keratin between cells.

PROGNOSIS

Aggressive salvage treatment of local recurrence is warranted because patients can achieve reasonable long-term survival after salvage therapy.[9] Patients who receive salvage treatment had a significantly better overall survival than those who did not receive salvage treatment.[9]

This review examines the various treatment options available, in particular the role of endoscopic nasopharyngectomy in the salvage of locally recurrent NPC.

MANAGEMENT OF RECURRENT NASOPHARYNGEAL CARCINOMA

Management of recurrent NPC remains challenging. Early detection of recurrent disease is essential for any form of salvage therapy to be successful.[10] Current treatment options include reirradiation, chemotherapy, or surgery. The role of chemotherapy alone is primarily reserved for palliation in patients not suitable for radical radiation therapy or a nasopharyngectomy.[9,11]

RADIOTHERAPY FOR RECURRENT NASOPHARYNGEAL CARCINOMA

Reirradiation options include external beam radiotherapy (conventional two-dimensional radiotherapy, three-dimensional [3D] conformal radiotherapy, IMRT, and stereotactic radiotherapy) with or without brachytherapy. Reirradiation of local recurrences using traditional external beam irradiation can result in further 5-year survival rates of 8% to 36%.[4,12–14] There is a significant correlation between the dose at reirradiation and the salvage rate; a higher local control rate is achieved with a dose of at least 60 Gy.[11,12] As a result of a high cumulative radiation dose, late complications are frequent and have been reported in 26% to 57% of patients.[5,14,15] Radiation-related complications included multiple cranial nerve palsies, temporal lobe necrosis, osteoradionecrosis, xerostomia, trismus, soft tissue fibrosis, hearing and visual impairment, endocrine dysfunction, and even carotid rupture. The treatment mortality ranged from 1.8% to 9.4% and was related mainly to neurologic damage.[14] Newer treatment modalities such as the 3D conformational radiation, IMRT, and stereotactic irradiation aim to deliver more precise tumor coverage and spare critical nearby structures, thereby reducing the incidence of late complications.

ANATOMY OF THE NASOPHARYNX

It is essential to understand the complex anatomic relationships of the nasopharynx regardless of the surgical approach used. The nasopharynx is a narrow space located posterior to the nasal cavity and sits above the soft palate. It is bounded superiorly by the sphenoid sinus and upper clivus and posteriorly by the lower clivus and the first cervical vertebra. Anterolaterally, it is bounded by the medial pterygoid plate. Posterior to the medial pterygoid plate is the sinus of Morgagni. Internally the nasopharynx is covered by mucosal, and the pharyngobasilar fascia lies deep to it. The pharyngobasilar or pharyngeal fascia is a tough fascia that connects the superior constrictor muscle to the skull base. It originates from the pharyngeal tubercle of the occipital bone posteriorly and attaches to the posterior edge of the medial pterygoid plates anteriorly.[16] The tensor veli palatini and the cartilaginous portion of the Eustachian tube pass through the sinus of Morgagni by traversing through the pharyngobasilar fascia. Posterior to the Eustachian tube along the lateral wall is the fossa of Rosenmuller, where NPC typically originates. When the tumor invades laterally through the sinus of Morgagni, it extends along the Eustachian tube and involves the parapharyngeal space and foramen ovale area. This situation results in a constellation of symptoms:

- Ipsilateral conductive hearing loss
- Ipsilateral akinesia of the soft palate
- Ipsilateral trigeminal (mandibular) neuralgia, also known as Trotter syndrome

The biggest risk in this surgery is the proximity of the parapharyngeal internal carotid artery (ICA) to the nasopharynx. Identification of key surgical landmarks and their relationship to the ICA minimizes the risk of injuring the carotid artery. Wen and colleagues[17] presented a detailed endoscopic anatomy of the nasopharynx and highlighted several landmarks. They found that osseous landmarks, such as the medial pterygoid plate, foramen lacerum, and the isthmus of the Eustachian tube, along with the muscular landmarks (longus capitis), all lead to the ICA.

PREOPERATIVE EVALUATION OF NASOPHARYNGEAL CARCINOMA

Patients are restaged using a combination of CT and MRI, each providing complementary information about bone erosion and soft tissue invasion (**Figs. 2** and **3**). The limiting factor for surgery is tumor involvement of the ICA in its petrous or parapharyngeal segment. When tumor is in contact with the ICA, surgical options include dissection of tumor from the artery with preservation of the ICA or sacrifice of the ICA to obtain a clear resection margin. The ability of the patient to tolerate sacrifice of the ICA is assessed with a balloon occlusion test with neuromonitoring (**Fig. 4**). If the patient tolerates temporary occlusion without a neurologic deficit or evidence of decreased cerebral perfusion, permanent occlusion can be performed with low risk of a delayed stroke. On the other hand, if the patient fails the balloon occlusion test, the goals of surgery need to be modified or alternative therapy should be considered.

SURGERY FOR RECURRENT NASOPHARYNGEAL CARCINOMA

Surgery presents a reasonable choice when the recurrent tumor is resectable. It gives satisfactory local control with a 5-year survival rate between 30% and 52%[9,18–21] and there is less morbidity than high-dose reirradiation.[11,18,21]

Access to the nasopharynx has always been difficult and is traditionally achieved with an open approach. Depending on the extent and site of the recurrent NPC, various approaches have been developed to facilitate adequate surgical resection, including transpalatal,[22,23] maxillary swing,[24] transmandibular,[25] facial translocation,[26] and transinfratemporal fossa[27] approaches. These approaches are complex and may result in considerable morbidity, including facial scarring, trismus, dental malocclusion, injury to cranial nerves (infraorbital nerve in the maxillary swing, lingual nerve in the mandibular swing, both in facial translocation, facial palsies with infratemporal fossa approaches), palatal defects, dysphagia, nasal regurgitation, osteonecrosis, osteomyelitis, and even rupture of the ICA.[18,19,28,29]

In an attempt to reduce the morbidities associated with open surgical approaches, minimally invasive techniques have emerged. To and colleagues[29] described a midfacial degloving transnasal approach, which avoided a facial incision. This approach was coupled with the use of stereotactic navigation for precise localization of the ICA. The investigators were able to achieve tumor clearance in 12 of 15 patients. The 3 remaining patients had their tumors stuck to the ICA. No follow-up data were available. In a follow-up publication,[30] To and colleagues compared this technique with a conventional open transfacial approach. There appeared to be fewer mortalities and morbidities in the

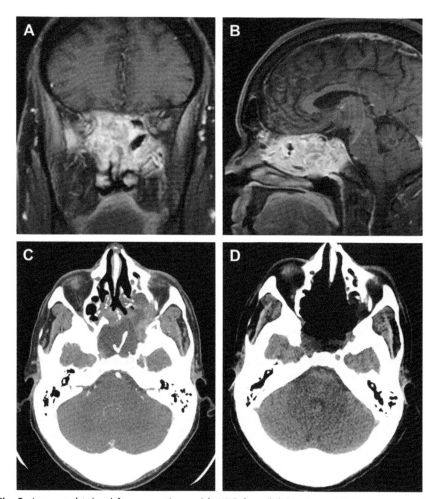

Fig. 2. Images obtained from a patient with NPC, keratinizing type. (*A*) MRI, coronal view, T1 with contrast. Observe the involvement of the nasal septum, turbinates, and dura. (*B*) MRI, sagittal view, T1 with contrast. The tumor presents a large anterior-posterior extension. Posterior, observe the involvement of the clivus. (*C*) Preoperative CT scan, axial view with contrast. The tumor extends to the left maxillary sinus. (*D*) CT scan, axial view with contrast, after endoscopic endonasal resection of the tumor with palliative intent.

minimally invasive group. However, the staging of the recurrent tumor in each group of patients was not indicated, and no follow-up data were available.

Roh and Park[31] described a transseptal approach similar to a conventional transseptal hypophysectomy to gain access to the nasopharynx. By inserting a bivalve speculum between the mucoperichondrial flaps, and with the aid of a microscope and CO_2 laser the investigators achieved complete resection of tumors in 3 patients with recurrent T1 NPC. There was no recurrence during a follow-up period of 12 to 28 months.

Endoscopes have revolutionized the approach to diseases involving the nasal cavity and the sinuses. The advantages include avoidance of a facial scar, less destruction of the surrounding tissues, and possibly better preservation of function.[32] With increasing experience and expertise, the indications have also expanded rapidly

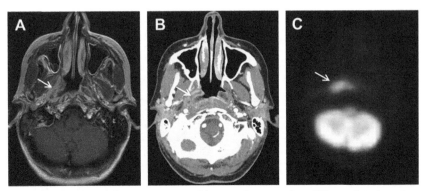

Fig. 3. Images obtained from a patient with nasopharyngeal undifferentiated carcinoma. (A) Preoperative MRI, axial view, T1 with contrast. Notice the thickness in the soft tissue around the right Eustachian tube (*white arrow*). (B) Preoperative CT scan shows tumor extension to the right ICA. (C) The PET scan confirms the presence of a suspicious lesion in the same region.

from dealing with benign pathologies to sinonasal malignancies. Anterior skull base tumors such as olfactory neuroblastoma can now be safely resected with an endoscopic craniofacial resection, maintaining the same oncologic principles as in open surgery. Early results on endoscopic resection of sinonasal malignancies are promising.[33] The limits of endoscopic surgical techniques are constantly evolving and now include diseases involving sites such as the infratemporal fossa and nasopharynx.

The endoscope is well suited for the nasopharynx. Improvement in the optics of the rod-lens endoscope, coupled with high-resolution cameras and monitors, have allowed excellent visualization of this area. Reliability of intraoperative navigational devices, the use of extended endonasal instruments, and better understanding of endoscopic anatomy of the nasopharynx have made endoscopic nasopharyngectomy safe and feasible.

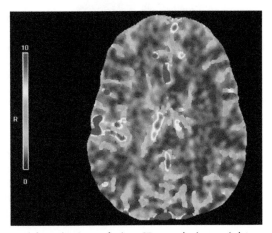

Fig. 4. Images obtained from brain perfusion CT scan during a right carotid artery balloon test occlusion (patient in **Fig. 3**). The test showed no significant drop of relative cerebral blood flow and no marked asymmetry during the occlusion. The artery was sacrificed with angiographic coils and resected intraoperatively.

PRINCIPLES OF ENDOSCOPIC NASOPHARYNGECTOMY

The surgical margin status is an important prognostic factor for both local control and overall survival for surgical salvage of recurrent NPC.[34–36] The ability to achieve clearance is dictated by the recurrent T stage, involvement of vital anatomic structures, and the ability to obtain adequate surgical exposure. The widest possible exposure offers the best opportunity to achieve complete resection with negative margins. This oncologic principle is also applicable to endoscopic surgery. Greater exposure can be achieved by resecting the posterior half of the septum (vomer) and reduction of the inferior turbinates.[30,37] This strategy allows the whole nasopharynx to be visualized. The need for further exposure depends on the site and extent of the tumor.

Castelnuovo and colleagues[38] described a modulated approach to the nasopharynx. Depending on the tumor extent, these investigators classified nasopharyngeal tumor resections into 3 types. Type 1 resection was the most conservative. The incision began superiorly from the nasopharyngeal vault, down along the posterior border of the torus into the fossa of Rosenmuller, and horizontally across at the level of the atlas. The Eustachian tube was preserved. Posteriorly the resection extended deep to the periosteum of the skull base, and the ventral part of the clivus was drilled out. This resection was suitable for small tumors centrally located in the nasopharynx. Type 2 was for tumors involving the roof of the nasopharynx, and the exposure was extended superiorly into the sphenoid sinus. Bilateral sphenoidectomies and removal of the rostrum allowed access into the sphenoid sinuses. The floor of the sinus was entirely drilled to the coronal plane of the clivus. The rest of the resection was similar to type 1. Type 3 was the most extensive, and the resection includes the lateral nasopharyngeal wall up to the parapharyngeal space and the ipsilateral cartilaginous portion of the Eustachian tube. A complete ethmoidectomy and a modified medial maxillectomy followed by drilling of the medial pterygoid plate were performed. An angled probe was placed into the Eustachian tube, and the cartilaginous portion was then removed up to its bony junction. This is a critical landmark because the parapharyngeal ICA lies just posterior to the bony Eustachian tube landmark and hence is at risk if the resection is carried beyond this point.

All-Sheibani and colleagues[39] also described a similar endonasal transpterygoid approach to the nasopharynx. An endoscopic medial maxillectomy supplemented by an endoscopic Denker approach allowed the removal of the posterior and lateral walls of the maxillary antrum. This procedure was followed by mobilization of the soft tissue contents of the pterygopalatine fossa laterally and removal of the pterygoid process and cartilaginous Eustachian tube. Again, this approach allowed control of the parapharyngeal and petrous segments of the ICA, thus allowing tumors in the fossa of Rosenmuller and infratemporal fossa to be safely resected.

If resection of the ICA is necessary to achieve a clear margin, this can be performed endoscopically if the artery is sacrificed preoperatively using endovascular techniques. Even so, this part of the operation may be facilitated by a combined open (infratemporal skull base) and endoscopic approach.

After a nasopharyngectomy, once the surgical margins are confirmed with frozen sections, consideration should be given to the reconstruction. The wound can be left to heal by secondary intention or alternatively it can be covered with either free mucosal or a pedicled turbinate graft. The latter allows for faster mucosalization. Coverage of heavily irradiated tissue with vascularized tissue speeds the healing process and decreases the risk of wound healing complications and postoperative headache. For large defects with an exposed ICA, a temporalis muscle transposition (combined approach) provides ample coverage.

RESULTS OF ENDOSCOPIC NASOPHARYNGECTOMY

There have been only a few publications in the literature reporting on the results of endoscopic nasopharyngectomy because the technique is relatively new (**Table 1**). Yoshizaki and colleagues[37] first reported on the use of a transseptal endoscopic naso-pharyngectomy for the treatment of 4 cases of recurrent T2 NPC and 1 case of sino-nasal malignant melanoma in 2005. Except for 1 case of rT2 NPC with massive parapharyngeal extension, the tumors were successfully resected without any surgical complications.

In 2007, Chen and colleagues[32] reported their experience of 6 cases of endoscopic nasopharyngectomy for recurrent T1-2a NPC using either diode laser or Harmonic scalpel. The extent of resection included laterally the cartilaginous portion of the Eustachian tube, superiorly, deep to the periosteum of the skull base and posteriorly deep to the prevertebral fascia. All cases were completely resected with clear margins. There were no complications. With an average of 29 months' follow-up (16–59 months), only 1 local recurrence was noted 33 months after surgery. One patient died of skull base osteoradionecrosis and bleeding 18 months after surgery. The early survival outcome appeared to be comparable with other salvage treatments.

Ko and colleagues[40] reported on the use of titanyl-phosphate laser in performing endoscopic nasopharyngectomy for early locally recurrent NPC in 28 patients. Twelve patients were classified as rT1N0, 14 as rT2aN0, and 2 as rT2aN1. All the rT1 tumors were in the central roof of the nasopharynx, whereas 12 of the 16 rT2a tumors grossly involved the fossa of Rosenmuller and Eustachian tube. The tumors were resected en bloc with a 2-mm surgical resection margins. The prevertebral muscles were also

Table 1
Results of recent series of endoscopic nasopharyngectomy for NPC

Authors	No. of Cases	Stage	Margins	Follow-up (mo)	Survival Results
Chen et al,[42] 2009	37	17 rT1N0M0, 4 rT2aN0M0 14 rT2bN0M0 2 rT3N0M0	36 (−) 1 (+)	6–45 (median: 24)	2-y OS 84.2% 2-y LRF 86.3% 2-y PFS 82.6%
Ko et al,[40] 2009	28	12 rT1N0 14 rT2aN0 2 rT2aN1	25(−) 3 (+)	3–48	2-y OS for rT1 90.9% 2-y OS for rT2a 38.5% 2-y LDF for rT1 100% 2-y LDF for rT2a 41.7%
Chen et al,[32] 2007	6	3 rT1, 3 rT2a	6 (−)	16–59 (mean: 29)	Local control rate 83.3% (1 recurrence)
Rohaizam et al,[41] 2009	6	6 rT1N0M0	6 (−)	3–14 mo	No recurrence
Castelnuovo et al,[38] 2009	8	4 rT1, 1rT2a 3 rT3	−	10–78 mo (mean: 28 mo)	No recurrence in rT1, rT2a rT3: 2 alive with disease 1 dead of disease

Abbreviations: LDF, local disease-free survival rate; LRF, local relapse-free survival rate; OS, overall survival rate; PFS, progression-free survival rate; +, positive; −, negative.

included in the resection if necessary. For tumors with lateral extension, the tumor was dissected from the lateral nasopharyngeal wall and from the cartilage of the Eustachian tube. Three patients required postoperative radiotherapy because of positive margins. The 2-year disease-free survival rate for these 28 patients was 57.6% and the 2-year overall survival rate was 59.4%. On further analysis, none of the 12 patients with rT1 tumor had locoregional recurrence, but 2 developed distant metastasis. Seven of the 16 patients with rT2a tumor had local recurrence and 2 patients had distant metastasis. This finding gave the 2-year local disease-free survival rates of the 12 patients with rT1 tumor and 16 patients with rT2a tumor to be 100% and 41.7%, respectively ($P = .007$).

Rohaizam and colleagues[41] also reported on their series of endoscopic nasopharyngectomy in 6 patients with recurrent NPC. All cases were staged as rT1N0M0. The resection was achieved with negative margins. With a short follow-up of 3 to 14 months, there was no recurrence.

In Castelnuovo and colleagues[38] series, there were 8 cases of recurrent NPC (1 also had regional recurrence): 4 rT1 cases, 1 rT2a case, and 3 rT3 cases. The mean follow-up was 28 months (10–78 months). There were no recurrences for the rT1 and rT2 groups. For the remaining 3 rT3 cases, 1 was dead of disease, whereas the other 2 were alive with disease.

Chen and colleagues[42] published the first large series of endoscopic nasopharyngectomy on locally recurrent NPC. They operated on 37 patients with tumors involving the:

1. Nasopharyngeal cavity (rT1)
2. Postnaris or nasal septum (rT2a)
3. Superficial parapharyngeal space (rT2b)
4. Base wall of the sphenoid sinus (T3).

The rT2b tumors had only limited invasion into the superficial part of the parapharyngeal space. They were staged as T1N0M0 (n = 17), rT2aN0M0 (n = 4), rT2bN0M0 (n = 14), and rT3N0M0 (n = 2), respectively. Thirty-five cases had a radical en bloc resection with negative surgical margins. In the remaining 2 patients, tumors were resected piecemeal because they had invaded deeply into the parapharyngeal space. One of these 2 patients had positive surgical margins. No patients received postoperative radiotherapy, including the patient with positive margins because the patient refused radiotherapy. All nasopharyngeal wounds healed within 1 to 6 months. Those with a pedicled middle turbinate flap healed faster than those without a flap (median of 4 weeks compared with 12 weeks).

The follow-up ranged from 6 to 45 months (median 24 months). None of the 17-rT1 patients developed a local recurrence or distant metastases. One of the 4 patients with rT2a tumor developed a soft palate recurrence 13 months after surgery and died of local failure and distant metastases 37 months after surgery and salvage radiotherapy. Of the 14 rT2b patients, 4 developed local recurrence between 6 and 26 months after surgery. Another 2 died of other causes. Of the 2 rT3 patients, 1 developed distant metastases without local recurrence. The overall 2-year overall survival, local relapse-free survival, and progression-free survival rate were 84.2%, 86.3% and 82.6%, respectively.

DISCUSSION: MINIMALLY INVASIVE NASOPHARYNGECTOMY

These studies show that the current role for endoscopic nasopharyngectomy is limited to early recurrent disease (see **Table 1**). All published studies report good early results with rT1 disease (grade C). There is no consensus yet on the role of this technique for rT2 tumor. Chen and colleagues[32] reported good results with rT2a, whereas Ko and colleagues[40] cautioned against it. They attributed the lower success rate for rT2a tumors to larger tumors with involvement of the fossa of Rossenmuller or the cartilage of the auditory tube and the fact that with an endoscopic nasopharyngectomy, the dissection could not be carried far enough laterally to yield adequate margins. In Chen and colleagues[42] series, the number of rT2a cases is limited and a conclusion cannot be drawn. For rT2b cases, they reported local recurrence developing in 4 of 14 patients (28.6%).

The most important factor governing a good outcome for T2 disease appeared to be related to the ability to achieve a negative margin laterally within the parapharyngeal space. For T2a tumors, although the tumors had by definition not involved the parapharyngeal space, the lesion may have involved the Eustachian tube or superficial parapharyngeal space microscopically. Wei[43] showed in serial sections of resected nasopharyngeal specimens that the tumor involved the Eustachian tube cartilage in 90% of specimens. Vlantis and colleagues[44] recommended the amount of resection to always include the residual or recurrent tumor, tissue previously involved by the primary tumor, and the ipsilateral Eustachian tube cushion.

For T2b tumor, the involvement of the parapharyngeal space has been shown to be an important prognostic factor for local control.[35] In Hao and colleagues' review of 53 patients undergoing open nasopharyngectomy, the local control of rT2 was only 27.8%. Given the proximity of the ICA, lateral dissection in this space to achieve negative margins becomes risky because of potential injury to the artery. Too much dissection laterally also leaves little supporting tissue adjacent to the artery, which predisposes it to delayed rupture.[28] If the artery becomes denuded during dissection, covering the carotid artery with a tissue flap may be necessary and require conversion to an open approach. Chen and colleagues[42] recommended the distance between the tumor and the ICA to be more than 1 cm for it to be considered for endoscopic nasopharyngectomy. Less than that requires an open approach such as the maxillary swing or a Fisch approach, which provide direct exposure and protection to the ICA.[32,42]

Advanced rT stage is another important prognostic factor governing survival or local control.[21,36] Local control and overall survival in rT3/T4 patients are worse than rT1/T2 patients.[45] In view of the extent of the recurrence, reirradiation using IMRT with and without chemotherapy is usually considered first.[45,46] Current evidence from the endoscopic nasopharyngectomy series suggests a limited role for endoscopic techniques. Only 2 rT3 cases were reported in Chen and colleagues'[42] series. with 1 patient developing distant metastases. Both cases had erosion of the base of the sphenoid sinuses. For these patients, the investigators recommended that the distance between the tumor and the posterior wall of the sphenoid sinus be at least 0.5 cm to achieve clear margins. Of the 3 patients in Casetelnuovo and colleagues'[38] series, 2 were alive with disease, and 1 was dead of disease. It was not clear if this finding represented local recurrence or distant metastases. Chang and colleagues[26] showed good early local control rate for rT3 and rT4 lesions (those with limited skull base, dura, or brain involvement) and attributed this to the commonly used open craniofacial procedures. The increasing experience gained from performing endoscopic craniofacial resection for anterior skull base tumors may be extended to carefully selected rT3 tumors with limited skull base erosion. More data in the future will further define the role of endoscopic nasopharyngectomy in rT3 tumors.

Patients with rT4 generally fail locally or die because of development of metastatic disease. The areas involved by the tumor that lead to it being classified as a T4 (ie, extracranial vs intracranial) have an impact on prognosis.[11] Although surgical salvage of patients with significant intracranial recurrence may be futile, those with infratemporal fossa recurrences may be more amenable to surgery. These recurrences are usually extensive and require open surgical approaches such as facial translocation or subtemporal-preauricular infratemporal fossa approaches.[35] In Hao and colleagues' series, the 5-year local control rates and overall survival rates for rT4 are 75% and 46.9%, respectively. However, there are only 8 rT4 patients in their series of 53 patients, and the investigators attributed the good outcome to carefully selected patients. There is also no comparison with a similar group of patients receiving reirradiation.

The results from currently available publications on endoscopic nasopharyngectomy indicate that the procedure is safe and carries low morbidity and no treatment-related mortality. This situation can be attributed to the careful selection of only patients with early-stage recurrence for this procedure. Common complications include headache, otitis media with effusion secondary to Eustachian tube resection, flap necrosis, and osteoradionecrosis. Headache is a common complaint postoperatively and usually occurs while the wound is healing. Covering the wound with a mucosal graft may accelerate wound healing and reduce the duration of headache. Osteonecrosis from radiotherapy can lead to bleeding, cervical spine abscess, or osteomyelitis. These complications may require long-term antibiotics or even debridement. Apart from the milder complications, endoscopic surgery is associated with less intraoperative blood loss, shorter operating time, and shorter hospital stay.

The same contraindications for open surgery also apply to endoscopic nasopharyngectomy. These contraindications include carotid artery encasement, tumors with extensive parapharyngeal space or infratemporal fossa involvement, dural, brain or cavernous sinus involvement, or severe perineural infiltration.

NEW DEVELOPMENTS

A new development regarding minimally invasive techniques for access to the nasopharynx is the use of robotic-assisted surgery.[47,48] Ozer and Waltonen[47] first described the feasibility of a transoral robotic approach to the nasopharynx. By incising the soft palate and retracting it, they showed the feasibility of exposing the whole nasopharynx, including bilateral Eustachian tubes, fossa of Rosenmuller, the clivus, and the choana. In addition, they were able to localize and dissect the ICA. Wei and Ho[48] reported the first case of transoral robotic resection of recurrent NPC. By using the palate split together with the surgical robot, the whole nasopharynx could be visualized, and the tumor located over the lateral wall of the nasopharynx was resected en bloc with a cuff of the medial crus of the Eustachian tube. Advantages of this approach include a 3D visualization and the maneuverability of the robotic instruments that allowed ease of resection. The main disadvantage remained the need for a palatal incision.

SUMMARY

Endoscopic nasopharyngectomy is a safe and feasible procedure for treatment of rT1 and selected rT2a NPCs (grade C recommendation). There is less convincing evidence for rT2b and rT3 cases (grade C). It may have a role for those with limited involvement of the superficial portion of the parapharyngeal space (rT2b) and base of the sphenoid sinus (rT3). For more extensive rT3 and T4 recurrences, concurrent chemoirradiation should be considered first (grade B). There is currently little evidence to suggest that open or endoscopic surgery for rT4 helps improve disease-free survival in these patients. The short-term outcome for endoscopic nasopharyngectomy is encouraging, but data from a larger cohort of patients with a longer follow-up are warranted.

EBM Question	Author's Reply
What is role of endoscopic surgery for recurrent NPC?	Endoscopic nasopharynectomy is a safe and feasible procedure for treatment of (post-radiotherapy) rT1 and selected rT2a nasopharyngeal carcinomas (Grade C recommendation). There is less convincing evidence for rT2b and rT3 cases (Grade C).

REFERENCES

1. Yu MC, Yuan JM. Epidemiology of nasopharyngeal carcinoma. Semin Cancer Biol 2002;12:421–9.
2. Barnes L, Eveson JW, Reichart P, et al, editors. World Health Organization classification of tumors. Pathology and genetics of head and neck tumors. Lyon (France): IARC Press; 2005.
3. Au JS, Law CK, Foo W, et al. In-depth evaluation of the AJCC/UICC 1997 Staging system of nasopharyngeal carcinoma: prognostic homogeneity and proposed refinements. Int J Radiat Oncol Biol Phys 2003;56:413–26.
4. Lee AW, Sze WM, Au JS, et al. Treatment results for nasopharyngeal carcinoma in the modern era: the Hong Kong experience. Int J Radiat Oncol Biol Phys 2005; 61:1107–16.
5. Leung TW, Tung SY, Sze WK, et al. Treatment results of 1070 patients with nasopharyngeal carcinoma: an analysis of survival and failure patterns. Head Neck 2005;27:555–65.
6. Cheng SH, Yen KL, Jian JJ, et al. Examining prognostic factors and patterns of failure in nasopharyngeal carcinoma following concomitant radiotherapy and chemotherapy: impact on future clinical trials. Int J Radiat Oncol Biol Phys 2001; 50:717–26.
7. Yen RF, Hung RL, Pan MH, et al. 18-Fluoro-2-deoxyglucose positron emission tomography in detecting residual/recurrent nasopharyngeal carcinomas and comparison with magnetic resonance imaging. Cancer 2003;98:283–7.
8. Kao CH, Tsai SC, Wang JJ, et al. Comparing 18-fluoro-2-deoxyglucose positron emission tomography with a combination of technetium 99m tetrofosmin single photon emission computed tomography and computed tomography to detect recurrent or persistent nasopharyngeal carcinomas after radiotherapy. Cancer 2001;92:434–9.
9. Yu KH, Leung SF, Tung SY, et al. Survival outcome of patients with nasopharyngeal carcinoma with first local failure: a study by the Hong Kong Nasopharyngeal Study Group. Head Neck 2005;27:397–405.
10. Wei WI, Kwong DL. Current management strategy of nasopharyngeal carcinoma. Clin Exp Otorhinolaryngol 2010;3:1–12.
11. Suarez C, Rodrigo JP, Rinaldo A, et al. Current treatment options for recurrent nasopharyngeal cancer. Eur Arch Otorhinolaryngol 2010;267:1811–24.
12. Teo PM, Kwan WH, Chan AT, et al. How successful is high-dose (>60 Gy) reirradiation using mainly external beams in salvaging local failures of nasopharyngeal carcinoma? Int J Radiat Oncol Biol Phys 1998;40:897–913.

13. Leung TW, Tung SY, Sze WK, et al. Salvage radiation therapy for locally recurrent nasopharyngeal carcinoma. Int J Radiat Oncol Biol Phys 2000;48:1331–8.

14. Chua DT, Sham JS, Kwong DL, et al. Locally recurrent nasopharyngeal carcinoma: treatment results for patients with computed tomography assessment. Int J Radiat Oncol Biol Phys 1998;41:379–86.

15. Lee AW, Foo W, Law SC, et al. Reirradiation for recurrent nasopharyngeal carcinoma: factors affecting the therapeutic ratio and ways for improvement. Int J Radiat Oncol Biol Phys 1997;38:43–52.

16. Hao SP, Tsang NM. Surgical management of recurrent nasopharyngeal carcinoma. Chang Gung Med J 2010;33:361–9.

17. Wen YH, Wen WP, Chen HX, et al. Endoscopic nasopharyngectomy for salvage in nasopharyngeal carcinoma: a novel anatomic orientation. Laryngoscope 2010;120:1298–302.

18. King WW, Ku PK, Mok CO, et al. Nasopharyngectomy in the treatment of recurrent nasopharyngeal carcinoma: a twelve-year experience. Head Neck 2000;22:215–22.

19. Fee WE Jr, Moir MS, Choi EC, et al. Nasopharyngectomy for recurrent nasopharyngeal cancer: a 2- to 17-year follow-up. Arch Otolaryngol Head Neck Surg 2002;128:280–4.

20. Wei WI. Salvage surgery for recurrent primary nasopharyngeal carcinoma. Crit Rev Oncol Hematol 2000;33:91–8.

21. Hsu MM, Hong RL, Ting LL, et al. Factors affecting the overall survival after salvage surgery in patients with recurrent nasopharyngeal carcinoma at the primary site: experience with 60 cases. Arch Otolaryngol Head Neck Surg 2001;127:798–802.

22. Fee WE Jr, Gilmer PA, Goffinet DR, et al. Surgical management of recurrent nasopharyngeal carcinoma after radiation failure at the primary site. Laryngoscope 1988;98:1220–6.

23. Tu GY, Hu YH, Xu GZ, et al. Salvage surgery for nasopharyngeal carcinoma. Arch Otolaryngol Head Neck Surg 1988;114:328–9.

24. Wei WI, Lam KH, Sham JS. New approach to the nasopharynx: the maxillary swing approach. Head Neck 1991;13:200–7.

25. Morton RP, Liavaag PG, McLean M, et al. Transcervico-mandibulo-palatal approach for surgical salvage of recurrent nasopharyngeal cancer. Head Neck 1996;18:352–8.

26. Chang KP, Hao SP, Tsang NM, et al. Salvage surgery for locally recurrent nasopharyngeal carcinoma–a 10 year experience. Otolaryngol Head Neck Surg 2004;131:497–502.

27. Fisch U. The infratemporal fossa approach for nasopharyngeal tumors. Laryngoscope 1983;93:36–44.

28. Shu CH, Cheng H, Lirng JF, et al. Salvage surgery for recurrent nasopharyngeal carcinoma. Laryngoscope 2000;110:1483–8.

29. To EW, Teo PM, Ku PK, et al. Nasopharyngectomy for recurrent nasopharyngeal carcinoma: an innovative transnasal approach through a mid-face deglove incision with stereotactic navigation guidance. Br J Oral Maxillofac Surg 2001;39:55–62.

30. To EW, Yuen EH, Tsang WM, et al. The use of stereotactic navigation guidance in minimally invasive transnasal nasopharyngectomy: a comparison with the conventional open transfacial approach. Br J Radiol 2002;75:345–50.

31. Roh JL, Park CI. Transseptal laser resection of recurrent carcinoma confined to the nasopharynx. Laryngoscope 2006;116:839–41.

32. Chen MK, Lai JC, Chang CC, et al. Minimally invasive endoscopic nasopharyngectomy in the treatment of recurrent T1-2a nasopharyngeal carcinoma. Laryngoscope 2007;117:894–6.

33. Ong YK, Solares CA, Carrau RL, et al. New developments in transnasal endoscopic surgery for malignancies of the sinonasal tract and adjacent skull base. Curr Opin Otolaryngol Head Neck Surg 2010;18:107–13.

34. Vlantis AC, Tsang RK, Yu BK, et al. Nasopharyngectomy and surgical margin status: a survival analysis. Arch Otolaryngol Head Neck Surg 2007;133:1296–301.

35. Hao SP, Tsang NM, Chang KP, et al. Nasopharyngectomy for recurrent nasopharyngeal carcinoma: a review of 53 patients and prognostic factors. Acta Otolaryngol 2008;128:473–81.

36. To EW, Lai EC, Cheng JH, et al. Nasopharyngectomy for recurrent nasopharyngeal carcinoma: a review of 31 patients and prognostic factors. Laryngoscope 2002;112:1877–82.

37. Yoshizaki T, Wakaisaka N, Murono S, et al. Endoscopic nasopharyngectomy in the treatment of recurrent T1-2a nasopharyngeal carcinoma. Laryngoscope 2005;115:1517–9.

38. Castelnuovo P, Dallan I, Bignami M, et al. Nasopharyngeal endoscopic resection in the management of selected malignancies: ten-year experience. Rhinology 2010;48:84–9.

39. Al-Sheibani S, Zanation AM, Carrau RL, et al. Endoscopic endonasal transpterygoid nasopharyngectomy. Laryngoscope. In press.

40. Ko JY, Wang CP, Ting LL, et al. Endoscopic nasopharyngectomy with potassium-titanyl-phosphate (KTP) laser for early locally recurrent nasopharyngeal carcinoma. Head Neck 2009;10:1309–15.

41. Rohaizam J, Subramaniam SK, Vikneswaran T, et al. Endoscopic nasopharyngectomy: the Sarawak experience. Med J Malaysia 2009;64:213–5.

42. Chen MY, Wen WP, Guo X, et al. Endoscopic nasopharyngectomy for locally recurrent nasopharyngeal carcinoma. Laryngoscope 2009;119:516–22.

43. Wei WI. Nasopharyngeal cancer: current status of management. Arch Otolaryngol Head Neck Surg 2001;127:766–9.

44. Vlantis AC, Yu BK, Kam MK, et al. Nasopharyngectomy: does the approach to the nasopharynx influence survival? Otolaryngol Head Neck Surg 2008;139:40–6.

45. Smee RI, Meagher NS, Broadley K, et al. Recurrent nasopharyngeal carcinoma: current management approaches. Am J Clin Oncol 2010;33:469–73.

46. Wei WI, Kwong DL. Recurrent nasopharyngeal carcinoma: surgical salvage vs. additional chemoradiation. Curr Opin Otolaryngol Head Neck Surg 2011;19:82–6.

47. Ozer E, Waltonen J. Transoral robotic nasopharyngectomy: a novel approach for nasopharyngeal lesions. Laryngoscope 2008;118:1613–6.

48. Wei WI, Ho WK. Transoral robotic resection of recurrent nasopharyngeal carcinoma. Laryngoscope 2010;120:2011–4.

Skull Base Chordomas

Maria Koutourousiou, MD[a], Carl H. Snyderman, MD[a,b,*],
Juan Fernandez-Miranda, MD[a], Paul A. Gardner, MD[a]

KEYWORDS

- Chordoma • Clivus • Endonasal skull base surgery
- Endoscopic skull base surgery

EBM Question	Level of Evidence	Grade of Recommendation
Is gross total resection of skull base chordomas better facilitated with a midline endoscopic endonasal approach?	4	C

Skull base chordomas are slowly growing tumors that originate from the clivus, infiltrate local bone, and extend to adjacent soft tissues. Although they are considered low-grade malignancies, their behavior is more malignant because of the difficulty of total removal, the high recurrence rate, and occasional metastasis.

The aim of this article is to present the epidemiologic and pathophysiologic characteristics of skull base chordomas, outline their anatomic localization and possible extension, describe their clinical features and imaging characteristics, discuss management options, and determine the optimal treatment for these rare but aggressive tumors.

EPIDEMIOLOGY

Chordomas are extra-axial tumors that originate from the remnants of notochord.[1–3] Approximately 50% develop in the sacrococcygeal region, 35% in the spheno-occipital region, and 15% in vertebrae.[3–5] Skull base chordomas account for less

The authors have nothing to disclose.
[a] Department of Neurological Surgery, University of Pittsburgh School of Medicine, 200 Lothrop Street, PUH 400, Pittsburgh, PA 15213, USA
[b] Department of Otolaryngology, University of Pittsburgh School of Medicine, 200 Lothrop Street, EEI 500, Pittsburgh, PA 15213, USA
* Corresponding author. Department of Otolaryngology, University of Pittsburgh School of Medicine, 200 Lothrop Street, EEI 500, Pittsburgh, PA 15213.
E-mail address: snydermanch@upmc.edu

than 0.2% of all intracranial neoplasms.[1–3] The overall incidence of chordomas is 0.08 to 0.5 cases per 100,000 individuals per year, and their incidence at the skull base location is 1 case per 2,000,000 individuals per year.[3,6] The incidence of skull base chordomas is higher in younger-age patients, often appearing in the second to fifth decades.[2,5]

HISTOPATHOLOGY

Chordomas are generally whitish soft multilobulated masses with a fibrous pseudo-capsule occasionally filled by a mucoid substance (secondary to hemorrhage) or with hemorrhage, necrosis, calcifications, and fragments of bone.[7] Microscopically they are characterized by physaliphorous cells, which are translucent cells of different sizes rich in mucin and glycogen.[7]

Chordomas are low-grade malignancies with low metastatic potential, divided into 3 overlapping and sometimes coexisting histopathologic types: conventional (typical), chondroid, and dedifferentiated (atypical). Typical chordomas are the most common; chondroid chordomas appear to confer a better prognosis,[8–10] although many pathologists believe this variant is actually a low-grade chondrosarcoma.[11] The aggressive "dedifferentiated" variety accounts for only 5% of cases and is considered a high-grade neoplasm.[9,12]

Evident in the immunoprofile of chordoma cells is reactivity for low-molecular-weight cytokeratins 7, 8, 18, and 19 (simple epithelium), as well as high-molecular-weight cytokeratins 4, 5, and 6 (mucosal epithelia),[8,13] S-100 protein, vimentin, and epithelial membrane antigen.[9,14–16] Loss of heterozygosity (LOH) of chromosomes 1p, 9p, 10q, and 17p was reported in chordomas.[16–18] Although chordomas are usually sporadic, a few familiar cases have been described and the deletion of 1p36 was found to be the most frequent genetic abnormality, occurring in 85% of both sporadic and familiar chordomas.[19] LOH at 10q, 17p, and 9p was identified in 57%, 52%, and 21% of skull base chordomas, respectively, with LOH at 9p being associated with a shorter overall survival.[20]

SURGICAL ANATOMY

Skull base chordomas arise in bone but may grow to involve multiple areas of the cranial base, and occasionally erode into the intradural space to encompass neuro-vascular structures and compress the brainstem. The selection of an operative approach depends on the tumor location and the relationship to the internal carotid, vertebral, and basilar arteries, cavernous sinus, and brainstem.[21] In the sagittal plane the clivus, the site of origin of skull base chordomas, can be divided for the purpose of surgical planning into 3 regions[22]:

- Upper clivus: above the crossing point of the trigeminal nerve root over the clivus, including the dorsum sellae (**Fig. 1**A)
- Mid clivus: from the trigeminal root inferiorly to the level of the glossopharyngeal nerve root (see **Fig. 1**B)
- Lower clivus: from glossopharyngeal nerve to foramen magnum (see **Fig. 1**C).

The real extension of skull base chordomas can exceed the clival anatomy and extend ventrally, to the anterior cranial fossa, or caudally, involving the upper cervical spine (**Fig. 2**).

Of significant surgical importance is the potential extension of the tumor in the coronal plane to involve the petrosphenoclival junction, petrous apex, occipital condyle, and

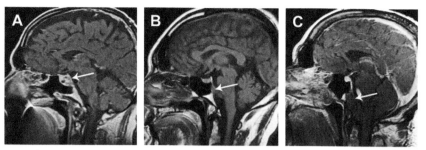

Fig. 1. (*A*) Sagittal T1-weighted magnetic resonance (MR) image with gadolinium (Gd) shows a mass involving the upper clivus/dorsum sellae (*arrow*). The chordoma extends into the pituitary fossa. The anterior stronger enhancement area represents the anteriorly displaced pituitary gland. (*B*) Sagittal T1-weighted MR image without Gd shows a mass in the region of the middle clivus (*arrow*). The tumor appears to emanate from the bone with projection into the prepontine cistern. It is inferiorly elongated and lies very close to the basilar artery. (*C*) Sagittal T1-weighted MR image with Gd demonstrates a mass of the lower clivus that extends down to the dens (*arrow*). It is an expansile destructive lesion, bulging and extending into the posterior fossa, where it abuts the cervicomedullary junction.

jugular foramen. For further lateralized tumors, the petrous ridge is divided into two areas:

- Medial area: medial to internal auditory canal (IAC) (**Fig. 3**A)
- Lateral area: lateral or posterior to the IAC (see **Fig. 3**B).

Most of the clival chordomas are completely extradural. However, some invade the outer layer of the dura mater, extend into the space between the outer and inner layers

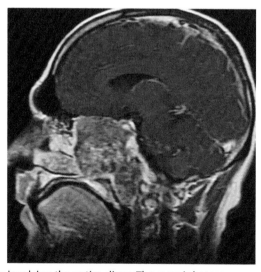

Fig. 2. A chordoma involving the entire clivus. The mass is heterogeneously hypointense on T1-weighted images and shows heterogeneous enhancement following contrast administration. Inferiorly, the mass destroys the anterior aspect of the clivus extending along the nasopharynx to the level of C1-C2. The chordoma extends anteriorly into the nasal cavity, and superiorly, remodels the planum sphenoidale and displaces the pituitary gland upward.

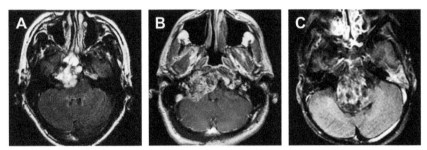

Fig. 3. (A) Axial T1-weighted MR image shows a large, lobulated mass centered on the right petroclival synchondrosis with heterogeneous signal. There is posterior extension with displacement of the posterior fossa and involvement of the right cerebellopontine angle. (B) Axial T1-weighted MR image demonstrates a larger clival chordoma extending more laterally compared with the previous image. The tumor extends into the cerebellopontine angle and beyond the internal auditory canal on the right with distortion of the cerebellum, lower pons, and medulla. (C) Axial T1-weighted MR image shows a large skull base chordoma with intradural extension that exerts severe mass effect on the pons and medulla. The fourth ventricle is narrowed, and displayed to the left and posteriorly. The basilar artery appears to be encased by the mass.

of the dura, or invade both layers of the dura and extend into the intradural space, resulting in direct brainstem compression (see **Fig. 3**C).[21]

CLINICAL PRESENTATION

Clinical presentation is related to tumor location and direct compression of the surrounding neural structures. Clival chordomas typically present with cranial neuropathies, most commonly visual deterioration (cranial nerve [CN] II) and CN III palsy with tumors confined to the upper clivus; diplopia (CN VI) with tumors of the mid clivus; and lower nerve palsies (CN IX, X, XII) when tumors involve the lower clivus.[6,21,23–25] Direct brainstem compression results in long tract dysfunction, and is accompanied by high morbidity and mortality. Headache due to direct dural invasion, trigeminal nerve compression, or increased intracranial pressure is another common complaint.

IMAGING FINDINGS

Both computed tomography (CT) and magnetic resonance (MR) imaging are required for the evaluation of skull base chordomas because of the bone involvement and the tumor proximity to critical soft-tissue structures.

The classic appearance of clival chordoma with high-resolution CT is that of a centrally located, well-circumscribed, expansile soft-tissue mass that arises from the clivus with associated extensive lytic bone destruction. Intratumoral calcifications usually represent bone destruction rather than dystrophic calcifications in the tumor itself (**Fig. 4**). However, the chondroid variant is more likely to demonstrate real intratumoral calcifications. There is moderate to marked enhancement following administration of iodinated contrast material.[26,27]

MR imaging is the single best modality for radiologic evaluation of skull base chordomas.[28] On conventional spin-echo T1-weighted MR images, chordoma has intermediate to low signal intensity and is easily recognized within the high signal intensity of the fat of the clivus. On T2-weighted images, chordoma has high signal

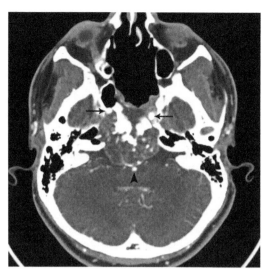

Fig. 4. High-resolution computed tomography following contrast administration demonstrates a heterogeneous enhancing, aggressive mass at the skull base. There is characteristic calcification and destruction of the clivus. The mass abuts both cavernous internal carotid arteries (ICAs) (*arrows*) and involves the right petrous apex. The mass indents the pons posteriorly and displaces the basilar artery (*arrowhead*).

intensity, a finding that likely reflects the high fluid content. The majority of chordomas demonstrate moderate to marked enhancement following contrast material injection (**Fig. 5**). The enhancement pattern of the tumor may have a "honeycomb" appearance.[29] Fat suppression is useful for differentiating enhanced tumor margins

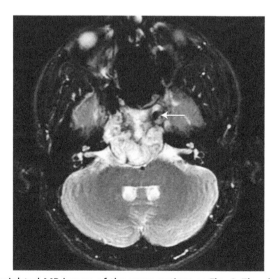

Fig. 5. Axial T2-weighted MR image of the same patient as **Fig. 4**. The chordoma is characteristically hyperintense to the brain. The intratumoral areas of calcification and a highly proteinaceous mucus pool give a heterogeneous appearance to the mass. The extension into the cavernous sinus bilaterally is more clearly demonstrated. The mass completely surrounds the left ICA (*arrow*). The basilar artery is compressed by the tumor.

from adjacent bright fatty bone marrow, and this technique is especially useful in detecting small intraclival chordomas. Chondroid chordomas may not be as bright as typical chordomas on T2-weighted images.[30] Also, T2-weighted imaging is excellent for differentiating tumor from adjacent neural structures.

Even though multiple synchronous tumors or drop metastases from an intracranial chordoma are very rare,[3] screening of the entire spine at the initial evaluation of a skull base chordoma patient should be considered.

MANAGEMENT

The therapeutic approach to skull base chordoma has traditionally relied on surgical resection. However, gross total resection (GTR) is not always possible because of the tumor extension, invasiveness, and proximity to critical structures. Radiation therapy has been demonstrated to be a valuable modality for local control in the postoperative setting, particularly with the advent of charged-particle radiotherapy and specifically with proton beam irradiation.[31–33] At present, the mainstay of therapy is surgical resection combined with high-dose radiation therapy.[10,31]

SURGICAL APPROACHES

In the absence of extenuating medical factors, the surgical goal should be a GTR with minimal morbidity.[10,21,34] The surgical approaches used are broadly classified as (1) anterior midline and (2) lateral approaches.[21,34] Anterior midline approaches consist of extended subfrontal, transmaxillary, transmandibular, transsphenoidal, endoscopic endonasal, transoral, and transcervical approaches.[25,35–39] Lateral open skull base approaches include frontotemporal transcavernous orbitozygomatic, anterior transpetrosal, preauricular infratemporal, combined supratentorial and infratentorial transtemporal, and extreme lateral transcondylar approaches.[40–44] Combined or staged surgeries are often necessary, depending on the size and anatomic distribution of the tumor.[21,23–25,34]

The following 4 transcranial approaches and the endoscopic endonasal approach (EEA) are the most frequently used, alone or in combination, for resection of skull base chordomas. For the purpose of this article the authors briefly outline the advantages and disadvantages of each of them, with emphasis on the advances of EEA, as it represents the most promising approach for total resection of skull base chordomas.

Extended Frontal Transbasal Approach

This approach is useful for midline tumors of the upper to lower clivus with extension into the sphenoethmoidal region, medial cavernous sinus (CS), petrous apex, occipital condyles, or foramen magnum.[39] The dorsum sella cannot be reached directly with this approach. Chordomas with extensive lateral components may not be totally resectable. The lateral limits of resection are the optic nerves, carotid arteries, CN VI, and CN XII. Accordingly, structures at highest risk of injury in this approach are the optic nerves, cavernous carotid artery, and CN VI.

Frontotemporal Transcavernous Approach

Combined with an orbitozygomatic osteotomy for better exposure, this approach provides excellent intradural access to the CS for chordomas extensively involving the CS. In combination with the subtemporal approach, it allows access to the upper clivus and petrous apex. It does not address any associated major bony involvement, so an auxiliary second approach may be needed to facilitate total tumor resection. Structures at highest risk of injury are the frontotemporal branch of CN VII, supraorbital nerves and vessels, and the optic nerves as well as CN III and IV during the resection of the clinoid. Large lacerations of the periorbita may result in muscle entrapment syndromes if not repaired.

Subtemporal and Subtemporal-Infratemporal Approach

The subtemporal approach provides access to the middle fossa, petrous apex, upper clivus, horizontal petrous internal carotid artery (ICA), and posterior CS. The subtemporal-infratemporal approach provides additional exposure of the clivus to the level of the foramen magnum, the CS, sphenoid, maxillary, and ethmoid sinuses, the infratemporal fossa, the retropharyngeal and parapharyngeal space, and the orbit. The latter approach is used when the petroclival bone is involved inferior to the level of the horizontal segment of the petrous ICA.[45] Cerebrospinal fluid (CSF) leak and associated meningitis are the most common complications of this approach. Almost all the CNs can be exposed and injured in the more extensive subtemporal-infratemporal approach. The ICA can also be injured during drilling. Mild trismus and malocclusion of the jaw may occur after distraction or resection of the condyle of mandible.

Extreme Lateral Transcondylar Approach

This approach is useful for chordomas involving the ventral upper cervical spine, lower clivus, foramen magnum, and occipital condyles.[43] For extradural resection of chordomas, the complete transcondylar approach is most commonly employed, which must be combined with an occipitocervical fusion to ensure stability of the occipitocervical junction. Lower CN dysfunction, CSF leak, and vascular injury to the vertebral artery or its branches, leading to brainstem or cerebellar infarction, are the most common complications of this approach.

Endoscopic Endonasal Approach

The binarial, purely endoscopic, 2-surgeon approach to the skull base has been described in detail.[46–54] For the purpose of a clival chordoma resection, image guidance and neurophysiological monitoring (monitoring of CNs in addition to brainstem-evoked responses and somatosensory evoked potentials) are substantial.[25] The vascularized nasoseptal flap[55–57] provides reconstruction of the skull base defect for tumors that extend beyond the margins of the clivus when dural penetration can be expected. The limitation of EEA is the extension of the tumor to anatomic areas that cannot be reached. However, the advent of endoscopic technologies and techniques (image guidance, angled endoscopes) has expanded the limits of conventional endoscopic approaches.[47–54,58] The EEA allows surgical access to the entire ventral skull base, from the frontal sinus to the second cervical vertebra in the sagittal plane, and from the midline to the roof of the orbit, the floor of the middle cranial fossa, and the jugular foramen in the coronal plane. Lateral extension of the chordoma at the level of the dorsum sella (upper clivus) requires a transposition of the pituitary gland superiorly with preservation of the pituitary stalk.[59] Lateral extension of the chordoma at the level of paraclival and petrous ICA (mid clivus) requires an endoscopic transpterygoid approach[60,61] with or without transposition of the vidian nerve.[62] Lateral extension of the tumor at the level of the lower clivus (from the foramen magnum across the occipital condyle and hypoglossal canal to the jugular foramen) requires an endoscopic medial maxillectomy with, if needed, a Denker maxillotomy and resection of the Eustachian tube.[54]

All of the CNs, but especially CN VI as it exits the Dorello canal and courses toward the CS, can be injured during EEA. The ICA or its branches can also be injured during drilling. EEAs for extreme lateral extended tumors that require manipulation of the ICA are considered the most difficult EEAs, as they demand incremental experience in managing the ICA endoscopically.[25] The potential complication of postoperative CSF leak can be avoided in most cases with the use of the vascularized nasoseptal flap.[55–57] Even in young patient populations, despite the smaller nares and nasal cavities, most patients older than 4 years are considered good candidates for EEA. A true limitation of EEA is the extension of tumor lateral to the optic nerves; in such cases, another approach is better considered.[58]

RADIATION THERAPY FOR CHORDOMAS

Postoperative radiotherapy can provide better control of the disease.[6,33] Chordomas respond best to high doses of radiation, in the range of 70 Gy. However, skull base chordomas represent a challenge for radiotherapy because nearby critical neural structures (optic apparatus, brainstem, and upper spinal cord) limit the doses that can be delivered.[63,64] Proton beam therapy appears to be more favorable than other irradiation techniques because it can deliver a higher dose to the tumor while sparing surrounding neural structures.[32,65] In a recent systematic review of the treatment of skull base chordomas with proton therapy and other irradiation techniques,[31] the average 5-year local control (LC) was 69.2% and the average 5-year overall survival (OS) was 79.8% after proton therapy. In comparison, the same study reported a 5-year LC and OS of 36% and 53.5%, respectively, after conventional radiotherapy; 50% and 82%, respectively, after stereotactic fractionated radiation therapy; and 56% and 75%, respectively, after radiosurgery. Although proton beam irradiation seems to extend the duration of survival and achieve better disease control in patients with residual chordoma, its effect on patients with no identifiable residual tumor is unclear.[21] No acute toxicity has been reported after proton beam therapy, while late toxicity is reported in a range of 8% to 17% and includes visual deficit, pituitary insufficiency, and radiation necrosis of the temporal lobe.[31] In both proton therapy and radiosurgery, a smaller tumor volume and an adequate distance from the brainstem and optic apparatus increases the likelihood of treatment success.[33,66] Conventional radiotherapy can still be considered for palliative management in advanced, unresectable, or multiple recurrent chordomas.[67]

RECURRENCE OF CHORDOMAS

Factors of importance in the recurrence of chordomas include the extent of resection, adjuvant radiation therapy, and histologic subtype.[10] According to individual surgical case series, tumor recurrence after total and near-total excision ranges from 16% to 45% at 10 years.[6,23,24,68] However, in a recent meta-analysis of patients treated for cranial chordomas,[10] the recurrence rate reached 68% with an average disease-free interval of 45 months (median, 23 months).

PROGNOSIS OF SKULL BASE CHORDOMAS

Patients' survival with skull base chordomas is generally considered to be poor,[3–5,69–71] with distant metastases that usually occur late during the natural history of the disease, mainly to the lungs, liver, and bones.

Age at onset of symptoms, previous surgery or radiotherapy, extent of resection, adjuvant radiotherapy, histopathological features of the tumor, and cytogenetic abnormalities are considered factors that influence the prognosis of patients with chordomas. According to a recent meta-analysis, younger patients, patients with chondroid histologic subtype of chordoma, and patients who have undergone surgery followed by adjuvant radiotherapy have a significantly lower recurrence rate than their respective counterparts.[10] Five-year survival varies from 52% to 90%[21,38] and when total tumor removal has been achieved, the 5-year survival climbs to greater than 80%.[6,21,24,68] The secondary surgery, after prior attempts at resection, is associated with a worse survival than that in patients who undergo only de novo surgery, and most investigators agree that the best outlook is associated with the greatest extent of tumor removal achieved during the first operation.[6,21,38]

SUMMARY: SKULL BASE CHORDOMAS

Skull base chordomas exhibit an insidious natural history and are difficult to eradicate. The combination of surgery and postoperative irradiation is the treatment of choice. Surgery is the mainstay of treatment, with the goal of total tumor resection. For unresectable chordomas, maximal tumor removal is desirable, as control rates with radiation improve when the residual tumor mass is small. The recurrence rate, even after complete resection, still remains high. Future molecular targeted therapies may be promising for the treatment of skull base chordomas.

EVIDENCE-BASED MEDICINE QUESTION: IS GROSS TOTAL RESECTION OF SKULL BASE CHORDOMAS BETTER FACILITATED WITH A MIDLINE ENDOSCOPIC ENDONASAL APPROACH?

The improvement of endoscopic technologies and techniques has expanded the indications of EEA. In this section, the authors present their personal experience in the management of skull base chordomas with 60 patients who underwent EEA (Koutourousiou M, Gardner PA, Tormenti MJ, et al. Endoscopic endonasal approach for resection of skull base chordomas: outcomes and learning curve. J Neurosurg 2011. Submitted for publication.). The outcomes are discussed in comparison with published surgical series that have employed other approaches.

Series Presentation

From April 2003 to March 2011, 60 patients with clival chordomas underwent EEA at the University of Pittsburgh Medical Center. The diagnosis was histologically confirmed in every case.

Sixty patients (70% male) with a median age of 41 years (range 4–84) underwent EEA for primary (n = 35) or recurrent (n = 25) skull base chordomas. In the group of primary tumors, total resection was achieved in 29 cases (82.9%), near total (>95% of tumor) in 4 (11.4%), and subtotal (>85%) in 2 (5.7%). With a mean follow-up of 17.8 months (range 1–71), 21 patients (60%) remain free of disease, 5 (14.3%) have stable or even decreased residual tumor after radiation therapy and are being closely monitored, and 9 (25.7%) showed tumor progression. Of the recurrences, 5 underwent reoperation, 3 are in close follow-up, and 1 died secondary to progression of disease. In the group of 25 patients that presented with recurrent chordomas, total resection was achieved in 11 (44%), near total in 5 (20%), subtotal in 4 (16%), and partial in 5 (20%). During the follow-up period, 10 (40%) of these patients are free of disease, 4 (16%) have stable residual tumor, and 11 (44%) showed recurrence with 9 being reoperated on. In total, 39 patients received adjuvant radiation therapy before (n = 14) or after surgery (n = 25). Surgical complications included 12 cases (20%) with CSF leakage, resulting in meningitis in 2 patients (3.3%). Carotid injuries occurred in 2 patients (3.3%), without any resulting deficit. One patient experienced quadriparesis and lower cranial neuropathies as a result of delayed pontine hemorrhage. New cranial neuropathies occurred postoperatively in 5 patients and remained unchanged in 4

Table 1
Resection rates and progress of disease in patients who underwent EEA for skull base chordomas during a mean follow-up period of 17.8 months

	GTR (%)	Near Total (%)	Subtotal (%)	Partial (%)	Free of Disease (%)	Stable Disease (%)	Progression of Disease (%)	Death from Disease (%)
Primary cases (n = 35)	82.9	11.4	5.7	0	60	14.3	25.7	2.8
Recurrent cases (n = 25)	44	20	16	20	40	16	44	20
Total (n = 60)	66.7	15	10	8.3	51.7	15	33.3	10

(6.7%). In total, the 60 patients underwent 101 surgical procedures. During the follow-up period 6 patients died, due to disease progression (**Table 1**).

Degree of Tumor Resection

Total tumor resection was the goal in every case, and was achieved in 66.7% of the patients. In patients with primary skull base chordomas, total resection was achieved in 82.9% and in recurrent cases in 44%.

Sen and colleagues,[21] in a study of 65 patients with clival chordomas, reported total tumor resection in 58%; 64% in primary and 48% in recurrent cases. In this study, both anterior midline and lateral approaches were employed, with similar results (62% total tumor resection with midline approaches, 57% with lateral approaches). However, the investigators, having used the EEA in some patients, have concluded that this technique is superior and less invasive, and therefore now prefer to use the EEA instead of the other anterior midline approaches.

Crockard and colleagues[6] have predominantly used anterior midline approaches in their 42 skull base chordomas. Their "radical" resection rate is more than 70%. However, they define "radical" as greater than 90% resection. The authors must exclude this series from any comparison, and remain strict in the definition of total resection to achieve comparable results.

Among publications from surgeons who preferred lateral approaches for skull base chordomas, the degree of total tumor resection varies. Colli and Al-Mefty[24] report total resection in 45.3% of the 53 patients with cranial chordomas; 44.1% in primary and 31.6% in recurrent cases. Gay and colleagues[23] managed total tumor resection in 47% of their 46 cranial chordoma patients. On the other hand, Tzortzidis and colleagues[68] reported total tumor resection in 71.6% of their 74 patients; total resection in primary cases was 83% and in recurrent cases 30%.

The comparison of the surgical series shows that EEA is superior to most of the approaches used in achieving total tumor resection. The selection of lateral or midline approach reflects differences in tumor location and the surgeon's preference. The tumor lateralization is not a limitation for EEA in most of the cases. Recent advances in endoscopic techniques have increased significantly the extent of exposure and have expanded the use of EEA for tumors that were considered unresectable a few years ago (**Fig. 6**). The surgeon's preference is a result of his or her training and experience. It is true that the long learning curve is one of the disadvantages of EEA.

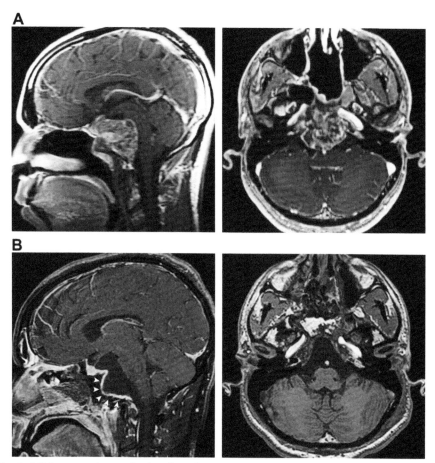

Fig. 6. (*A*) Preoperative sagittal and axial T1-weighted MR images. A large heterogeneous enhancing mass is located within the clivus and completely replaces the normal fat signal within the clivus. The mass extends into the suprasellar cistern and is retrochiasmatic. It also extends posteriorly and causes mass effect on the pons, and extends into both petrous apices. It surrounds the basilar artery and extends into both cavernous sinuses. It completely surrounds the left ICA. The mass extends inferiorly to the bottom of the occiput. (*B*) Postoperative sagittal and axial T1-weighted MR images demonstrate a complete resection of the tumor. There appears to be intrinsic decompression of the components of pons and decompression of the basilar artery, as well as decompression of components of the suprasellar cistern and optic system. Note mucosal enhancement of the septal flap reconstruction.

Table 2 summarizes the GTR rates achieved by different approaches and the main surgical complications.

Surgical Complications

The most common complications after surgery for skull base chordomas are CSF leakage and new cranial neuropathies. Although clival chordomas are primarily extradural tumors, the dura may be violated either by the tumor itself or by the surgical technique, resulting in an increased risk of CSF leak postoperative. Therefore, it is important to reconstruct the skull base defect primarily. CSF leak after EEA occurred

Table 2
Comparison of GTR and complications after surgery for skull base chordomas with different approaches

	No. of Patients	Preferred Approach	Overall GTR (%)	GTR in Primary Tumor (%)	GTR in Recurrent Tumor (%)	CSF Leak (%)	Meningitis (%)	New CN Deficit (%)	Operative Mortality (%)
UPMC	60	EEA	66.7	82.9	44	20	3.3	6.7	0
Sen et al[21]	65	Lateral & midline (EEA)	58	64	48	21.5	10.8	N/A	N/A
Colli and Al-Mefty[24]	53	Lateral	45.3	44.1	31.6	12.2	1.9	20.6	1.9
Gay et al[23]	46	Lateral	47	N/A	N/A	30	10	80	5
Tzortzidis et al[68]	74	Lateral	71.6	83	30	1.35	N/A	4	2.7
Crockard et al[6]	42	Midline (transoral)	4.7	4.1	5.5	21	8	11.9	4.3

Abbreviations: N/A, data not available; UPMC, University of Pittsburgh Medical Center.

in 20% of the authors' patients. However, this rate has decreased significantly in recent years after the evolution of the vascularized nasoseptal flap. New cranial neuropathies developed in 5 patients and remained unchanged in 4 (6.6%).

Postoperative CSF leak rate was 21% in the series of Crockard and colleagues[6] and 21.5% in that of Sen and colleagues,[21] similar to the authors' results.

Gay and colleagues[23] reported CSF leak in 30% of their patients and new CN deficits in 80%. Colli and Al-Mefty[24] noted CSF leak in 12.2%, but the incidence of permanent CN deficits was 20.6%. The increase in cranial neuropathies in lateral approaches is expected because working through spaces between CNs increases the likelihood of manipulation of the nerves and functional impairment postoperatively. However, Tzortzidis and colleagues,[68] using mainly lateral approaches, reported the remarkably low CSF leak rate of 1.3% and new CN deficit rate of 4%.

More severe complications have been reported, including hemiparesis, monoparesis, and cerebral and brainstem infraction leading to severe functional deterioration and poor survival results, and have been usually associated with aggressive or recurrent chordomas.[21,23,24,68] Besides one patient who developed delayed pontine hemorrhage resulting in quadriparesis, the authors experienced no major complications. The carotid injuries that occurred in 2 patients during EEA were managed without any resulting deficit.

Summary: Level of Evidence

The degree of tumor resection has proved to be the only independent factor for tumor recurrence and the strongest determinant of survival. Recent technological advancements have expanded the indications of EEA, allowing surgical access to the entire ventral skull base and better facilitating the goal of total tumor removal. Anterior approaches, as compared with lateral approaches, lead to better postoperative CN function, and this is especially true for the EEA given the excellent visualization offered by the endoscope along with the use of intraoperative image guidance and neuromonitoring. In addition, rapid recovery and decreased hospitalization improves patients' outcomes. Ultimately, the EEA tends to allow for less morbid procedures and more extensive tumor resection.

However, all of the authors' results are based on individual case series, level 4b evidence. Much of the data regarding outcomes following treatment has been reported by small case series and case reports that lack statistical power to derive significant conclusions about appropriate management of these tumors. Given the rarity of skull base chordomas, it would be difficult to develop randomized studies that could prove the superiority of EEA over other approaches in the treatment of skull base chordomas. Uniform reporting of data and pooling of data from multiple institutions will be necessary to answer these questions.

EBM Question	Author's Reply
Are oncological outcomes the same with EES compared to open craniofacial surgery?	The comparison of the surgical series shows that EEA is superior to most of the approaches used in achieving total tumor resection. Disease free survival for primary cases (60%, overall survival 97.2%) and all cases (51.7%, overall survival 80%) compares favourably to other approaches (Grade c)

REFERENCES

1. Burger PC, Scheithauer BW, Vogel SF. Surgical pathology of the nervous system and its coverings. 3rd edition. New York: Churchill Livingstone; 1991. p. 503–36.

2. Huvos AG. Bone tumors. diagnosis, treatment, and prognosis. 2nd edition. Philadelphia: WB Saunders Co; 1991. p. 599–616.

3. McMaster ML, Goldstein AM, Bromley CM, et al. Chordomas: incidence and survival patterns in the United States, 1973–1995. Cancer Causes Control 2001;12:1–11.

4. Dahlin DC, MacCarty CS. Chordoma: a study of 59 cases. Cancer 1952;5: 1170–8.

5. Higinbotham NL, Phillips RF, Farr HW, et al. Chordoma. Thirty-five-year study at Memorial Hospital. Cancer 1967;20:1841–50.

6. Crockard HA, Steel T, Plowman N, et al. A multidisciplinary approach to skull base chordomas. J Neurosurg 2001;95:175–83.

7. Batsakis JG. Tumors of the head and neck. Baltimore (MD): Williams and Wilkins; 1979.

8. Mitchell A, Scheithauer BW, Unni KK, et al. Chordoma and chondroid neoplasms of the spheno-occiput. An immunohistochemical study of 41 cases with prognostic and nosologic implications. Cancer 1993;72:2943–9.

9. Hoch BL, Nielsen GP, Liebsch NJ, et al. Base of skull chordoma in children and adolescents: a clinicopathologic study of 73 cases. Am J Surg Pathol 2006;30: 811–8.

10. Jian BJ, Bloch OG, Yang I, et al. Adjuvant radiation therapy and chondroid chordoma subtype are associated with a lower tumor recurrence rate of cranial chordoma. J Neurooncol 2010;98:101–8.

11. Brooks JJ, LiVolsi VA, Trojanowski JQ. Do chondroid chordomas exist? Acta Neuropathol (Berl) 1987;72:229–35.

12. Barnes L. The biology and pathology of selected skull base tumors. J Neurooncol 1994;20:213–40.

13. Heikinheimo K, Persson S, Kindblom LG, et al. Expression of different cytokeratin subclasses in human chordoma. J Pathol 1991;164:145–50.

14. Coindre JM, Rivel J, Trogiani M, et al. Immunohistological study in chordomas. J Pathol 1986;150:61–3.

15. Abenoza P, Sibley RK. Chordoma: an immunohistologic study. Hum Pathol 1986; 17:744–7.

16. Larizza L, Mortini P, Riva P. Update on the cytogenetics and molecular genetics of chordoma. Hered Cancer Clin Pract 2005;3:29–41.

17. Dalpra L, Malgara R, Miozzo M, et al. First cytogenetic study of a recurrent familiar chordoma of the clivus. Int J Cancer 1999;81:24–30.

18. Riva P, Crosti F, Orzan F, et al. Mapping of candidate region for chordoma development to 1p36.13 by LOH analysis. Int J Cancer 2003;107:493–7.

19. Longoni M, Orzan F, Stroppi M, et al. Evaluation of 1p36 markers and clinical outcome in a skull base chordoma study. Neuro Oncol 2008;10:52–60.

20. Horbinski C, Oakley GJ, Cieply K, et al. The prognostic value of Ki-67, p53, epidermal growth factor receptor, 1p36, 92.21, 10q23, and 17p13 in skull base chordomas. Arch Pathol Lab Med 2010;134:1170–6.

21. Sen C, Triana AI, Berglind N, et al. Clival chordomas: clinical management, results, and complications in 71 patients. J Neurosurg 2010;113:1059–71.

22. Sekhar LN, Raso J, Schessel DA. The presigmoid petrosal approach. In: Sekhar LN, Oliveira ED, editors. Cranial microsurgery: approaches and techniques. New York: Thieme; 1999. p. 432–63.

23. Gay E, Sekhar LN, Rubinstein E, et al. Chordomas and chondrosarcomas of the cranial base: results and follow up of 60 patients. Neurosurgery 1995;36: 887–97.

24. Colli B, Al-Mefty O. Chordomas of the craniocervical junction: follow up review and prognostic factors. J Neurosurg 2001;95:933–43.
25. Stippler M, Gardner PA, Snyderman CH, et al. Endoscopic endonasal approach for clival chordomas. Neurosurgery 2009;64:268–77.
26. Meyer JE, Oot RF, Lindorfs KK. CT appearance of clival chordomas. J Comput Assist Tomogr 1986;10:34–8.
27. Whelan MA, Reede DL, Meisler W, et al. CT of the base of the skull. Radiol Clin North Am 1984;22:177–217.
28. Larson TC, Houser W, Laws ER. Imaging of cranial chordomas. Mayo Clin Proc 1987;62:886–93.
29. Doucet V, Peretti-Viton P, Figarella-Branger D, et al. MRI of intracranial chordomas: extent of tumour and contrast enhancement—criteria for differential diagnosis. Neuroradiology 1997;39:571–6.
30. Sze G, Uichanco LS III, Brant-Zawadzki MN, et al. Chordomas: MR imaging. Radiology 1988;166:187–91.
31. Amichetti M, Cianchetti M, Amelio D, et al. Proton therapy in chordoma of the base of the skull: a systematic review. Neurosurg Rev 2009;32:403–16.
32. Munzenrider JE, Liebsch NJ. Proton therapy for tumors of the skull base. Strahlenther Onkol 1999;175(Suppl 2):57–63.
33. Hug EB, Loredo LN, Slater JD, et al. Proton radiation therapy for chordomas and chondrosarcoma of the skull base. J Neurosurg 1999;91:432–9.
34. Rostomily RC, Sekhar LN, Elahi F. Chordomas and chondrosarcomas. In: Sekhar LN, Fessler RG, editors. Atlas of neurosurgical techniques. New York: Thieme Medical Publishers, Inc; 2006. p. 778–810.
35. Delgado TE, Garrido E, Harwick RD. Labiomandibular transoral approach to chordomas in the clivus and the upper cervical spine. Neurosurgery 1981;8: 675–9.
36. DeMonte F, Diaz E Jr, Callender D, et al. Transmandibular circumglossal retropharyngeal approach for chordomas of the clivus and upper cervical spine. Technical note. Neurosurg Focus 2001;10(3):E10.
37. Couldwell WT, Weiss MH, Rabb C, et al. Variations on the standard transsphenoidal approach to the sellar region, with emphasis on the extended approaches and parasellar approaches: surgical experience in 105 cases. Neurosurgery 2004;55:539–47.
38. Choi D, Melcher R, Harms J, et al. Outcome of 132 operations in 97 patients with chordomas of the craniocervical junction and upper cervical spine. Neurosurgery 2010;66(1):59–65.
39. Sekhar LN, Nanda A, Sen CN, et al. The extended frontal approach to tumors of the anterior, middle and posterior skull base. J Neurosurg 1992;76: 198–206.
40. Margalit NS, Lesser JB, Singer M, et al. Lateral approach to anterolateral tumors at the foramen magnum: factors determining surgical procedure. Neurosurgery 2005;56(Suppl 2):ONS324–36.
41. Salas E, Sekhar LN, Ziyal IM, et al. Variations of the extreme-lateral craniocervical approach: anatomical study and clinical analysis of 69 patients. J Neurosurg 1999;90(Suppl 2):206–19.
42. Sekhar LN, Schramm VL, Jones NF. Subtemporal-preauricular infratemporal fossa approach to large lateral and posterior cranial base neoplasms. J Neurosurg 1987;67:488–99.
43. Sen CN, Sekhar LN. An extreme lateral approach to intradural lesions of the cervical spine and foramen magnum. Neurosurgery 1990;27:197–204.

44. Sen CN, Sekhar LN. The subtemporal and preauricular infratemporal approach to intradural structures ventral to the brain stem. J Neurosurg 1990;73:345–54.

45. Cass SP, Sekhar LN, Pomeranz S, et al. Excision of petroclival tumors by a total petrosectomy approach. Am J Otol 1994;15:474–84.

46. Carrau R, Kassam A, Snyderman C, et al. Endoscopic transnasal anterior skull base resection for the management of sinonasal malignancies. Op Tech Otolaryngol 2006;17:102–10.

47. Kassam A, Carrau RL, Snyderman CH, et al. Evolution of reconstructive techniques following endoscopic expanded endonasal approaches. Neurosurg Focus 2005;19:E8.

48. Kassam AB, Gardner P, Snyderman C, et al. Expanded endonasal approach: fully endoscopic, completely transnasal approach to the middle third of the clivus, petrous bone, middle cranial fossa, and infratemporal fossa. Neurosurg Focus 2005;19:E6.

49. Kassam AB, Mintz AH, Gardner PA, et al. The expanded endonasal approach for an endoscopic transnasal clipping and aneurysmorrhaphy of a large vertebral artery aneurysm: technical case report. Neurosurgery 2006;59(Suppl 1):ONS162–5.

50. Kassam A, Snyderman C, Carrau R, et al. Endoscopic, expanded endonasal approach to the jugular foramen. Op Tech Neurosurg 2005;8:35–41.

51. Kassam A, Snyderman CH, Carrau RL, et al. Endoneurosurgical hemostasis techniques: lessons learned from 400 cases. Neurosurg Focus 2005;19:E7.

52. Kassam AB, Snyderman C, Gardner P, et al. The expanded endonasal approach: a fully endoscopic transnasal approach and resection of the odontoid process: technical case report. Neurosurgery 2005;57:E213.

53. Kassam A, Snyderman CH, Mintz A, et al. Expanded endonasal approach: the rostrocaudal axis. Part I. Crista galli to the sella turcica. Neurosurg Focus 2005; 19:E3.

54. Kassam A, Snyderman CH, Mintz A, et al. Expanded endonasal approach: the rostrocaudal axis. Part II. Posterior clinoids to the foramen magnum. Neurosurg Focus 2005;19:E4.

55. Hadad G, Bassagasteguy L, Carrau RL, et al. A novel reconstructive technique after endoscopic expanded endonasal approaches: vascular pedicle nasoseptal flap. Laryngoscope 2006;116:1882–6.

56. Kassam AB, Thomas A, Carrau RL, et al. Endoscopic reconstruction of the cranial base using a pedicled nasoseptal flap. Neurosurgery 2008;63(Suppl 1): ONS44–53.

57. Zanation AM, Carrau RL, Snyderman CH, et al. Nasoseptal flap reconstruction of high flow intraoperative cerebral spinal fluid leaks during endoscopic skull base surgery. Am J Rhinol Allergy 2009;23:518–21.

58. Snyderman CH, Pant H, Carrau RL, et al. What are the limits of endoscopic sinus surgery?: the expanded endonasal approach to the skull base. Keio J Med 2009; 58:152–60.

59. Kassam AB, Prevedello DM, Thomas A, et al. Endoscopic endonasal pituitary transposition for a transdorsum sellae approach to the interpeduncular cistern. Neurosurgery 2008;62(Suppl 1):ONS57–74.

60. Kassam AB, Vescan AD, Carrau RL, et al. Expanded endonasal approach: vidian canal as a landmark to the petrous internal carotid artery. J Neurosurg 2008;108: 177–83.

61. Fortes FS, Sennes LU, Carrau RL, et al. Endoscopic anatomy of the pterygopalatine fossa and the transpterygoid approach: development of a surgical instruction model. Laryngoscope 2008;118:44–9.

62. Prevedello DM, Pinheiro-Neto CD, Fernandez-Miranda JC, et al. Vidian nerve transposition for endoscopic endonasal middle fossa approaches. Neurosurgery 2010;67(2 Suppl Operative):478–84.
63. Tai PT, Craighead P, Bagdon F. Optimization of radiotherapy for patients with cranial chordoma. A review of dose-response ratios for photon techniques. Cancer 1995;75:749–56.
64. Mendenhall WM, Mendenhall CM, Lewis SB, et al. Skull base chordoma. Head Neck 2005;27:159–65.
65. Suit HD, Goitein M, Munzenrider J, et al. Definitive radiation therapy for chordoma and chondrosarcoma of base of skull and cervical spine. J Neurosurg 1982;56: 377–85.
66. Debus J, Hug EB, Liebsch NJ, et al. Brainstem tolerance to conformal radiotherapy of skull base tumors. Int J Radiat Oncol Biol Phys 1997;39:967–75.
67. Catton C, O'Sullivan B, Bell R, et al. Chordoma: long-term follow-up after radical photon irradiation. Radiother Oncol 1996;41:67–72.
68. Tzortzidis F, Elahi F, Wright D, et al. Patient outcome at long term follow up after aggressive microsurgical resection of cranial base chordomas. Neurosurgery 2006;59:230–7.
69. Eriksson B, Gunterberg B, Kindblom LG. Chordomas: a clinicopathologic and prognostic study of a Swedish National Series. Acta Orthop Scand 1981;52: 49–58.
70. Forsyth PA, Cascino TL, Shaw EG, et al. Intracranial chordomas: a clinicopathological and prognostic study of 51 cases. J Neurosurg 1993;78:741–7.
71. O'Neill P, Bell BA, Miller JD, et al. Fifty years of experience with chordomas in southeast Scotland. Neurosurgery 1985;16:166–70.

Proton Beam Therapy in Skull Base Pathology

Michelle Alonso-Basanta, MD, PhD[a],*, Robert A. Lustig, MD[a],
David W. Kennedy, MD[b]

KEYWORDS

• Chordoma • Proton therapy • Photon therapy • Skull base

EBM Question	Level of Evidence	Grade of Recommendation
Is proton beam therapy superior to other radiation techniques in patients with chordoma?	4	C

Chordomas are rare tumors with an incidence of less than 0.1 per 100,000 per year.[1,2] Originating from the remnant of embryonal notochord, such lesions can occur along the spinal axis, including the base of skull.[3] Optimal treatment consists of maximal surgical resection followed by local radiation therapy. Given the increased experience with endoscopic skull-based techniques; improved instrumentation; and, when necessary, the use of arterially based mucosal flaps for cerebrospinal fluid leak closure,[4] the ability to approach resections of these lesions has significantly improved. However, obtaining a complete surgical resection, given the anatomic constraints and infiltrative nature of the lesion, is challenging in this region. Accordingly, the role of radiation therapy in this location is ever important. Data have shown an increase in local control and survival with the use of proton therapy, although several radiation techniques have been used to improve local control. Although the senior surgeon (D.W.K) has had a patient with a 19-year disease-free period after combined endoscopic resection and proton therapy, the question arises whether, in the era of more modern techniques, the additional cost of proton therapy is validated by outcomes.

The authors have nothing to disclose.
[a] Department of Radiation Oncology, Perelman School of Medicine, University of Pennsylvania, Philadelphia, PA, USA
[b] Department of Otorhinolaryngology: Head and Neck Surgery, Perelman School of Medicine, University of Pennsylvania, Philadelphia, PA, USA
* Corresponding author. Department of Radiation Oncology, University of Pennsylvania Health System, 3400 Civic Center Boulevard, TRC-2 West, Philadelphia, PA 19104.
E-mail address: michelleab@uphs.upenn.edu

Radiation therapy can be delivered with several techniques. Most therapies use photons. The dose distribution of photons enters the body, delivers the dose, and then has a long tail dose (**Fig. 1**). In the era of intensity-modulated radiation therapy (IMRT), the dose distribution of photons remained the same; however, technology in the linear accelerator allowed modulation of the photon beam. This modulation allowed better conformality (shaping of the dose to the tumor) around critical structures by using several beams or angles to deliver dose. However, this technology came at a price because the integral dose received by the body was greater than that in the 3-dimensional (3D) era.

Stereotactic radiation (photon) therapy involves immobilization and image guidance to decrease treatment margins and better spare normal tissue, all while delivering high doses in 1 to 5 treatment fractions. There are several delivery systems available, including the Gamma Knife (Elekta, Sweden) and the CyberKnife (Accuray, Sunnyvale, CA, USA). Given the increased number of beam angles available, conformality was greater with this technique, allowing delivery of high doses of radiation.

Proton beam therapy is a particle beam therapy that has a different dosimetric distribution of dose (see **Fig. 1**). Although the photon beam has a tail that delivers dose past the tumor target, the beam has a sharp steep falloff with no dose to tissues past the range of tumor. Theoretically, this falloff allows for delivery of high doses, yet allows sparing of tissue beyond the tumor. In the skull base, this feature is critical, given the critical structures at risk after treatment. The critical structures at risk include the optic nerves, optic chiasm, cranial nerves, cochlea, brainstem, pituitary gland, and temporal lobes. The goal of radiation therapy is to deliver high enough doses to the tumor while maintaining low dose to critical structures. The close proximity of the tumor to critical structures at the skull base makes this location one of the most difficult to treat.

Because of the significant potential advantages of proton therapy, the University of Pennsylvania elected to invest in a proton facility (the Roberts Proton Therapy Center,

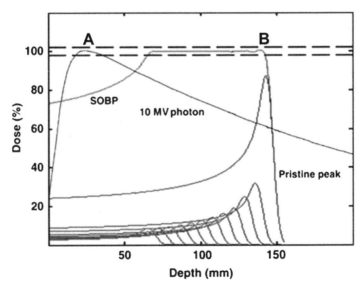

Fig. 1. Relative contribution of a photon x-ray (A) and the spread out Bragg peak for protons (B). (*Data from* available at: www.wikipedia.com. Accessed August 1, 2011.)

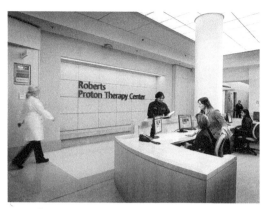

Fig. 2. Main hallway at the Roberts Proton Therapy Center. (*Courtesy of* Scott Nibauer, Philadelphia, PA.)

Figs. 2 and 3). Such technology does not come cheaply, with a total investment of approximately $250 million ($140 million for the proton component and $110 million for the remaining radiation equipment, software, and facility). The cyclotron required to produce the proton beam weighs more than 250 metric ton, and, when combined with the system required to distribute the beam to the gantries; this occupies an area the size of a football field and is surrounded by 17 ft of shielding concrete. However, because proton therapy is frequently combined with conventional photon therapy, the Penn facility was designed with a unique advantage of having both modalities on the same site (**Fig. 4**).

Early treatment of chordomas (1950–1980) with radiation therapy included photon radiation therapy delivered at a total dose of 55 Gy using conventional 2-dimensional techniques.[5] In this early report, 25 patients treated had a freedom from progression of 32 months with an overall survival at 5 and 10 years of 44% and 17%, respectively. At Princess Margaret Hospital, the median survival was 62 months, with a pain response of 85% and a neurologic response of 45%.[6] The median time to progression was 35 months, and, when the investigators examined the role of hypofractionated regimens, they found no benefit. The importance of a maximal safe resection was documented in a study from the Mallinckrodt Institute of 21 patients with chordoma. Although

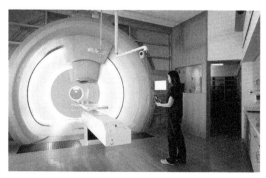

Fig. 3. Proton gantry room at the Roberts Proton Therapy Center. (*Courtesy of* Scott Nibauer, Philadelphia, PA.)

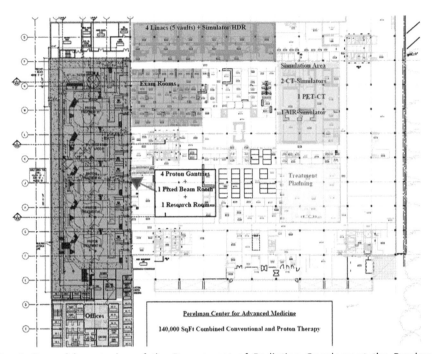

Fig. 4. General layout plan of the Department of Radiation Oncology at the Perelman Center for Advanced Medicine including the Roberts Proton Therapy Center. (*Courtesy of* Stephen M. Hahn, MD, Philadelphia, PA.)

disease-free survival was not different among the groups reviewed, those with surgery alone compared with those with biopsy and radiation therapy had an improvement in the 10-year survival.[7] The Mayo Clinic reviewed the role of postoperative radiation therapy after various surgical modalities and found an increase in disease-free survival and an increase in overall survival dependent on the extent of surgical resection (55% resection vs 36% for biopsy only).[8] Multivariate analysis showed that younger age and diplopia were prognostic of longer survival.

Given the poor outcomes with photon therapy alone in the 1960s and 1970s, proton therapy was evaluated, with the first proton references in the literature regarding treating primary brain tumors appearing in the 1960s in murine models.[9–11] Early work was done in skull base tumors,[12,13] in which the benefit of proton therapy was best seen in chordomas and chondrosarcomas of the base of skull. Reports in 1982 showed that treatment of 10 patients with doses of 76 cobalt Gray equivalent (CGE) were feasible without significant morbidity.[14] Massachusetts General Hospital (MGH) reported on the use of fractionated proton radiation therapy in 1989 in 68 patients who received postoperative radiation therapy at a median dose of 69 CGE, with a 5-year actuarial local control rate of 82% and disease-free survival of 76%.[15] Some temporal lobe damage was reported by the same institution in 1998 in a study of 96 patients with chordomas and chondrosarcomas of the base of skull.[16] All patients were treated with either 66.6 or 72 CGE with conventional fractionation. Ten patients developed temporal lobe damage with a cumulative damage incidence of 13.2% at 5 years. Despite the different temporal lobe damage rates related to age, tumor volume, number of surgical procedures before radiation therapy, and prescribed doses to the tumor, only gender was a significant predictor of damage ($P = .0155$) using a univariate (log-rank) test. In a stepwise Cox regression that included gender as a variable, no other baseline variable improved the prediction of damage.

A review of cases at MGH published in 1999 showed a 10-year local control rate of combined proton-photon therapy that was highest for chondrosarcomas, intermediate for chordomas in men, and lowest for chordomas in women (94%, 65%, and 42%, respectively).[17] A similar review at the Loma Linda University Medical Center in 58 patients with skull base chordomas and chondrosarcomas treated with total doses between 64.8 and 79.2 CGE showed local control rates of 92% for chondrosarcoma and 76% for chordomas.[18] Actuarial 5-year survival rates were 100% for patients with chondrosarcoma and 79% for patients with chordoma. Grade 3 and 4 late toxicities (those requiring increased medical intervention or hospital admission, **Table 1**) were observed in 4 patients (7%) and were symptomatic in 3 patients (5%).

The Centre de Protontherapie D'Orsay France treated 45 patients with a median total dose delivered within the gross tumor volume of 67 CGE (range, 60–70 CGE).[19] With a mean follow-up of 30.5 months, the 3-year local control rates for chordomas and chondrosarcomas were 83.1% and 90%, respectively, and 3-year overall survival rates were 91% and 90%, respectively. Young age at the time of radiotherapy influenced local control positively ($P<.03$) in univariate analysis but not in multivariate analysis. Only 2 patients presented grade 3 or 4 complications. A further review of 67 patients (including some cervical spine) treated showed 3-year local control rates of 71% and 85% for chordomas and chondrosarcomas, respectively, and 3-year overall survival rates of 88% and 75%, respectively.[20] Once again, on multivariate analysis, only age was an independent prognostic factor of local control.

Although promising, given the limited availability of protons and the inability of many patients to travel long distances, there is clearly a need to consider other radiation options. In the 1980s, there were series published examining the role of brachytherapy in the treatment of chordomas. In patients requiring reirradiation, iodine 125 was used to treat 5 chordomas. Of the 5 patients, 3 had stable disease or regression of their disease.[21] In treating recurrent clival chordomas with iodine 125, a dose of 40 Gy was given, and, although the patient numbers were small, there was a regression to tumor as well as symptomatic relief of symptoms.[22]

In the 1990s, the era of 3D conformal photon therapy, an increase in dose to 66.6 Gy brought an increase in overall survival to 80%.[23] Although these results were

| Table 1 |
| Common Terminology Criteria for Adverse Events version 4.0 general guidelines |

Grade 1	Mild, asymptomatic or mild symptoms, clinical or diagnostic observations only, intervention not indicated
Grade 2	Moderate; minimal, local, or noninvasive intervention indicated; limiting age-appropriate instrumental activities of daily living
Grade 3	Severe or medically significant but not immediately life-threatening, hospitalization or prolongation of hospitalization indicated, disabling, limiting self-care activities of daily living
Grade 4	Life-threatening consequences, urgent intervention indicated
Grade 5	Death related to adverse event

US Department of Health and Human Services, National Institutes of Health, National Cancer Institute.

Grade refers to the severity of the adverse event. The Common Terminology Criteria for Adverse Events displays grades 1 through 5 with unique clinical descriptions of severity for each adverse event based on this general guideline.

promising, around the same time, the increased use of stereotactic radiosurgery was heralding a new technique for the treatment of base of skull chordomas. The University of Pittsburgh documented a small series in 1991 using Gamma Knife radiosurgery in patients with recurrent chordomas after surgery alone. The volume was small (<3 cm), and a dose of 20 Gy was given at the tumor margin.[24] With a mean follow-up of 20 months, two-thirds did not have progressive tumor, whereas one-third had a reduction in tumor size. Of the 6 patients, half had improvement in neurologic deficit, whereas the others remained stable.

The North American Gamma Knife Consortium recently published their review of 6 institutions treating base of skull chordomas with Gamma Knife radiosurgery as the primary, adjuvant, or salvage management.[25] With a median follow-up of 5 years, of the 71 patients treated, 23 had died of tumor progression. Overall survival at 5 years was 93% for patients who had not received prior radiation therapy and 43% for those who had received prior therapy. Patients of younger age and with longer disease-free interval before Gamma Knife radiosurgery, no prior radiation therapy, less than 2 cranial nerve deficits, and small tumor volume were associated with a longer survival. Tumor control rate at 5 years was 69% in the group without prior radiation and 62% for those with prior radiation. As expected, older age, prior radiation therapy, recurrence, and large tumor volume were associated with worse tumor control. Most patients went on to get other modalities of therapy after Gamma Knife radiosurgery.

The use of CyberKnife for stereotactic treatment has introduced a new treatment technique particularly useful for chordomas when they occur in the spinal region, although there are literature reports also for its use in skull base lesions.[26] These techniques are typically fractionated regimens (1–5 fractions) that facilitate treatment of larger tumors with high doses per fraction. As expected, patients with prior radiation therapy were at a higher risk of complications and poorer tumor control. In 18 patients treated with a median follow-up of 65 months, the local control was 59% and overall survival was 74%, with a disease-specific survival of 88.9%.

As 3D photon therapy continued to evolve, so did the software as well as technology for photon treatment delivery. Multiple institutions examined the role of IMRT in the treatment of chordomas and chondrosarcomas. However, there are several abstracts published that have examined the role of IMRT alone in the treatment of base of skull chordomas. IMRT offers the advantage of the ability to shape the dose around critical structures such as the optic apparatus and brainstem.[27–29] To date, these have not been published in a full article form, likely because of short follow-up. However, IMRT also shows promise in providing local control. Although traditional proton therapy has been able to spare normal tissue via a "patching" technique, this is time consuming and laborious. Given the feasibility of IMRT and its widespread availability across the country, the need to consider IMRT as a treatment option is now surfacing more than ever.

As photon technology has evolved, so has the proton beam, and, in the next generation of treatment, the use of spot scanning (single pencil proton beams that can be modulated or conformed, ie, IMRT) to mimic current photon technique is taking precedence. The Paul Scherrer Institut, Switzerland, treated 29 patients with chordomas and chondrosarcomas using spot-scanning proton radiotherapy with a median dose of 74 and 68 CGE, respectively.[30] With a median follow-up of 29 months, the 3-year local control rates were 87.5% and 100% for chordoma and chondrosarcoma, respectively. At 3 years, actuarial progression-free survival and overall survival was 90% and 93.8%, respectively. Actuarial 3-year complication-free survival was 82.2%. Radiation-induced pituitary dysfunction was observed in 4 (14%) patients (Common Terminology Criteria for Adverse Events grade 2). No patient presented with postradiation brainstem or optic pathway necrosis or dysfunction. In univariate analysis, age ($\leq$40 years at the time of proton therapy) favorably affected the progression-free survival ($P = .09$). An update in 2009 showed actuarial 5-year local control rates of 81% for chordomas and 94% for chondrosarcomas.[31] Five-year rates of overall survival were 62% for chordomas and 91% for chondrosarcomas. High-grade late toxicity consisted of 1 patient with grade 3 and 1 patient with grade 4 unilateral optic neuropathy and 2 patients with grade 3 central nervous system necrosis. No patient experienced brainstem toxicity. Actuarial 5-year freedom from high-grade toxicity was 94%. These results compare favorably to those of other combined proton-photon therapy (**Table 2**).

For many of these institutions, the treatment of chordomas and chondrosarcomas remains a combination of both protons and photons. Torres and colleagues[32] reviewed the optimal treatment plan for treatment of tumors located at the skull base. Five patients with skull base chordomas were included to generate 4 plans: an IMRT photon plan with a 1-mm planning target volume (PTV) for stereotactic treatment, an IMRT photon plan with a 3-mm PTV for standard treatment, a proton plan targeted at the clinical target volume (CTV), and a combination plan using the 3-mm PTV for photons and the CTV for protons. The primary objective was to achieve a PTV-prescribed dose coverage of 95% or more. Proton plans were the least homogeneous and conformal. Dosimetric advantages were seen using either a 1-mm PTV for stereotactic treatment or a combined plan, with this yielding the best target coverage and most conformality.

In addition to proton therapy, heavy ion beams have been used to treat chordomas, and its use has been increasing, especially in Europe and Asia. The use of heavy ions, such as carbon ions, has been theoretically postulated to have a biological advantage over proton therapy, particularly in slow-growing tumors. The relative biological effectiveness is a number that expresses the relative amount of damage that a fixed amount of ionizing radiation of a given type can inflict on biological tissues. The higher that number, the more damaging is that type of radiation, for the same amount of absorbed energy. There is a current randomized phase 3 trial examining the role of carbon ion

Table 2 Summary of radiation treatment outcomes for chordomas			
Treatment Modality	**Dose**	**Local Control Rate**	**Overall Survival**
Surgery (subtotal resection)	—	<20%/5 y	—
Royal Marsden (photons)	55 Gy	—	44%/5 y
Princess Margaret Hospital (photons)	50 Gy	—	50%/5 y
Mayo Clinic (photons)	—	—	51%/5 y
Mallinckrodt Institute (photons)	—	—	32%/10 y
Debus et al, Heidelberg (photons)	66.6 Gy	50%/5 y	82%/5 y
University of Pittsburgh (SRS)	20 Gy	59%/5 y	56%/5 y
Munzenrider and Leibsch, MGH (proton + photon)	66–83 GyE	73%/5 y	—
Hug et al, Loma Linda (protons)	70.7 GyE	76%/3 y	79%/5 y
Noel et al, Orsay (proton + photon)	67 GyE	83%/3 y	91%/3 y
NAGKC (SRS)	—	69%/5 y	93%/5 y
Paul Scherrer Institut (IMPT)	74 GyE	87.5%/3 y	93.8/3 y

Abbreviations: GyE, gray equivalent; NAGKC, North American Gamma Knife Consortium; SRS, stereotactic radiosurgery.

radiation therapy compared with proton beam for chordomas of the skull base.[33] There are currently no carbon ion centers in the United States. However, as we attempt to determine the optimal treatment technique for chordomas of the skull base, such a trial is helpful in determining level 1 evidence among the particle beam treatment modalities (**Table 3**).

To best answer the question at hand, there needs to be a continued follow-up with adequate surveillance of not only tumor control and survival but also normal tissue toxicity, including neurocognitive function and fatigue levels. At the University of Pennsylvania, a current study follows up patients after proton therapy to the base of skull, including chordomas, for neurocognitive as well as magnetic resonance imaging changes. The goal is to determine a correlation and comparison among patients receiving proton therapy versus IMRT. Only long-term and detailed follow-up will determine if protons, whether in their current form or with intensity-modulated proton therapy (IMPT), can indeed be proved to be superior. Although adequate surgery and radiation therapy have shown improvement in local control and survival, as with most tumors, genetic and biological approaches will be a third and important partner in the future management of these tumors. A current trial at the University of Virginia is examining the role of imatinib (platelet-derived growth factor receptor inhibitor) and

Table 3
Radiation therapy trials in chordomas

Study	Institution	Title	Status
NCT00496119	MDACC	Proton Beam Therapy for Chordoma Patients	Active, not recruiting
NCT00496522	MDACC	Proton Beam Therapy for Chondrosarcoma	Recruiting
NCT00797602	U Florida	Proton Therapy for Chordomas and/or Chondrosarcomas Outcomes Protocol	Recruiting
NCT00713037	MGH	Hypoxia-Positron Emission Tomography (PET) and Intensity Modulated Proton Therapy (IMPT) Dose Painting in Patients with Chordomas	Recruiting
NCT00592748	MGH	Charged Particle RT for Chordomas and Chondrosarcomas of the Base of Skull or Cervical Spine	Active, not recruiting
NCT01182779	U Heidelberg	Trial of Proton vs Carbon Ion Radiation Therapy in Patients with Chordoma of the Skull Base (HIT-1)	Recruiting
NCT01346124	MGG/MDACC	High Dose Intensity Modulated Proton Radiation Treatment +/− Surgical Resection of Sarcomas of the Spine, Sacrum and Base of Skull	Not yet opened

Abbreviations: MDACC, M. D. Anderson Cancer Center; U Florida, University of Florida; U Heidelberg, University of Heidelberg.
Data from available at: www.clinicaltrials.gov. Accessed August 1, 2011.

a histone deacetylase inhibitor in the treatment of newly diagnosed or recurrent chordomas (www.clinicaltrials.gov).

SUMMARY

Proton therapy has significant dosimetric advantages in the management of these patients. However, additional data are required to further delineate the role of proton therapy vis-à-vis advanced photon techniques. The optimal radiation technique for a patient depends largely on the extent of surgery, the biological profile, and the availability of resources. Although the number of proton therapy centers in the United States is growing, more definitive answers to determine which patients are best served by which radiation technique are best developed through collaboration with other institutions performing other advanced techniques. Given the most recent literature, until the proton pencil beam delivery system is fully developed (ie, IMPT) to conform to the delicate normal tissue organs in the base of skull, the most appropriate treatment will likely continue to be a combination approach of proton-photon radiation therapy.

EBM Question	Author's Reply
Is proton beam therapy superior to other radiation techniques in patients with chordoma?	There are significant dosimetric advantages in proton therapy and favorable outcomes in case series (level 4). However, there have been advancements in photon therapy (Gamma Knife, CyberKnife, and IMRT) that have helped to overcome excessive dosing to surrounding skull base tissues that are yet to be compared with proton therapy.

REFERENCES

1. McMaster ML, Goldstein AM, Bromley CM, et al. Chordoma: incidence and survival patterns in the United States, 1973–1995. Cancer Causes Control 2001;12(1):1–11.
2. Jemal A, Siegel R, Xu J, et al. Cancer statistics, 2010. CA Cancer J Clin 2010; 60(5):277–300.
3. Chugh R, Tawbi H, Lucas DR, et al. Chordoma: the nonsarcoma primary bone tumor. Oncologist 2007;12(11):1344–50.
4. Harvey RJ, Stamm AC, Vellutini E, et al. Closure of large skull base defects after endoscopic trans-nasal craniotomy. J Neurosurg 2009;111(2):371–9.
5. Fuller DB, Bloom JG. Radiotherapy for chordoma. Int J Radiat Oncol Biol Phys 1988;15(2):331–9.
6. Catton C, O'Sullivan B, Bell R, et al. Chordoma: long-term follow-up after radical photon irradiation. Radiother Oncol 1996;41(1):67–72.
7. Keisch ME, Garcia DM, Shibuya RB. Retrospective long-term follow-up analysis in 21 patients with chordomas of various sites treated at a single institution. J Neurosurg 1991;75(3):374–7.
8. Forsyth PA, Cascino TL, Shaw EG, et al. Intracranial chordomas: a clinico-pathological and prognostic study of 51 cases. J Neurosurg 1993;78(5): 741–7.
9. Nystrom SH. Some aspects of the use of protons in the treatment of experimental brain tumors. Naturwissenschaften 1966;53(6):159–60.

10. Nystrom SH. Effects of high energy protons on brain and glioma of mice. Acta Radiol Ther Phys Biol 1966;5:133–48.

11. Stratton K, Anderson A, Koehler AM. Effects of radiation mediating agents on the response of a murine ependymoma to proton irradiation. Radiology 1966;87(1): 68–73.

12. Kjellberg RN, Shintani A, Frantz AG, et al. Proton-beam therapy in acromegaly. N Engl J Med 1968;278(13):689–95.

13. Proton radiation for acromegaly. N Engl J Med 1968;278(13):732.

14. Suit HD, Goitein M, Munzenrider J, et al. Definitive radiation therapy for chordoma and chondrosarcoma of base of skull and cervical spine. J Neurosurg 1982; 56(3):377–85.

15. Austin-Seymour M, Munzenrider J, Goitein M, et al. Fractionated proton radiation therapy of chordoma and low-grade chondrosarcoma of the base of the skull. J Neurosurg 1989;70(1):13–7.

16. Santoni R, Liebsch N, Finkelstein DM, et al. Temporal lobe (TL) damage following surgery and high-dose photon and proton irradiation in 96 patients affected by chordomas and chondrosarcomas of the base of the skull. Int J Radiat Oncol Biol Phys 1998;41(1):59–68.

17. Munzenrider JE, Liebsch NJ. Proton therapy for tumors of the skull base. Strahlenther Onkol 1999;175(Suppl 2):57–63.

18. Hug EB, Loredo LN, Slater JD, et al. Proton radiation therapy for chordomas and chondrosarcomas of the skull base. J Neurosurg 1999;91(3):432–9.

19. Noel G, Habrand JL, Mammar H, et al. Combination of photon and proton radiation therapy for chordomas and chondrosarcomas of the skull base: the Centre de Protontherapie D'Orsay experience. Int J Radiat Oncol Biol Phys 2001; 51(2):392–8.

20. Noel G, Habrand JL, Jauffret E, et al. Radiation therapy for chordoma and chondrosarcoma of the skull base and the cervical spine. Prognostic factors and patterns of failure. Strahlenther Onkol 2003;179(4):241–8.

21. Gutin PH, Leibel SA, Hosobuchi Y, et al. Brachytherapy of recurrent tumors of the skull base and spine with iodine-125 sources. Neurosurgery 1987;20(6):938–45.

22. Kumar PP, Good RR, Skultety FM, et al. Local control of recurrent clival and sacral chordoma after interstitial irradiation with iodine-125: new techniques for treatment of recurrent or unresectable chordomas. Neurosurgery 1988;22(3): 479–83.

23. Debus J, Schulz-Ertner D, Schad L, et al. Stereotactic fractionated radiotherapy for chordomas and chondrosarcomas of the skull base. Int J Radiat Oncol Biol Phys 2000;47(3):591–6.

24. Kondziolka D, Lunsford LD, Flickinger JC. The role of radiosurgery in the management of chordoma and chondrosarcoma of the cranial base. Neurosurgery 1991;29(1):38–45 [discussion: 45–6].

25. Kano H, Iqbal FO, Sheehan J, et al. Stereotactic radiosurgery for chordoma: a report from the North American Gamma Knife Consortium. Neurosurgery 2011;68(2):379–89.

26. Henderson FC, McCool K, Seigle J, et al. Treatment of chordomas with Cyber-Knife: Georgetown university experience and treatment recommendations. Neurosurgery 2009;64(Suppl 2):A44–53.

27. Burnet NG, Foweraker KL, Burton KE, et al. High-dose radiotherapy in the management of chordoma chondrosarcoma of the skull base and cervical spine: part 1—clinical outcomes. Clin Oncol (R Coll Radiol) 2007;19(7):509–16.

28. Foweraker KL, Burton KE, Jena R, et al. High dose photon radiotherapy in the management of chordoma and chondrosarcoma of the skull base and cervical spine. Clin Oncol (R Coll Radiol) 2007;19(3):S28.
29. Foweraker KL, Chantler HJ, Geater AR, et al. Conformal versus IMRT for chordoma of the skull base and cervical spine. Clin Oncol (R Coll Radiol) 2007;19(3):S28–9.
30. Weber DC, Rutz HP, Pedroni ES, et al. Results of spot-scanning proton radiation therapy for chordoma and chondrosarcoma of the skull base: the Paul Scherrer Institut experience. Int J Radiat Oncol Biol Phys 2005;63(2):401–9.
31. Ares C, Hug EB, Lomax AJ, et al. Effectiveness and safety of spot scanning proton radiation therapy for chordomas and chondrosarcomas of the skull base: first long-term report. Int J Radiat Oncol Biol Phys 2009;75(4):1111–8.
32. Torres MA, Chang EL, Mahajan A, et al. Optimal treatment planning for skull base chordoma: photons, protons, or a combination of both? Int J Radiat Oncol Biol Phys 2009;74(4):1033–9.
33. Nikoghosyan AV, Karapanagiotou-Schenkel I, Munter MW, et al. Randomised trial of proton vs. carbon ion radiation therapy in patients with chordoma of the skull base, clinical phase III study HIT-1-Study. BMC Cancer 2010;10:607.

Functional Outcomes for Endoscopic and Open Skull Base Surgery: An Evidence-Based Review

John R. de Almeida, MD, MSc, FRCS(C)[a],
Ian J. Witterick, MD, MSc, FRCS(C)[b], Allan D. Vescan, MD, FRCS(C)[c],*

KEYWORDS

- Skull base surgery • Endoscopic • Open • Transcranial
- Transfacial • Functional outcomes • Quality of life

EBM Question	Level of Evidence	Grade of Recommendation
Is functional outcome from endonasal surgery better to open craniofacial surgery?	4-2a	C-B

Evaluation of new medical technologies requires a careful comparison of outcomes for existing treatment strategies. The advent of endoscopic techniques for the management of skull base neoplasms over the past decade has spawned much enthusiasm; however, outcomes comparing endoscopic approaches and traditional open

Financial Disclosures: Dr de Almeida has no financial disclosures to declare. Drs Ian Witterick and Allan Vescan are members of the advisory boards for Merck and Ethicon/Acclarent. Dr Ian Witterick is a member of the advisory boards for GlaxoSmithKline and Pharmascience Inc and is a consultant for Alcon.

[a] Department of Otolaryngology-Head and Neck Surgery, University of Toronto, Toronto, Canada
[b] Department of Otolaryngology-Head and Neck Surgery, Mount Sinai Hospital 600 University Avenue, Room 413, Toronto, Ontario, Canada M5G 1X5
[c] Department of Otolaryngology-Head and Neck Surgery, Mount Sinai Hospital, 600 University Avenue, Room 401, Toronto, Ontario, Canada M5G 1X5
* Corresponding author.
E-mail address: avescan@mtsinai.on.ca

Otolaryngol Clin N Am 44 (2011) 1185–1200
doi:10.1016/j.otc.2011.06.017
0030-6665/11/$ – see front matter © 2011 Elsevier Inc. All rights reserved.

approaches still need to be studied. Proponents of endoscopic skull base surgery suggest that this technique offers improved visualization, shorter hospital stays, reduced complication rates, comparable tumor control rates, and improved functional outcomes.

Most studies in skull base surgery have focused on local tumor control and improving disease-specific survival. Despite advances in instrumentation and surgical technologies, no significant improvements in these specific outcome measures have been made. Longitudinal studies with long-term follow-up are being undertaken to compare the oncologic results between endoscopic and open techniques, and the early results seem to be promising, with comparable and even improved local control rates.[1–4]

As long-term survival and tumor control outcomes data are awaited, much attention has shifted toward functional outcomes. The interest in functional outcomes is particularly relevant to patients with skull base neoplasms, because both the disease process and the treatment can be highly morbid to the nose and sinuses and adjacent vital structures, including the orbit, brain, and carotid arteries. Injury to these structures can result in temporary or permanent functional limitations. This article reviews the available evidence for functional outcomes after skull base surgery to determine how these differ for endoscopic and open approaches. The Oxford Centre for Evidence-based Medicine Levels of Evidence are used to provide recommendations (**Tables 1** and **2**) for each functional outcome.[5]

DEFINING FUNCTIONAL OUTCOMES

Starfield[6] defines functional status as "the capacity to engage in activities of daily living and social role activities." Physical morbidity incurred by skull base neoplasms directly impacts one's functional status. Functional status is often the result of

Table 1 The Oxford Centre for Evidence-based Medicine—levels of evidence	
Level	**Therapy/Prevention/Etiology/Harm**
1a	Systematic review (with homogeneity) of randomized controlled trials
1b	Individual randomized controlled trial (with narrow CI)
1c	All or none[a]
2a	Systematic review (with homogeneity) of cohort studies
2b	Individual cohort study (including low-quality randomized controlled trials; eg, <80% follow-up)
2c	"Outcomes" research; ecological studies
3a	Systematic review (with homogeneity) of case-control studies
3b	Individual case-control studies
4	Case-series (and poor-quality cohort and case-control studies)
5	Expert opinion without explicit critical appraisal, or based on physiology, bench research or "first principles"

[a] Met when all patients died before the treatment became available, but now some survive on it; or when some patients died before the treatment became available, but now none die on it.

Adapted from Phillips B, Ball C, Sackett D, et al. Oxford Centre for Evidence-based Medicine—levels of evidence (March 2009). Available at: http://www.cebm.net/index.aspx?o51025. Accessed November 25, 2010; with permission.

Table 2	
The Oxford Centre for Evidence-based Medicine—grades of recommendation	
A	Consistent level 1 studies
B	Consistent level 2 or 3 studies or extrapolations from level 1 studies
C	Level 4 studies or extrapolations from level 2 or 3 studies
D	Level 5 studies or troublingly inconsistent or inconclusive studies of any level

Adapted from Phillips B, Ball C, Sackett D, et al. Oxford Centre for Evidence-based Medicine—levels of evidence (March 2009). Available at: http://www.cebm.net/index.aspx?o51025. Accessed November 25, 2010; with permission.

a combination of factors, some of which may include the disease, the treatment, coping strategies of the individual, and the individual's support network.

Many quality-of-life instruments contain items to measure functional status. However, outcomes collected from instruments are often subjective and may vary based on the individual patient or the method of administration. A variety of functional outcomes are specific to skull base surgery. Collecting information about these outcomes requires good follow-up of postoperative patients and, in certain instances, objective measurement of various outcomes.

FUNCTIONAL OUTCOMES

The following functional outcomes relating to skull base pathology are described and the evidence for endoscopic and open approaches are compared and discussed:

1. Endocrine outcomes
2. Nasal outcomes
3. Neurologic outcomes
4. Visual outcomes
5. Quality of life outcomes.

Between 1998 and 2008, the authors performed a retrospective review at the University Health Network in Toronto of 138 patients who underwent skull base surgery.[7] Of these patients, 73 underwent open approaches and 65 endoscopic approaches. The median follow-up for open cases was 48 months compared with 17 months for endoscopic cases, suggesting a more recent switch to endoscopic approaches. Postoperative physical morbidity leading to functional limitation was categorized into endocrine, nasal, neurologic, visual, and "other" outcomes. These outcomes were compared according to surgical approach (**Table 3**). Patients who underwent endoscopic approaches had more postoperative nasal morbidity (80% vs. 68.5%; $P = .003$), whereas patients treated with open approaches had more visual morbidity (28.8% vs. 9.2%; $P = .02$) after adjusting for tumor location and preoperative symptoms. However, these results are retrospective; prospective comparative studies are needed to confirm these findings.

ENDOCRINE OUTCOMES
Hormonal Stabilization

Endocrine outcomes are particularly relevant as they relate to skull base tumors in the sella, suprasellar region, and surrounding areas. Endocrine outcomes can be divided into improvement in preoperative endocrinopathies or the development of new

Table 3			
Postoperative functional outcomes by surgical approach			
Postoperative Symptom Type	Endoscopic Approach (%)	Open Approach (%)	Adjusted *P* Value
Endocrine	4.6	1.4	.52
Nasal	80	68.5	.003
Neurologic	16.9	24.7	.45
Visual	9.2	28.8	.02
Other[a]	13.8	13.7	.86

[a] Other symptoms include those that do not directly fit into one of the above, such as dry mouth, fatigue, and weight loss.
Data from de Almeida JR, Vescan A, Witterick I, et al. Physical morbidity by tumour location and surgical approach in skull base surgery. Skull Base 2011;21(Suppl 1):143.

endocrinopathies as a result of surgical intervention. Rotenberg and colleagues.[8] performed a systematic review of studies comparing open (transseptal microscopic or transnasal microscopic) and endoscopic approaches for pituitary pathology. In this review of 11 studies, 3 of them, 1 of which was a randomized trial[9] and 2 of which were cohort studies,[10,11] compared effectiveness of hormonal stabilization between endoscopic and microscopic approaches. None of these studies reported statistical differences between the groups.

Dorward[12] reviewed endocrinologic outcomes of endoscopic and microscopic approaches for all pituitary adenomas using methodology applied in a previous systematic review.[13] The details of the search strategy used are unclear; however, the results compared pooled hormonal stabilization rates from 20 studies using endoscopic approaches to an undisclosed number of pooled microscopic studies. The definitions for endocrinologic cures vary by primary study, but the pooled cure rates favor endoscopic approaches (75% vs. 73%) for all adenomas. The authors of this article suggest that the benefit is incremental for macroadenomas (70% vs. 45% cure rate) compared with microadenomas (84% vs. 77% cure rate). Most of the primary studies included in this review include retrospective cohort studies. **Fig. 1**

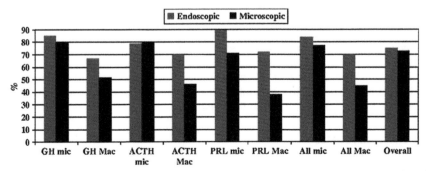

Fig. 1. Review of endocrinological cures for endoscopic and microscopic approaches for pituitary adenomas. (*From* Dorward NL. Endocrine outcomes in endoscopic pituitary surgery: a literature review. Acta Neurochir 2010;152:1275–9; with permission.)

depicts endocrinologic cure rates in various functioning adenomas. All functioning adenomas except for adrenocorticotropic hormone–secreting microadenomas had better cure rates using the endoscopic approach. However, no statistical meta-analyses were performed.

Dorward[12] also examined the rates of anterior pituitary dysfunction in his review of the endoscopic and microscopic literature. In the analysis of 1980 cases of endoscopic resection of pituitary tumors, the overall rates of anterior pituitary dysfunction were 5.4%. For microscopic studies, the rate of anterior pituitary dysfunction was 5%; however, the methods of meta-analysis and the included studies are unclear. The author notes that a survey administered to surgeons using the microscopic approach for resection of pituitary adenomas suggests a 19.4% rate of anterior pituitary dysfunction.[12,14]

Level of Evidence: 2a

Recommendation

1. For pituitary macroadenomas, endoscopic approaches may offer better endocrinologic cure rates compared with microscopic (open) approaches (grade B).
2. For pituitary microadenomas, whether endoscopic approaches are superior to microscopic approaches or vice versa for endocrinologic cure is unclear (grade B).
3. Whether endoscopic approaches are superior to microscopic approaches or vice versa for minimization of anterior pituitary dysfunction is unclear (grade B).

Diabetes insipidus

In a systematic review of comparative studies between endoscopic and microscopic approaches for pituitary adenomas,[8] seven studies were reviewed that compared either transient or permanent diabetes insipidus (DI), one of which was a randomized trial, five of which were cohort studies, and one was a case-series.[9,15–20] One study noted increased rates of DI in the microscopic group immediately postoperatively (<2 weeks), but no significant difference was seen at 6 months.[20] Another study showed a higher rate of DI for the sublabial microscopic approach (33%) compared with the endoscopic (7%) and transnasal microscopic (5%) approaches.[18] However, no statistical analyses were performed. The authors of the review conclude that endoscopic approaches are associated with fewer cases of transient postoperative DI, but these differences equalize over time.

Level of Evidence: 2a

Recommendation

No conclusive evidence exists that either endoscopic or microscopic approaches for skull base neoplasms offer better rates of DI (grade B).

Nasal Outcomes

Rotenberg and colleagues[8] describe six studies that compare nasal outcomes of endoscopic and open (transnasal microscopic and sublabial microscopic) approaches for pituitary adenomas.[9,10,15–17,19] In three of these studies, rates of septal perforations were insignificant between the groups.[10,15,19] One group reported more septal perforations in the microscopic group, although no statistical analysis was performed.[16] Another group reported significantly more epistaxis in the microscopic group,[19] and another group reported more rhinologic complications in the microscopic group in a randomized trial.[17] These data conflict with data obtained by the authors of this article in a retrospective analysis adjusting for tumor location and preoperative symptoms that suggest that open approaches are associated with significantly fewer nasal complications compared with endoscopic approaches.[7]

In a prospective cohort study, the authors prospectively collected rhinologic outcome data for 1 year for a total of 63 patients who underwent endoscopic skull base surgery for various tumors.[21] Nasal crusting was the most common (98%) symptom reported, followed by nasal discharge (46%), whereas loss of smell was reported by only 9.5% of patients. Crusting was short-lived, with half of the patients achieving a crust-free nose by 101 days (95% CI, 87.8–114.2 days). More complex operations (defined by surgical manipulation of more than one anatomic module) had significantly longer times to achieve absence of crusting. However, no independent risk factors were seen in a multivariable analysis predisposing patients to longer periods of postoperative crusting. These data are corroborated by another study that suggests nasal morbidity, as indicated by the SinoNasal Outcome Test 22 (SNOT-22) questionnaire, gradually improves with time.[22] These prospective data suggest that crusting may in fact be underreported in other trials and reviews. No large-scale functional outcome studies have reported nasal outcomes for patients undergoing open skull base surgery.

Level of Evidence: 1b–2b

Recommendation
Conflicting evidence exists regarding whether open approaches or endoscopic approaches have superior nasal outcomes, and a paucity of studies have compared these approaches for nasal outcomes. Further good-quality studies are needed (grade D).

Neurologic Outcomes

In a single institution, neurologic outcomes were compared between patients undergoing endoscopic approaches and those undergoing open approaches for clival tumors.[23] In this study, 17 patients underwent endoscopic approaches and 48 underwent open approaches, including anterior (transfacial or transoral) approaches or lateral approaches (pterional, fronto-orbito zygomatic approaches). On patient (6%) who underwent endoscopic approaches experienced neurologic worsening (new hemiparesis), compared with 33% who underwent open approaches. These neurologic symptoms included worsening hemiparesis, brainstem compression, and new cranial nerve deficits. Another series of chordomas resected endoscopically reported no neurologic deficits postoperatiely,[24] and a report of chordomas resected through open approaches (retrosigmoid, pterional, subtemporal) noted a 28% rate of neurologic complications, including cranial nerve palsies, hemiparesis, and hemiplegia.[25]

Reports of poor neurologic outcomes, however, are not universal for open skull base surgery. In a series of 81 olfactory groove meningiomas resected with open approaches, one group reported no new neurologic deficits except for anosmia.[26] Similarly, endoscopic approaches for anterior cranial base meningiomas may be associated with a low complication rate, with only 1 patient of 35 experiencing neurologic compromise (new hemiparesis and cognitive impairment) after endoscopic resection.[27]

Level of Evidence: 4

Recommendation
There is some suggestion in poorly designed cohort studies and case-series that endoscopic approaches may have better neurologic outcomes. However, selection

biases for endoscopic approaches and heterogeneity in outcomes by location and pathology make these results difficult to interpret (grade C).

Visual Outcomes

In a review of visual outcomes in microscopic versus endoscopic pituitary surgery, Schaberg and colleagues[28] describe two studies in which complete visual recovery from preoperative visual deficits was experienced by 50% and 70% of patients, respectively, after endoscopic surgery.[29,30] They compare this to a large-scale microscopic series in which complete visual recovery is experienced by only 40% of patients.[31]

Stamm and colleagues[32] recently reviewed the published series for endoscopic and transcranial management of craniopharyngiomas. The rate of visual recovery in seven small series (between 1 and 10 patients) ranged from 56% to 100%,[32–39] whereas the rate of visual recovery in the transcranial studies ranged from 64% to 89%.[40–44] Although none of the endoscopic series reported visual worsening, two of the microscopic series reported visual worsening (3% and 8%).[41,43]

The authors compared the incidence of postoperative visual complaints in 65 patients undergoing endoscopic approaches and 73 patients undergoing open approaches for skull base pathology, and noted that patients with open approaches had more postoperative visual complaints (28.8% vs. 9.2%, adjusted $P = .02$) after adjusting for confounders such as preoperative symptoms and tumor location.[7]

Level of Evidence: 4

Recommendation

There is some suggestion in poorly designed cohort studies and case-series that endoscopic approaches may have better visual outcomes. However, selection biases for endoscopic approaches and heterogeneity in outcomes according to location and pathology make these results difficult to interpret (grade C).

Quality of Life

A recent movement has occurred toward better elucidating the quality of life in patients who undergo skull base surgery. Much of this impetus is rooted in the fact that oncologic outcomes have reached a relative plateau, and that surgery in this anatomic region can be fraught with significant impairments in functional status. The goals of therapy are now balanced between maximizing oncologic control and minimizing functional disability.

Despite this new interest, no large multi-institutional studies have examined quality of life in patients undergoing skull base surgery. However, some single institutional experiences with quality of life for endoscopic surgery[22,45] and open skull base surgery have been reported.[46–49] However, the current data are limited in that no direct comparative studies have been performed in the form of either randomized trials or matched case-control series.

In a cross-sectional study of 54 patients after endoscopic pituitary surgery with follow-up ranging from 4 to 20 months, Karabatsou and colleagues[45] studied quality of life using the SF-36. When compared with normative data, patients who underwent surgery for pituitary adenomas only differed from healthy individuals in the general health domain ($P = .002$) but were no different with respect to all other domains (physical functioning, role limitations physical, role limitations emotional, energy, emotional well-being, social functioning, bodily pain). Among patients undergoing surgery, those with Cushing disease had significantly lower scores in role-limitations emotional ($P = .02$). The only published report of disease-specific quality of life for endoscopic surgery used the anterior skull base quality of life instrument to prospectively follow 51 patients who underwent skull base surgery.[22] The data from this study suggest that overall quality of life and functional status tend to improve over the course of the year after surgery. These data corroborate those for patients who have undergone open approaches for skull base neoplasms.[46]

Gil and colleagues[46] studied quality of life for patients undergoing open skull base surgery using the anterior skull base surgery disease-specific quality of life in a cross-sectional study. Forty patients completed the anterior skull base questionnaire at various time points (minimum of 3 months) after surgery. Overall, a trend seemed to be present toward improved outcomes starting 6 months after surgery. The only risk factor for poorer overall quality of life scores in this study was whether the tumor was malignant versus benign (P<.05).

Although no head-to-head studies have compared open and endoscopic approaches, when comparing the data from Gil and colleagues[46] and Pant and colleagues[22] using the same disease-specific quality of life questionnaire (**Figs. 2 and 3**),[22,46] the authors of this article note that the open surgical patients have mean scores between 2 and 3 (on a scale from 1 to 5), whereas the patients who underwent endoscopic approaches have mean scores greater than 4. This comparison is necessarily fraught with limitations given the heterogeneity of tumors, the different indications for surgery, and the various rates of malignancy. Also, the ASB questionnaire was not designed nor validated for patients undergoing endoscopic approaches.

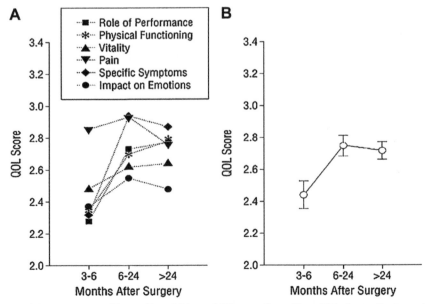

Fig. 2. (A) Domain-specific quality of life and (B) overall quality of life for patients undergoing open skull base surgery using the anterior skull base surgery quality-of-life questionnaire. (*From* Gil Z, Abergel A, Spektor S, et al. Quality of life following surgery for anterior skull base tumors. Arch Otolaryngol Head Neck Surg 2003;129(12):1303–9; with permission.)

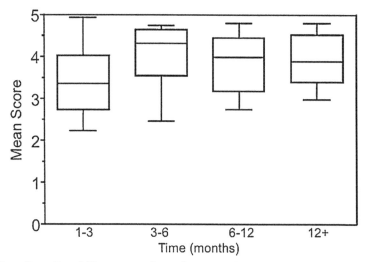

Fig. 3. Overall quality of life expressed as a function of time (months) postoperatively for patients undergoing endoscopic skull base surgery using the anterior skull base surgery quality-of-life questionnaire. (*From* Pant H, Bhatki AM, Snyderman CH, et al. Quality of life following endonasal skull base surgery. Skull Base 2010;20(1):35–40; with permission.)

Level of Evidence: 4

Recommendation

Although two of these studies are described as cohort studies, neither includes both endoscopic and open approaches. The conclusions regarding differences in quality of life can only be as strong as comparing individual case series. Therefore, the authors have rated the evidence as level 4. There is some suggestion in these studies that endoscopic approaches may have better quality-of-life outcomes. However, selection biases for endoscopic approaches and heterogeneity in outcomes according to location and pathology make these results difficult to interpret (grade C).

Challenges in measuring functional outcomes

Several challenges exist with regards to measuring functional outcomes in skull base surgery. Patients with skull base neoplasms may experience cognitive impairments from direct tumor involvement of frontal lobes and other parts of the brain responsible for executive function. As many as 80% of patients undergoing radiotherapy for skull base neoplasms may experience memory loss or difficulty with frontal lobe executive function.[50] Self-reporting of functional limitations is less reliable with patients who experience cognitive impairments.

Furthermore, the measurement of functional outcomes varies among studies, with health care providers, caregivers, and patients themselves all involved in reporting functional outcomes. A discrepancy is apparent between what each of these groups perceives as important functional outcomes. Gil and colleagues[47] report a poor correlation between the self-ratings of quality of life among patients who underwent skull base surgery and the reports of the physicians involved in their care ($r = 0.23$; $P = .60$). This discrepancy makes functional outcomes from heterogeneous studies difficult to compare.

Another challenge in measuring functional outcomes is that deficits related to treatment may be difficult to decipher from those related to the disease process itself. In measuring postoperative morbidity after endoscopic or open skull base surgery, one must account for preoperative morbidity. Furthermore, oncologic goals often conflict with functional goals. Achieving gross-total tumor extirpation may come at the expense of increased morbidity. This concept is particularly relevant when comparing surgical approaches for which the indications are different. Many larger tumors, for example, require open approaches as opposed to endoscopic. Achieving a good oncologic result can thus be associated with a poor functional result.

Lastly, skull base neoplasms are heterogeneous in terms of both pathology and location. A lesion in the sella or clivus may be associated with vastly different functional deficits than a lesion in the anterior skull base, for example. Therefore, tumor location and surgical pathology should be accounted for when measuring functional outcomes for various surgical approaches.

Quality-of-life instruments and prospective large-scale multi-institutional studies are needed to better measure functional outcomes.

Quality-of life instruments

Much of the early work in quality of life for skull base surgery was measured using generic quality-of-life questionnaires. The SF-36, the Sickness Impact Profile, the Karnofsky Performance Scale, and the Glasgow Outcome scale are all generic quality-of-life questionnaires used to gauge general health states.[51–53] Although these instruments are extensively validated in different disease states and have the ability to differentiate disparate diseases, they may lack the ability to discriminate similar disease entities.[54] Disease-specific quality-of-life instruments are helpful for differentiating between similar disease entities. With these instruments, the greater the amount of disease-specific questions, the better the instrument's ability to differentiate like entities.[55]

This concept can be illustrated using the bandwidth-fidelity dilemma in communications theory. A general quality-of-life scale is akin to having a wide bandwidth but low fidelity. It would be able to measure several types of pathology, but no one pathology can be measured well. A disease-specific scale, on the other hand, is akin to having low bandwidth but high fidelity. These instruments can measure similar diseases and discriminate among them because little noise is present in the information obtained.

Some authors have used quality-of-life instruments specific to head and neck cancer to measure quality of life for skull base neoplasms.[56] These instruments include the European Organisation for Research and Treatment of Cancer Quality of Life Questionnaire–Head and Neck module (EORTC-QLC-H&N35), the University of Washington Quality of Life questionnaire (UW-QOL), and the Functional Assessment of Cancer Therapy–Head and Neck module (FACT-H&N). These instruments have undergone extensive psychometric testing.[57] However, even though skull base neoplasms are considered head and neck tumors, the range of functional limitations incurred by skull base neoplasms differ dramatically from the deficits incurred from most other head and neck cancers.

The authors performed a systematic review of multiple electronic databases to identify quality-of-life instruments relevant to skull base neoplasms. The initial search yielded 3250 articles, of which 9 contained instruments relating to quality of life for skull base neoplasms.[58–66] **Table 4** lists the quality-of-life instruments identified. Of the 9 instruments, 7 relate to pituitary pathology and 2 to all anterior skull base pathology. The anterior skull base surgery quality-of-life questionnaire[59] and the Midface

Table 4
Items derived from systematic review

References	Instrument	Target Patient Population	Domains	Number of Items	Number of Response Categories
Badia et al[58]	AcroQOL	Acromegaly	Physical, psychological appearance, psychological relations	22	5
Gil et al[59]	ASB-QOL	Anterior skull base cancer	Performance, physical function, vitality, pain, specific symptoms, influence on emotions	35	5
Herschbach et al[60]	QLS-H	Growth hormone deficiency	Physical, emotional	9	5
Kan et al[61]	Pituitary adenoma	Pituitary adenoma	General health, emotional, social, family, health problems, physician relations	54	7
Lovas et al[62]	AddiQoL	Addison disease	Physical, emotional	36	5
McKenna et al[63]	QOL-AGHDA	Growth hormone deficiency	n/a	25	2
McMillan et al[64]	HDQOL	Hypopituitary	Work, family, social, sex, appearance, self-confidence, physical capabilities, leisure, travel, motivation, spiritual, society's reaction, future worries, finances, dependence, others fussing, living conditions, diet	20	7
Palme et al[65]	Midface Dysfunction Scale	Anterior skull base	n/a	4	5
Webb et al[66]	CushingQoL	Cushing disease	n/a	12	5
	Totals	9	—	217	—

Abbreviations: AcroQOL, Acromegaly Quality of Life; AddiQOL, Addison's Quality of Life; ASB-QOL, Anterior Skull Base Quality of Life; Cushing QOL, Cushing Quality of Life; HDQOL, Hormone Deficiency Quality of Life; QLS-H, Quality of Life Satisfaction: Hypopituitarism; QOL-AGHDA, Quality of Life Assessment for Growth Hormone Deficiency in Adults.

Dysfunction Scale[65] both contain items relevant to anterior skull base pathology; however, the latter has only four items and has not undergone any reliability or validity testing.

The anterior skull base questionnaire was developed using a cohort of 35 patients with a combination of benign and malignant skull base neoplasms treated with open skull base surgery.[59] Items for this questionnaire were derived through a composite approach. The SF-36, SF-12, Glasgow Benefit Inventory, Center for Epidemiology Studies Depression Scale, European Organisation for Research and Treatment of Cancer Quality of Life Questionnaire (EORTC-QLQ-C30), and the UW-QOL questionnaire were reviewed to identify some items, and others were further generated from interviews with surgeons, patients, and caregivers. The questionnaire has been tested for psychometric properties among patients undergoing open surgical approaches but has not been validated in those undergoing endoscopic approaches. It is also limited in that it contains only seven disease-specific items.

The authors' group is currently developing a 41-item disease-specific multidimensional quality-of-life questionnaire for anterior and central skull base surgery: the Skull Base Inventory (SBI).[67] It contains 26 disease-specific items, including five physical subdomains (endocrine, nasal, neurologic, visual, other) and a domain containing cognitive items. The instrument was developed with input from 34 patients, 18 of whom underwent endoscopic approaches and 16 of whom underwent open approaches. With several disease-specific items, the SBI will be well suited to compare quality of life for endoscopic and open approaches. Early psychometric evaluation is still underway, but large-scale validation will be required to test the reliability and validity of the SBI.

Prospective large-scale multi-institutional studies

Because of the relative paucity of skull base pathology, large-scale multi-institutional prospective studies are required to better delineate quality of life and functional outcomes. Self-reported quality-of-life questionnaires must be administered both preoperatively and postoperatively, and standardized assessment and collection of information regarding functional outcomes is required. In a special issue of *Skull Base* dedicated to quality of life, Shah[68] suggests a need for new instruments and rigorous multi-institutional data collection. A previous, large, international collaborative effort for anterior skull base surgery focusing on oncologic outcomes has been published.[69] A similar endeavor is necessary to better understand functional outcomes for both open and endoscopic surgery. This type of effort is inherently plagued with obstacles, such as managing large volumes of data and achieving standardization of data collection. Patel[70] suggests an Internet-based database to overcome many of these hurdles.

SUMMARY

Although functional status is arguably one of the most important outcomes to patients, a paucity of good prospective functional status outcome data is available for skull base surgery. Particularly with the advent of new technologies for skull base surgery, such as endoscopic approaches and robotics,[71–73] rigorous measurement of functional outcomes and quality of life is of paramount importance. Future longitudinal studies must standardize measurement of endocrine, nasal, neurologic, and visual outcomes for all surgical approaches. Furthermore, longitudinal studies of quality of life are required using a standardized quality-of-life instrument to compare open and endoscopic approaches and other emerging technologies.

EBM Question	Author's Reply
Is endocrine cure rate from endonasal surgery better to open craniofacial surgery?	For pituitary macroadenomas, endoscopic approaches may offer better endocrinologic cure rates compared with microscopic (open) approaches (grade B, level 2a)
Is DI outcome from endonasal surgery better to open craniofacial surgery?	No conclusive evidence exists that either endoscopic or microscopic approaches for skull base neoplasms offer better rates of DI (grade B, level 2a).
Is nasal outcome from endonasal surgery better to open craniofacial surgery?	Conflicting evidence exists regarding whether open approaches or endoscopic approaches have superior nasal outcomes, and a paucity of studies have compared these approaches for nasal outcomes. (grade D, level 1b-2b)
Is visual outcome from endonasal surgery better to open craniofacial surgery?	Endoscopic approaches may have better visual outcomes. However, selection biases for endoscopic approaches and heterogeneity in outcomes according to location and pathology make these results difficult to interpret (grade C, level 4).
Is quality-of-life outcome from endonasal surgery better to open craniofacial surgery?	Quality of life outcomes are better for endoscopic approaches (Grade C, level 4)

REFERENCES

1. Busquets JM, Hwang PH. Endoscopic resection of sinonasal inverted papilloma: a meta-analysis. Otolaryngol Head Neck Surg 2006;134:476–82.
2. Nicolai P, Berlucchi M, Tomenzoli D, et al. Endoscopic surgery for juvenile angiofibroma: When and how. Laryngoscope 2003;113:775–82.
3. Devaiah AK, Lee MK. Endoscopic skull base/sinonasal adenocarcinoma surgery: what evidence exists. Am J Rhinol Allergy 2010;24(2):156–60.
4. Hanna E, DeMonte F, Ibrahim S, et al. Endoscopic resection of sinonasal cancers with and without craniotomy: oncologic results. Arch Otolaryngol Head Neck Surg 2009;135(12):1219–24.
5. Phillips B, Ball C, Sackett D, et al. Oxford Centre for Evidence-based Medicine—levels of evidence (March 2009). Available at: http://www.cebm.net/index.aspx?o=1025. Accessed November 25, 2010.
6. Starfield B. Basic concepts in population health and health care. J Epidemiol Community Health 2001;55(7):452–4.
7. de Almeida JR, Vescan A, Witterick I, et al. Physical morbidity by tumour location and surgical approach in skull base surgery. Skull Base 2011;21(Suppl 1):143.
8. Rotenberg B, Tam S, Ryu W, et al. Microscopic versus endoscopic pituitary surgery: a systematic review. Laryngoscope 2010;120:1292–7.
9. Cho DY, Liau WR. Comparison of endonasal endoscopic surgery and sublabial microsurgery for prolactinomas. Surg Neurol 2002;58:371–5.
10. Choe JH, Lee Ks, Jeun SS, et al. Endocrine outcome of endoscopic endonasal transsphenoidal surgery in functioning pituitary adenomas. J Korean Neurosurg Soc 2008;44:151–5.
11. Cappabianca P, Alfieri A, Colao A, et al. Endoscopic endonasal transsphenoidal approach: an additional reason in support of surgery in the management of pituitary lesions. Skull Base Surg 1999;9:109–17.
12. Dorward NL. Endocrine outcomes in endoscopic pituitary surgery: a literature review. Acta Neurochir 2010;152:1275–9.

13. Tabaee A, Anand VK, Barron Y, et al. Endoscopic pituitary surgery: a systematic review and meta-analysis. J Neurosurg 2009;111(3):545–54.
14. Ciric I, Ragin A, Baumbartner C, et al. Complications of transsphenoidal surgery: results of a national survey, review of the literature and personal experience. Neurosurgery 1996;40(2):225–37.
15. Higgins TS, Courtemanche C, Karakla D, et al. Analysis of transnasal endoscopic versus transseptal microscopic approach for excision of pituitary tumors. Am J Rhinol 2008;22:649–52.
16. Casler JD, Doolittle AM, Mair EA. Endoscopic surgery of the anterior skull base. Laryngoscope 2005;115:16–24.
17. Jain AK, Gupta AK, Pathak A, et al. Excision of pituitary adenomas: randomized comparison of surgical modalities. Br J Neurosurg 2007;21:328–31.
18. Neal JG, Patel SJ, Kulbersch JS, et al. Comparison of techniques for transsphenoidal pituitary surgery. Am J Rhinol 2007;21:203–6.
19. White Dr, Sonnenburg RE, Ewend MG, et al. Safety of minimally invasive pituitary surgery (MIPS) compared with a traditional approach. Laryngoscope 2004;114: 1945–8.
20. Shah S, Har-El G. Diabetes insipidus after pituitary surgery: incidence after traditional versus endoscopic transsphenoidal approaches. Am J Rhinol 2001;15: 377–9.
21. de Almeida JR, Snyderman CH, Gardner PA, et al. Nasal morbidity following endoscopic skull base surgery: a prospective cohort study. Head Neck 2011; 33(4):547–51.
22. Pant H, Bhatki AM, Snyderman CH, et al. Quality of life following endonasal skull base surgery. Skull Base 2010;20(1):35–40.
23. Carrabba G, Dehdashti AR, Gentili F. Surgery for clival lesions: open resection versus expanded endoscopic endonasal approach. Neurosurg Foc 2008; 25(6):E7.
24. Fatemi N, Dusick JR, Gorgulho AA, et al. Endonasal microscopic removal of clival chordomas. Surg Neurol 2008;69(4):331–8.
25. Samii A, Gerganov VM, Herold C, et al. Chordoma of the skull base: surgical management and outcome. J Neurosurg 2007;107:319–24.
26. Spektor S, Valarezo J, Fliss DM, et al. Olfactory groove meningiomas from neurosurgical and ear, nose, and throat perspectives: approaches, techniques and outcomes. Neurosurg 2005;57(Suppl 4):268–80.
27. Gardner PA, Kassam AB, Thomas A, et al. Endoscopic endonasal resection of anterior cranial base meningiomas. Neurosurgery 2008;63(1):36–52.
28. Schaberg MR, Anand VK, Schwartz TH, et al. Microscopic versus endoscopic transnasal pituitary surgery. Curr Opin Otolaryngol Head Neck Surg 2010;18:8–14.
29. Zhang Y, Want Z, Liu Y, et al. Endoscopic transsphenoidal treatment of pituitary adenomas. Neurol Res 2008;30:581–6.
30. Dehdashti AR, Ganna A, Karabatsou K, et al. Pure endoscopic endonasal approach for pituitary adenomas: early surgical results in 200 patients and comparison with previous microsurgical series. Neurosurg 2008;62:1006–15.
31. Montini P, Losa M, Barzaghi R, et al. Results of transsphenoidal surgery in a large series of patients with pituitary adenoma. Neurosurgery 2005;56:1222–33.
32. Stamm AC, Vellutini E, Harvey RJ, et al. Endoscopic transnasal craniotomy and the resection of craniopharyngioma. Laryngoscope 2008;118:1142–8.
33. De Divitiis E, Cavallo LM, Cappabianca P, et al. Extended endoscopic endonasal transsphenoidal approach for the removal of suprasellar tumors: part 2. Neurosurg 2007;60:46–58.

34. Laufer I, Anand VK, Schwartz TH. Endoscopic, endonasal extended transsphenoidal, transplanum transtuberculum approach for resection of suprasellar lesions. J Neurosurg 2007;106:400–6.
35. Frank G, Pasquini E, Doglietto F, et al. The endoscopic extended transsphenoidal approach for craniopharyngiomas. Neurosurg 2006;59(Suppl 1):ONS75–83.
36. Rudnick EF, DiNardo LJ. Image-guided endoscopic endonasal resection of a recurrent craniopharyngioma. Am J Otolaryngol 2006;27:266–7.
37. Rudnick A, Zawadzki T, Wojtacha M, et al. Endoscopic transnasal transsphenoidal treatment of pathology of the sellar region. Minim Invasive Neurosurg 2005;48:101–7.
38. Jho HD, Carrau RL. Endoscopic endonasal transsphenoidal surgery: experience with 50 patients. J Neurosurg 1997;87:44–51.
39. Cappabianca P, Cavallo LM, Colao A, et al. Endoscopic endonasal transsphenoidal approach: outcome analysis of 100 consecutive procedures. Minim Invasive Neurosurg 2002;45:193–200.
40. Zada G, Kelly DF, Cohan P, et al. Endonasal transsphenoidal approach for pituitary adenomas and other sellar lesions: an assessment of efficacy, safety, and patient impressions. J Neurosurg 2003;98:350–8.
41. Chakrabarti I, Amar AP, Couldwell W, et al. Long-term neurological, visual, and endocrine outcomes following transnasal resection of craniopharyngioma. J Neurosurg 2005;102:650–7.
42. Dusick JR, Esposito F, Kelly DF, et al. The extended direct endonasal transsphenoidal approach for non-adenomatous suprasellar tumors. J Neurosurg 2005; 102:832–41.
43. Laws ER, Kanter AS, Jane JA, et al. Extended transsphenoidal approach. J Neurosurg 2005;102:825–7.
44. Maira G, Anile C, Albanese A, et al. The role of transsphenoidal surgery in the treatment of craniopharyngiomas. J Neurosurg 2004;100:445–51.
45. Karabatsou K, O'Kelly C, Ganna A, et al. Outcomes and quality of life assessment in patients undergoing endoscopic surgery for pituitary adenomas. Br J Neurosurg 2008;22(5):630–5.
46. Gil Z, Abergel A, Spektor S, et al. Quality of life following surgery for anterior skull base tumors. Arch Otolaryngol Head Neck Surg 2003;129(12):1303–9.
47. Gil Z, Abergel A, Spektor S, et al. Patient, caregiver, and surgeon perceptions of quality of life following anterior skull base surgery. Arch Otolaryngol Head Neck Surg 2004;130:1276–81.
48. Woertgen C, Rothoerl RD, Hosemann W, et al. Quality of life following surgery for malignancies of the anterior skull base. Skull Base 2007;17(2):119–23.
49. Kelleher MO, Fernandes MF, Sim DW, et al. Health-related quality of life in patients with skull base tumors. Br J Neurosurg 2002;16:16–20.
50. Meyers CA, Geara F, Wong PF, et al. Neurocognitive effects of therapeutic irradiation for base of skull tumors. Int J Radiat Oncol Biol Phys 2000;46(1):51–5.
51. McHorney CA, Ware JE, Lu JF, et al. The MOS 36-item Short-Form Health Survey (SF-36): III: test of data quality, scaling assumptions, and reliability across diverse patient groups. Med Care 1994;32(1):40–66.
52. McHorney CA, Ware JE, Raczek AE. The MOS 36-item Short-Form Health Survey (SF-36): II. Psychometric and clinical tests of validity in measuring physical and mental health constructs. Med Care 1993;31(3):247–63.
53. Bergner M, Bobbitt RA, Pollard WE, et al. The sickness impact profile: validation of a health status measure. Med Care 1976;14(1):57–67.
54. Fitzpatrick R, Fletcher A, Gore S, et al. Quality of life measures in health care, I: applications and issues in assessment. BMJ 1992;305:1074–7.

55. Cronbach LJ. Essentials of psychological testing. 5th edition. New York: Harper and Row; 1990.
56. DeMonte F. Functional outcomes in skull base surgery. What is acceptable. Clin Neurosurg 2001;48:340–50.
57. Ringash J, Bezjak A. A structured review of quality of life instruments for head and neck cancer patients. Head Neck 2001;23:201–13.
58. Badia X, Webb SM, Prieto L, et al. Acromegaly quality of life questionnaire (Acro-QOL). Health Qual Life Outcomes 2004;2:13.
59. Gil Z, Abergel A, Spektor S, et al. Development of a cancer-specific anterior skull base quality of life questionnaire. J Neurosurg 2004;100:813–9.
60. Herschbach P, Henrich G, Strasburger CJ, et al. Development and psychometric properties of a disease-specific quality of life questionnaire for adult patients with growth hormone deficiency. Eur J Endocrinol 2001;145:255–65.
61. Kan P, Cusimano M. Validation of a quality of life questionnaire for patients with pituitary adenoma. Can J Neurol Sci 2006;33:80–5.
62. Lovas K, Curran S, Oksnes M, et al. Development of a disease-specific quality of life questionnaire in Addison's disease. J Clin Endocrinol Metab 2010;95(2):545–51.
63. McKenna SP, Doward LC, Alonso J, et al. The QoL-AGHDA: an instrument for the assessment of quality of life in adults with growth hormone deficiency. Qual Life Res 1999;8:373–83.
64. McMillan CV, Bradley C, Gibney J, et al. Preliminary development of the new individualized HDQOL questionnaire measuring quality of life in adult hypopituitarism. J Eval Clin Pract 2006;12(5):501–14.
65. Palme CE, Irish JC, Gullane PJ, et al. Quality of life analysis in patients with anterior skull base neoplasms. Head Neck 2009;31:1326–34.
66. Webb SM, Badia X, Barahona MJ, et al. Evaluation of health-related quality of life in patients with Cushing's syndrome with a new questionnaire. Eur J Endocrinol 2008;158:623–30.
67. de Almeida JR, Vescan AD, Ringash J, et al. Development of the University of Toronto Skull Base Inventory (UT-SBI) quality of life questionnaire. Skull Base 2009; 19(Suppl 3):043.
68. Shah J. Quality of life after skull base surgery: the patient's predicament. Skull Base 2010;20(1):3–4.
69. Patel SG, Singh B, Polluri A, et al. Craniofacial surgery for malignant skull base tumors: report of an international collaborative study. Cancer 2003;98:1179–87.
70. Patel SG. Internet-based multi-institutional clinical research: a new method to conduct and manage quality of life studies. Skull Base 2010;20(1):23–6.
71. O'Malley BW, Weinstein GS. Robotic skull base surgery: preclinical investigations to human clinical application. Arch Otolaryngol Head Neck Surg 2007;133(12): 1215–9.
72. O'Malley BW, Weinstein GS. Robotic anterior and midline skull base surgery: preclinical investigations. Int J Radiat Oncol Biol Phys 2007;69(Suppl 2):S125–8.
73. Hanna EY, Holsinger C, DeMonte F, et al. Robotic endoscopic surgery of the skull base: a novel surgical approach. Arch Otolaryngol Head Neck Surg 2007; 133(12):1209–14.

Reconstructive Options for Endoscopic Skull Base Surgery

Adam M. Zanation, MD[a],*, Brian D. Thorp, MD[a],
Priscilla Parmar, MD[b], Richard J. Harvey, MD[b]

KEYWORDS

- Reconstruction • Nasoseptal Flap • Endoscopic • Endonasal
- Skull Base • Septal • Septum • Local flap

EBM Question	Level of Evidence	Grade of Recommendation
How does endoscopic compare to open reconstruction of the skull base?	3a	C

Over the past 10 years, significant anatomic and technical advances coupled with improvements in instrumentation have facilitated the exposure and resection of a multitude of extradural and intradural skull base lesions via fully endoscopic expanded endonasal approaches (EEA). Endonasal skull base surgery encompasses a wide range of surgical pathology including everything from extradural benign tumors to sinonasal cancers to intradural primary brain tumors. When the outcomes of successful endonasal resection were first reported, the primary disadvantage documented was postoperative cerebrospinal fluid (CSF) leak secondary to intraoperative dural violation.

This article describes the sequential learning from initial free tissue grafting reconstructive techniques to the current use of vascularized flaps. Outcomes and limitations of current endoscopic reconstructive techniques are discussed. The pathophysiology

Disclosure Statement: The authors have no conflicts of interest.
[a] Department of Otolaryngology/Head and Neck Surgery, University of North Carolina at Chapel Hill, CB 7070, Physicians Office Building Manning Drive, Chapel Hill, NC 27599, USA
[b] Department of Otolaryngology and Skull Base Surgery, University of New South Wales and Macquarie University, St Vincent's Hospital, 354 Victoria Street, Sydney 2010, New South Wales, Australia
* Corresponding author.
E-mail address: adam_zanation@med.unc.edu

of idiopathic CSF leak as treatment is well documented and differs from that of surgical skull base defects, thus is not discussed here.

PATHOPHYSIOLOGY

Reconstruction of the skull base directly relates to the nature of the surgical defect with differing goals between surgical groups. For example, many extradural tumor resections necessitate reconstruction to promote healing (especially in the setting of radiation therapy). In these cases, primary reconstructive goals are not avoidance of postoperative CSF leak and potential intracranial infection, but rather defect coverage to facilitate healing. This is in contrast to intradural surgery, as postoperative CSF leak and potential intracranial infection must be taken into consideration. Intradural tumor surgery can be divided into 2 main groups:

1. Intradural, but extra-arachnoidal, as is the case with pituitary surgery when the diaphragm is not violated
2. Intra-arachnoidal surgery where by definition an intraoperative CSF leak is appreciated 100% of the time.

Intra-arachnoidal surgery can be further divided into high-flow and low-flow leaks depending on whether a cistern was directly opened into the sinonasal defect. In addition to anatomic considerations, other important factors that must be noted when approaching reconstruction are the size of the dural defect, the nature of the patient's CSF pressure, obesity, and states of poor healing such as Cushing disease and prior irradiation.

The underlying, foundational goals of surgical defect reconstruction in endonasal skull base surgery are identical to those of conventional external approaches, ie, to completely separate the cranial cavity from the sinonasal tract, eliminate dead space, and preserve neurovascular and ocular function.[1] The principle of a multilayered reconstruction to reestablish tissue barriers is also preserved. Using endonasal pedicled vascular flaps and a reconstruction based on the aforementioned principles, postoperative CSF leak rates are now below 5%, a figure comparable to that reported for open cranial base reconstructive techniques.

CLINICAL PRESENTATION

Postoperative CSF leaks are typically noted within a week following surgery. The patient's history is most suggestive and often diagnostic. Primary symptoms include persistent, often salty tasting, rhinorrhea. Primary physical examination findings include a positive reservoir sign and increased rhinorrhea with Valsava maneuver. Sinonasal endoscopy should be performed and at times the leak can be confirmed or localized; however, in the early postoperative period absorbable packing often remains in place rendering visualization of the skull base defect difficult. Mental status changes are not common findings unless the patient has worsening pneumocephalous, a finding identified on computed tomography (CT) scan. It is important to note that Beta-2 transferrin can be used as a confirmatory test; however, in the early postoperative period the history and physical examination are diagnostic. Intermediate timed CSF leaks (2 to 6 weeks postoperative) are less common and usually present with intermittent low flow leaking episodes from a pinpoint dural opening. Late CSF leaks (more than 6 weeks postoperative) are very rare and are usually seen with patient noncompliance (hard nose blowing) or radionecrosis.

MANAGEMENT
Endoscopic Reconstruction with Free Tissue Grafts

Before the adoption of vascularized tissue flaps as our primary reconstructive technique (see later in this article) skull base reconstruction after EEA was limited to the use of free tissue grafts. These techniques were adapted from experience accumulated with the endoscopic repair of CSF leaks associated with endoscopic sinus surgery and trauma,[2] and then expanded to repair larger dural defects as well as defects over high-flow intraoperative CSF leaks. As with any reconstruction, a multilayer approach with complete defect coverage is the key to an endoscopic dural reconstruction.

First, a subdural inlay graft (between the brain and the dura) of collagen matrix (Duragen, Integra Life Sciences, Plainsboro, NJ, USA) is placed; this helps to obliterate the intradural dead space. Its pliability and texture allows for safe manipulation around neurovascular structures. Ideally, this subdural graft should extend 5 to 10 mm beyond the dural margins in all directions. A subsequent inlay graft of acellular dermis (AlloDerm Life Cell, Branchburg, NJ, USA) is then placed in the epidural space (between the dura and the skull base). Occasionally, the bony ledges of the defect are not adequate to support an inlay graft; therefore, the acellular dermal graft is placed extracranially (at the nasal side of the defect) as an onlay graft. All the edges of the defect should be denuded of mucosa to allow for revascularization of the graft and to avoid mucocele formation. Alternatively, this graft can be sutured to the dura with nitinol U-clips (Medtronic U-Clips, Memphis, TN), placement of which is technically challenging. Importantly, U-clips provide anchor points to prevent migration of the graft, but do not result in a water-tight suture line.

Although this is an off-label indication for the acellular dermal graft, we have found that the handling characteristics, availability (no need for skin graft harvesting), and ingrowth of the patient's own tissue with rapid epithelialization are advantages that outweigh its cost. When using this technique, it is important to use a single graft with dimensions extending beyond the defect margins in all directions, and ensure the graft is adequately hydrated in normal saline solution before its insertion. In our experience, a thinner graft offers the best take, although it is somewhat difficult to manipulate endonasally.

Once both grafts are in place, the edges of the AlloDerm are bolstered intranasally with oxidized cellulose (absorbable packing). A biologic or synthetic glue is then sprayed or applied over the edges and absorbable gelatin sponge squares are used to further bolster the reconstruction. These layers of absorbable packing accomplish 3 goals. First, they fix the grafts in place and protect them from changes in airflow within the nose. Second, these layers allow for "filling" of the concavities and convexities of the skull base to better distribute the pressure of removable packing on the underlying grafts. Third, the absorbable packing protects the grafts from movement during removal of nonabsorbable packing that typically occurs 3 to 5 days postoperatively, as later described. We then use the balloon of a 12-French Foley catheter or 10-cm expandable sponge packing to stabilize and bolster the inlay/onlay grafts, further preventing early brain herniation. Placement and inflation of the balloon catheter using 10 mL of saline is performed under direct endoscopic visualization. Care is taken to avoid overinflation, as this may result in compressive effects over the intracranial structures. Moreover, if the optic nerves or chiasm are exposed during the dissection, Foley placement is avoided, as the balloon may exert too much pressure on these structures. Instead, expandable sponge packing is used. Any nonabsorbable nasal packing or balloon is removed 3 to 5 days after the EEA.

For moderate-sized skull base defects, we have also used an onlay free mucosal graft harvested from the resected middle turbinate instead of an AlloDerm graft. The remainder of the reconstructive procedure is as described previously. The take of the free mucosal grafts is excellent; however, use is limited by size and the fact that they can be used only as onlay grafts. Last, abdominal free fat is mainly used as a bolster or biologic dressing to the multilayered reconstruction. Fat can also be used to obliterate spaces such as the clival recess or a nasopharyngeal defect after a transnasal approach to the anterior spine. Harvesting abdominal fat has the added morbidity of an abdominal incision, scar, and the potential for infection, hematoma, or seroma formation.

Endoscopic reconstruction with multilayered free tissue grafts for larger dural defects during skull base tumor cases historically resulted in postoperative CSF leak rates of 20% to 30%.[3] These leaks were usually managed with further endoscopic bolstering and some required CSF diversion for 3 to 5 days with lumbar drainage (see later in this article for further details). It is important to note that when managed with endoscopic revisions, it was clear that most of the CSF leaks were a result of graft migration or CSF fistula formation in the most dependent area of the flap. Given the unacceptably high CSF leak rate of 20% to 30% for skull base tumor resections with grafting reconstruction, vascularized tissue options were sought to reduce this incidence.

Endoscopic Reconstruction with Vascular Pedicled Flaps

Technique: nasoseptal flap (Hadad-Bassagastegay flap)

In most recent months, the use of a vascular pedicle flap has become the preferred skull base reconstruction. The most commonly used technique is a vascular flap of the nasal septum mucoperiosteum and mucoperichondrium that is pedicled on the nasoseptal artery, a branch of the posterior septal artery, which is one of the terminal branches of the internal maxillary artery.[3]

The nasal cavity is decongested with 0.05% oxymetazoline on pledgets and the nasal septum is infiltrated with 0.5% to 1.0% lidocaine with 1:100,000 to 1:200,000 epinephrine. The inferior and middle turbinates are out-fractured to allow visualization of the entire height of the nasal septum from the olfactory sulcus to the nasal floor.

To facilitate a bimanual technique during the EEA, we usually elect to remove one of the middle turbinates, usually the right. Additionally, resection of the middle turbinate facilitates visualization of the nasoseptal flap (NSF) vascular pedicle and ipsilateral elevation of the septal flap.

The side of the flap (right or left) is determined by several factors:

- If the lesion requires dissection of the lateral pterygoid recess or the pterygomaxillary fossa, then the vascular supply of the flap will be compromised; thus, a flap on the opposite side is used.
- Similarly, lesions that invade the rostrum of the sphenoid or the septal mucoperiosteum will mandate harvesting a contralateral NSF.
- If the lesion is in the midline, and no significant lateral dissection is required, then sharp or large septal spurs (conferring a risk for perforation of the flap during dissection) may dictate the side from which the flap is harvested.
- Last, all things being equal, the right side is usually an easier dissection for the right-handed surgeon, especially in the setting of right middle turbinate removal.

The flap is designed according to the size and shape of the anticipated defect, although it is best to overestimate the size and then trim the flap if needed.

Two parallel incisions are performed following the sagittal plane of the septum, one over the maxillary crest and the other 1 to 2 cm below the most superior aspect of the septum, thereby preserving the olfactory epithelium (**Figs. 1** and **2**A, B). These

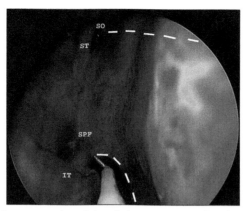

Fig. 1. Planned incisions around pedicle of the nasoseptal flap (*dashedline*). IT, inferior turbinate; ST, superior turbinate; SO, sphenoid ostium; SPF, mucosa over the sphenopalatine foramen.

incisions are joined anteriorly by a vertical incision at a level that is anterior to the plane of the anterior head of the inferior turbinate (see **Fig. 2C**). These incisions may be modified to account for the specific area of reconstruction or to allow for adequate oncologic margins.

At the posterior septum, the superior incision is extended laterally with an inferior slant over the rostrum of the sphenoid sinus, crossing it horizontally at the level of the natural ostium (see **Fig. 1**).

The inferior incision is extended superiorly along the free posterior edge of the nasal septum and then laterally to cross the posterior choana below the floor of the sphenoid sinus.

Elevation of the NSF begins anteriorly with a Cottle dissector or a small suction dissector (see **Fig. 2D, E**). It is advantageous to complete all incisions before elevating the flap because it becomes difficult to orient the tissue and maintain it at tension once it has been elevated. Septal incisions may be completed with scissors or other sharp instruments as necessary. Elevation of the flap from the anterior face of the sphenoid sinus is completed with preservation of its posterolateral neurovascular pedicle (see **Fig. 2F**).

The flap is then placed in the nasopharynx or maxillary sinus until it is needed at the end of the procedure for reconstruction. Multiple dimensional modifications are possible. The entire ipsilateral mucoperiosteum and mucoperichondrium may be harvested to cover anterior skull base defects as extensive as those that include the area from the posterior wall of the frontal sinus to the sella turcica and from orbit to orbit.

Additionally, a wider flap may be harvested by extending the incision to include the mucoperiosteum of the floor of the nose.

A radioanatomic study of the nasoseptal flap compared the relative size of the anterior skull base to the size of potential nasoseptal flaps, and demonstrated that most anterior skull base defects can be completely covered with the nasoseptal flap (**Fig. 3**).[4,5]

Additional considerations must be taken into account when reconstructing pediatric skull base defects with the NSF. It is clear that before age 10 years, the NSF area is significantly smaller than the area of larger, age-corresponding skull base defects (such as a transcribriform defect). Between the ages of 10 and 14, the NSF area approaches 100% of the size but not larger.[5] This size discrepancy is because cranial

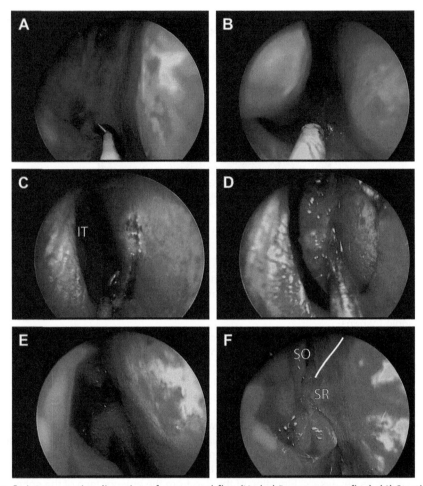

Fig. 2. Intraoperative dissection of nasoseptal flap (Hadad-Bassagastegay flap). (*A*) Starting the incision crossing the posterior choana. (*B*) Continuing the inferior incision along the nasal floor. (*C*) Connecting the inferior and superior incisions via a vertical incision anterior to the inferior turbinate (IT). (*D*) Starting to dissect the anterior nasoseptal flap. (*E*) Continuing to dissect the nasoseptal flap from the underlying septal cartilage. (*F*) Final posterior dissection of the flap along area of the pedicle over the sphenoid rostrum (SR). The white line represents the area of the superior incision as it continues right below the sphenoid ostium (SO).

growth occurs earlier in life and septal growth does not occur until puberty when mid-face growth accelerates.[5] Bilateral flaps are conceptually possible; however, they are rarely used. During surgery, it is important to be careful with bone removal lateral to the pterygoid canal so that the vascular pedicle is not injured.

Once the extirpative portion of the procedure is complete (**Fig. 4**A), a multilayer cranial base repair is performed (see **Fig. 4**). An inlay collagen matrix (Duragen, Integra Life Sciences or DuraMatrix Onlay, Styker, Kalamazoo, MI, USA) is placed as described previously (see **Fig. 4**B). The NSF is then placed as an onlay, over the bony edges of the cranial base defect (see **Fig. 4**C). All mucosa is removed from around the defect before the flap is placed to promote healing and prevent mucocele

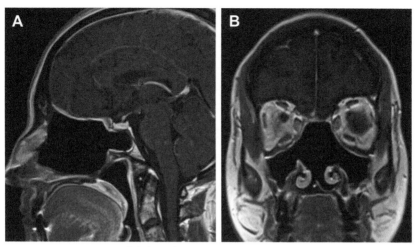

Fig. 3. Postoperative sagittal (*A*) and coronal (*B*) T1 with contrast magnetic resonance imaging (MRI). An anterior transcribriform skull base resection with excellent NS flap reconstruction.

formation. After the collagen graft and flap are in place, the edges of the flap are bolstered intranasally with oxidized cellulose absorbable packing (see **Fig. 4D**); Duraseal (Confluent Surgical Inc, Waltham, MA, USA) is then placed (see **Fig. 4E**). It is critical to separate the grafts from the nonabsorbable packing using some type of nonadherent material, such as absorbable gelatin sponge or absorbable gelatin film, as this will prevent traction on the grafts when the packing is removed (see **Fig. 4F**). Shifting of the underlying inlay/onlay grafts may occur during the placement of the packing; thus, the surgeon must be vigilant and perform placement under direct visualization with the endoscope. Packing materials include either a Foley balloon or expandable tampon-type packing sponges as described previously. Sealants are never used between the grafts or under the flap, as this prevents direct tissue contact and healing. Packing is kept in place for 3 to 5 days postoperatively.

After adoption of the NSF for the reconstruction of EEA defects, postoperative CSF leak rates dropped considerably to less than 5% for all endonasal defects, a rate that compares with that of traditional open techniques.[3,6] In fact, in a prospective series of 70 NSF skull base reconstructions for high-flow leaks with large dural defects (either the cistern or ventricle was widely opened into the nasal cavity during the dissection), the observed postoperative leak rate was 5.7% (4/70).[7] A clear advantage of the NSF as a reconstructive option is endoscopic graft harvest, thereby avoiding a second approach or incision. A major drawback of the NSF is that its need must be anticipated before embarking on the resection, as the vascular pedicle of this flap is frequently compromised during sphenoidotomy and/or posterior septectomy. In addition, if a revision procedure is necessary, the flap may have been used previously or the pedicle previously damaged; therefore, 2 other pedicled flap options have been described and are reviewed later in this article. In selected revision cases, the NSF can be dissected from the defect and reused. In a series of 20 NSF takedowns and reuses for staged procedures or recurrence, 1 (5%) of 20 reconstructions leaked.[8] There were no flap deaths during takedown and reuse. Healing of the intranasal dissection and nasoseptal flap reconstruction is usually completed in 6 to 12 weeks (see **Fig. 3**, **Fig. 5**).

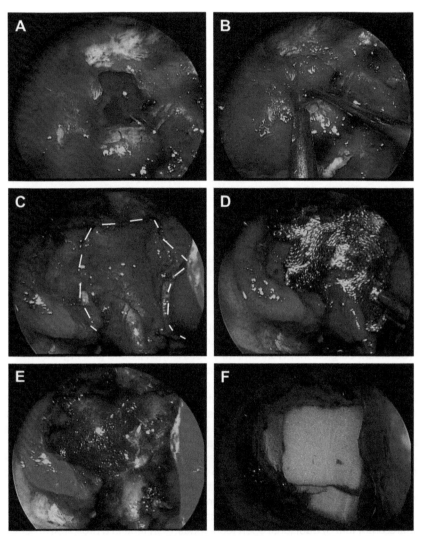

Fig. 4. Placement of nasoseptal flap (Hadad-Bassagastegay flap). (*A*) A transsellar and transplanar skull base defect over the area of the suprasellar cistern. (*B*) A collagen matrix inlay graft. (*C*) Placement of the nasoseptal flap over the entire defect and over the denuded surrounding bone (*dashedline*). (*D*) The edges of the flap are bolstered intranasally with oxidized cellulose absorbable packing. (*E*) Duraseal placement. (*F*) Absorbable gelatin sponge placed. This will prevent traction on the repair when the nonabsorbable packing is removed.

Technique: posterior pedicled inferior turbinate flap

In patients with prior septectomy or prior wide sphenoidotomies, the NSF blood supply has been interrupted and this option cannot be used. Other options such as free grafting or other locoregional vascular pedicle flaps have to be considered. The posterior pedicle inferior turbinate flap (PPITF) is based on the inferior turbinate artery, a terminal branch of the posterior lateral nasal artery (PLNA), which arises from the sphenopalatine artery (SPA).[9] For the design and harvesting of the PPITF, the anatomic course of the PLNA has to be understood.[9] The PLNA runs in a descending

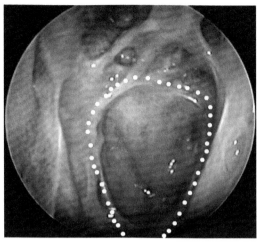

Fig. 5. Healed nasoseptal flap over a transsellar and transclival defect (*dotted line*).

vertical or anteroinferior course over the perpendicular plate of the ascending process of the palatine bone, giving a branch medially to supply the middle turbinate. As the artery courses inferiorly, it enters the inferior turbinate on the superior aspect of its lateral attachment, approximately 1.0 to 1.5 cm from its posterior tip.[10] Some have found that the artery may lie within the bone (50%), within the soft tissue (14%), or follow a mixed pattern (36%).[11] The artery runs for some distance (mean of 1.2 cm) before piercing the bone and soft tissue and splitting off into between 2 and 6 branches.[11]

The nasal cavity is decongested and the lateral nasal wall, just anterior to the inferior turbinate, is injected with a solution of 1% lidocaine with 1:100,000 epinephrine. We harvest the PPITF after completion of the EEA. This should be performed ipsilateral to the defect whenever possible to minimize the distance of the pedicle to the defect. Initially, the inferior turbinate is gently medialized to better expose the entire medial surface of the inferior turbinate. Given that this flap is substantially smaller when compared with the NSF, it is best to harvest the entire turbinate to ensure adequate coverage (**Fig. 6**A). A wider flap may be harvested by extending the lower incision to include the lateral mucoperiosteum of the turbinate and even the middle meatus. The first step is to identify the SPA as it exits the sphenopalatine foramen and follow it distally to identify the PLNA. The flap will be based solely on this vascular pedicle. Two parallel incisions are performed endoscopically following the sagittal plane of the inferior turbinate, one superiorly just above the inferior turbinate and the other inferiorly following the caudal margin of the inferior turbinate (see **Fig. 6**A). A vertical incision, placed over the anterior head of the inferior turbinate, connects the 2 previously performed incisions (see **Fig. 6**B). The mucoperiosteum is then elevated, starting at the anterior aspect of the inferior turbinate. A variable amount of bone may also be elevated, depending on the ease of dissecting the mucoperiosteum from the underlying bone. Care must be taken to avoid injuring the vascular pedicle as it enters at the superior aspect of its lateral attachment, approximately 1.0 to1.5 cm from its posterior tip. In addition, it is important to preserve the lateral nasal artery as it descends vertically over the ascending process of the palatine bone. It may course anteriorly to the posterior wall of the maxillary sinus; therefore, this should be considered when extending the maxillary antrostomy posteriorly. Once harvested, the flap is

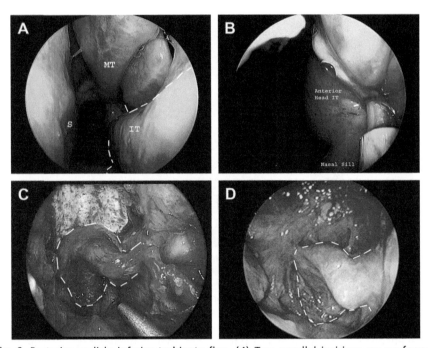

Fig. 6. Posterior pedicle inferior turbinate flap. (*A*) Two parallel incisions are performed endoscopically following the sagittal plane of the inferior turbinate, the superior one just above the inferior turbinate and the inferior one following the caudal margin of the turbinate (*dashed line*). IT, inferior turbinate; MT, middle turbinate; S, septum. (*B*) A vertical incision, placed over the anterior head of the inferior turbinate, connects the 2 previous incisions. (*C*) Posterior pedicle inferior turbinate flap placed over a clival defect (*dashed line*). (*D*) Healed posterior pedicle inferior turbinate flap (*dashed line*).

gently unrolled and mobilized to cover the skull base defect (see **Fig. 6**C). The PPITF can be applied directly to dura or denuded bone or may be used over a fat graft. However, it is critical that the vascularized flap be in direct contact with the margins of the defect and any nonvascularized tissue between the margins of the defect and the flap must be meticulously removed. Biologic glue is applied over the flap, absorbable gelatin sponges are placed, and sponge nasal packing or the balloon of a 12-French Foley catheter is inserted to press the PPITF against the defect. Silicone nasal splints are used to protect the denuded lateral wall and are left in place for approximately 10 to 21 days postoperatively. According to an anatomic analysis of the anteriorly based inferior turbinate flap, the mucosal surface area is approximately 4.97 cm^2 (2.8 cm length with 1.7 cm width).[12] Endoscopic analysis of the PPITF reveals that approximately 60% of the anterior cranial fossa can be covered.[13] Although this may represent suboptimal coverage in some, the ability to bring vascular tissue into the repair and augment with free grafts may be sufficient in many cases (**Fig. 7**). Bilateral flaps can be harvested to cover larger defects.

The flap's shorter length and limited arch of rotation in comparison with the NSF limits its use. The PPITF is best suited for posterior defects of the sella or parasellar and midclival areas, as far anterior skull base reconstructions are limited by flap size. Another disadvantage of using the PPITF is the formation of crusting over the inferior turbinate bone in the postoperative period. Mucosalization of the donor site was observed after a period of 3 to 4 weeks (see **Fig. 6**D).[5]

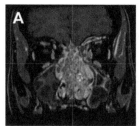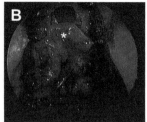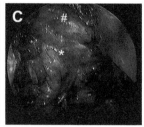

Fig. 7. Posterior pedicle inferior turbinate flap (ITPF). A SCC of the nasal septum with anterior cranial fossa involvement (*A*). The ITPF (#) manages to cover 60% of the defect (*B*) with free mucosal grafts (*) augmenting the repair (*C*). The pericranial flap would be used if this was not sufficient or failed. Bringing vascularized tissue (*) to the repair may be as important as the concept of complete coverage.

Technique: posterior pedicled middle turbinate flap

The posterior pedicled middle turbinate flap (PPMTF) is another local flap available for reconstruction of anterior skull base defects. The middle turbinate (MT) attaches to the lateral nasal wall at its anterior and posterior segments. Between these insertions, it attaches to the skull base at the vertical lamella of the cribriform plate. The anatomic description of the vasculature around the lateral nasal wall has been described previously. Cadaver studies have shown that the MT draws its blood supply from a branch of the sphenopalatine artery that courses through the posterior attachment.[14] It is this artery that serves as the pedicle for the PPMTF.

The flap is harvested by first making a vertical incision along the anterior face of the MT head. A second incision is made horizontally along the vertical attachment of the turbinate just below the skull base, in an anterior to posterior direction. The mucoperiosteum is then raised from the medial face of the MT in a superior to inferior direction. Thin bone of the middle turbinate is carefully removed from the inner aspect of the flap. The bony vertical attachment of the turbinate is then transected from the skull base. Once the bone is removed, the lateral attachment of the flap to the skull base is sharply released. Further elevation of the flap posteriorly and the transection of the basal lamella yields a posteriorly pedicled flap. The pedicle is further dissected to allow for a better arc of rotation and extended length.

One of the limitations of the PPMTF is the technical difficulty associated with elevating the flap. It becomes a more challenging task when anatomic variations, such as concha bullosa, paradoxic turbinate, or hypoplasia are seen. The dimensions of middle turbinates vary greatly. The mean area of the PPMTF is somewhat limited at 5.6 cm^2, which is comparable with the PPITF.[14] However, further comparison of the PPMTF with the PPITF reveals that the more superior position of its pedicle allows the PPMTF to reach defects of the planum sphenoidale, sella, and fovea ethmoidalis better than the PPITF. To date, the PPMTF has been used sparingly as a secondary option if an NSF is not available and the defect is not too large. The middle turbinate flap is most useful for reconstruction of limited defects of the planum sphenoidale, cribriform plate, or sella, but can be also be used to reconstruct defects of the clivus.

Technique: endoscopic-assisted pericranial flap

The pericranial flap (PCF) has been one of the most commonly used reconstructive options for traditional open anterior cranial base procedures. It is an axial flap based on the supraorbital and supratrochlear arteries, which yields large, durable vascularized tissue that can cover the entire skull base (**Fig. 8**A). However, the use of the

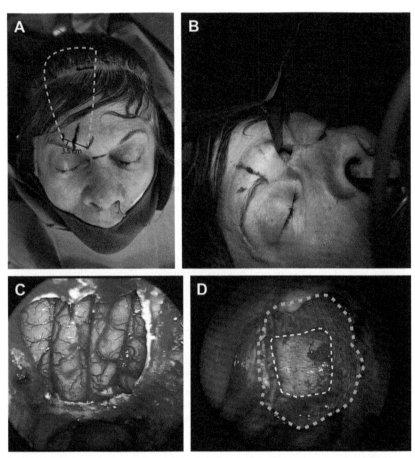

Fig. 8. Minimally invasive pericranial flap. (*A*) Planned endoscopic pericranial flap incisions from a unilateral 3-cm pedicle (*dashed line*). (*B*) Pericranial flap rotated from beneath the scalp out a 1-cm glabellar incision. (*C*) Transcribriform defect from esthesioneuroblastoma. (*D*) Reconstruction of the defect with significant overlay of the defect in Fig. 8C (*dashed line*).

PCF became limited with the advent of endoscopic skull base techniques, because of an inability to incorporate the externally harvested flap into the nasal cavity. By developing a technique that allows endoscopic harvest and transposes the flap through a bony window at the nasion, the PCF was reintroduced into the armamentarium of skull base reconstruction options.[15]

A 2-cm midline incision and a 1-cm lateral port incision are made along the coronal plane of the scalp (see **Fig. 8**A). The supraorbital and supratrochlear arteries are located by Doppler ultrasound, and a 3-cm-wide flap pedicle is marked at the level of the supraorbital rim (see **Fig. 8**A). A subgaleal plane dissection is performed through the vertex incisions extending to the vascular pedicle. The pericranium is incised with electrocautery to the desired width and then elevated from the underlying bone down to the level of the pedicle.

A 1-cm transverse glabellar incision is made and dissection down to the level of the periosteum of the nasion is performed. A subperiosteal plane is developed, communicating it with the subperiosteal plane of the flap dissection. The bone over the nasion is then drilled to form a horizontal channel that enters into the nasal cavity. The PCF is transposed through the glabellar incision (see **Fig. 8**B) and then into the endonasal surgical field via the nasionectomy. Care must be taken not to twist the flap as it passes through the glabellar incision. The flap should be applied to the skull base defect as it would in an open approach with the superficial surface of the flap in contact with the dural defect (see **Fig. 8**C, D). The flap is then bolstered into place as described previously for the nasoseptal flap reconstruction. Additionally, the PCF may be harvested with a bicoronal incision instead of with endoscopic assistance to avoid a glabellar incision.

The endoscopic-assisted PCF is ideal for endoscopic reconstruction of the anterior cranial base given its pedicle location. It is well suited for reconstruction of cribriform and planar defects and can be extended to cover defects of the sella. The length of the flap can be extended by placing the incisions further posterior on the scalp or by dissecting posterior to the incisions.

From April 2008 (when the first endoscopic PCF was performed) until December 2008, 10 cases of endonasal skull base reconstruction with the pericranial flap have been performed without a postoperative leak.[16] Moreover, the pericranial flap healed without any complication in 3 patients who had previous radiation treatment. Additionally, the reconstruction withstood treatment in 5 patients who required postoperative radiation.

Technique: temporoparietal fascial flap

The temporoparietal fascia flap (TPFF) has been used extensively in various head and neck reconstructive procedures and its anatomy is well described. This section describes the use of the TPFF in endoscopic skull base reconstruction.[17] This flap is used when no viable endonasal options are available for reconstruction of clival and parasellar defects.

The temporoparietal fascia (TPF) is a strong fascial layer that is connected to the overlying fibrous septae of subcutaneous tissue. Blood supply for the TPF comes from the superficial temporal artery (STA), one of the terminal branches of the external carotid artery. It courses through the retromandibular parotid gland, crosses the posterior root of the zygomatic process, and becomes incorporated into the temporal fascia at the level of the zygomatic arch. The average diameter of the vessel is 2.73 mm over the zygomatic arch, and the mean distance between the STA and the tragus is 16.68 mm.[10] In most patients, the STA divides into an anterior frontal and a posterior parietal branch at the level of the zygomatic arch (61%–88%); however, the bifurcation point can vary considerably with branching occurring superior to the arch (4%–26%) or inferior to the arch (7%–12%).[17–19] One or 2 veins accompany the STA, which lies deep to these venous structures.[10] The frontal branch of the facial nerve courses just under the TPF after it crosses the superficial surface of the zygomatic arch.[20] The TPF is 2 to 3 mm in thickness over the parietal region and extends in a fanlike manner from the preauricular region, comprising a surface area as large as 17 $\times$ 14 cm.[21]

Harvesting and transposition of the TPFF to the nasal cavity is performed after the EEA dissection is complete so the defect size is known. It may be harvested from either side of the scalp, but we most commonly use the side that is ipsilateral to the defect. Previous incisions over the area of the flap may alter the laterality of harvest.

If not performed previously as a part of the EEA, an anterior and posterior ethmoidectomy and a large maxillary antrostomy are performed. Then, the SPA and posterior nasal artery are clipped at the level of the sphenopalatine foramen. A retrograde dissection of the SPA serves to remove the posterior wall of the maxillary sinus, thus exposing the pterygopalatine fossa (PPF). In addition, a portion of the lateral wall of the maxillary sinus is removed to open a wide communication with the infratemporal fossa (ITF). The descending palatine artery is identified in its inferior vertical trajectory from the internal maxillary artery (IMA) and is dissected from its canal. This allows inferior and lateral displacement of the contents of the upper PPF, thereby exposing the pterygoid plates. The pterygopalatine ganglion may be preserved, but the vidian nerve must be divided to allow displacement of the ganglion. The anterior aspect of the pterygoid plates is then reduced with a high-speed drill to enlarge the space for transposition of the TPFF.

A TPFF is harvested from the ipsilateral side using a conventional technique. A hemicoronal incision is carried down to the level of the hair follicles. Care must be taken to avoid injuring the pedicle during the hemicoronal incision as the STA lies directly under the skin within the subcutaneous tissues. Dissection of the TPF from the subcutaneous tissue effectively elevates the flap. Once enough surface area is exposed, the fascia is incised at its lateral margins and elevated from the cranium and deep temporal fascia down to its pedicle. The superficial layer of the deep temporal fascia is incised vertically, and the fascia is separated from the muscle following this plane of dissection inferiorly to elevate the periosteum from the surface of the zygomatic arch. This creates a wide tunnel beneath the superficial layer of the deep temporalis fascia that will accept the passage of the pedicle without compression. To help the transposition of the TPFF, a lateral canthotomy incision is used to expose and separate the temporalis muscle from the lateral orbital wall and pterygomaxillary fissure, creating a tunnel that communicates the temporal, infratemporal fossa, and endoscopic transpterygoid approach. The soft tissue tunnel is sequentially dilated by passing a guide wire into the nose under endonasal endoscopic visualization and then advancing percutaneous tracheotomy dilators over the wire. After an adequate tunnel is created, the dilators are removed, and the flap is tied to the external end of the guide wire. As the nasal end of the guide wire is pulled out through the nostril, the flap follows in tow through the tunnel into the nasal cavity. The mobilization of the flap through the tunnel is assisted with external manipulation with care taken to avoid rotation of the flap because this may compromise its blood supply. The external incisions are closed with a running nylon stitch after insertion of a suction drain. The reconstruction of the skull base begins with the placement of an inlay graft of a collagen matrix. The edges of the defect are refreshed, and the TPFF is placed over the defect. A sealant may be used after the flap is in position. The flap is then covered with absorbable gelatin sponges, and a sponge packing is placed to stabilize the flap. Packing is removed 3 to 5 days later.

Advantages of the TPFF include a large tissue area, vascularized tissue from a nonradiated field in the setting of sinonasal or skull base radiotherapy, and pliability with sufficient thickness for ample reconstruction. Disadvantages of this technique include the need for an external approach and a surgical scar, risk of alopecia, risk to the frontal branch of the facial nerve, and the need for an associated EEA access to the infratemporal fossa.

Pedicled palatal mucosal flap

The intranasal pedicled flaps described thus far use terminal branches of the sphenopalatine artery arising from the internal maxillary artery system. We have recently described a pedicled flap based on the descending palatine artery, which also arises from the internal maxillary artery. The pedicled palatal flap can be used in skull base reconstruction by transposing the vascularized mucoperiosteal tissue of the hard palate into the nasal cavity through the greater palatine foramen.[22] This flap is considered a last resort if other tissue options are not available, owing to the potential donor site morbidity and current clinical inexperience.

Patient Factors for High-Risk Postoperative CSF Leak Potential

1. Body habitus of the patient. Large body mass is associated with high ventricular pressure.
2. Pathology being treated, especially craniopharyngiomas and lesions involving the cisterns.
3. Entry into arachnoid cisterns or ventricles.
4. Site and size of the defect. Defects in the anterior cranial base are much more likely to leak than clival defects.
5. Patients with Cushing disease with extrasellar adrenocorticotropic hormone–secreting tumors, likely owing to the poor state of tissue healing in these patients.
6. Patients with no vascularized tissue reconstructive options owing to prior surgery or chemoradiotherapy.

Lumbar CSF Drainage

Lumbar spinal drains are not routinely used in the postoperative period after EEA except in cases of a significant intraoperative high-flow CSF leak. Patients with postoperative leak are routinely taken directly back to the operating room for endoscopic exploration and repair. If at that time, the patient is noted to have a high-flow leak, a spinal lumbar drain is considered. CSF diversion is usually continued for 3 to 5 days, using intermittent drainage of 50 mL of CSF every 8 hours. This is preferable to leaving the lumbar drain open to gravity, as excessive CSF drainage may occur with changes in patient position. Rarely, patients have a refractory CSF leak that persists after endoscopic reexploration, repair, and spinal lumbar drain. In these situations, the CSF pressure is measured, and if high-pressure hydrocephalus is noted, permanent CSF shunting is considered.

Skull Base Reconstructive Algorithm

Clearly there are a significant number of free graft and vascularized tissue options for reconstruction of large skull base defects. So the question is: How to choose? Following is a brief description of a more complex algorithm[23] that guides the surgeon through which options are most ideal.

First, if there is an intraoperative CSF leak, the quality of the leak must be determined. If the leak is a low-flow leak, then the defect site and size will determine the vascular tissue flap needed. If the leak is a high-flow leak, then the defect site alone guides reconstruction.

The advantages of each vascular tissue flap based on the size and site are discussed later in this article and are outlined in **Table 1**. The NSF may be applied to any skull base defect and size. The PPITF excels in the reconstruction of small clival defects. If the surgeon is forced to reconstruct defects larger than 1 cm, then a fat bolster is needed. Because of limitations in pedicle length, the PPITF cannot reach the anterior cranial fossa or sella area. The PCF has an extended pedicle that supports reconstruction from the anterior cranial fossa to the sella, but reconstruction of the posterior skull base is limited. The TPFF is ideal for clival and parasellar defects. The TPFF is an inadequate choice for anterior skull base defects owing to limitations in the arc of rotation necessary to tunnel the pedicle through the pterygopalatine fossa. The 2 remaining vascular tissue flaps are more difficult to harvest and have specific indications. The first is the PPMTF. The flap is small, difficult to elevate, and

Table 1
Intranasal and regional vascular flaps available for skull base reconstruction

Location	Vascular Tissue Flap	Pedicle	Comments/Limitations
Intranasal Vascular Tissue Flap	NSF	Sphenopalatine artery	• Ideal for all skull base reconstructions
	ITF	Inferior turbinate artery[a]	• Good for small clival defects • Cannot reach ACF or sella
	MTF	Middle turbinate artery[a]	• Good for small ACF or transphenoidal defects • Small in size • Thin mucosa • Difficult to elevate
Regional Vascular Tissue Flap	PCF	Supraorbital & supratrochlear artery	• Hearty flap with versatile dimensions • Extends from ACF to sella, but not to posterior skull base
	TPFF	Superficial temporal artery	• Good for clival or parasellar defects • 90° pedicle rotation limits reconstruction of ACF
	PF	Greater palatine artery	• Theoretical flap that reaches all areas of skull base • 3-cm pedicle, but difficult to dissect • Experience

Abbreviations: ACF, anterior cranial fossa; ITF, inferior turbinate flap; MTF, middle turbinate flap; NSF, nasoseptal flap; PCF, pericranial flap; PF, palatal flap; TPFF, temporoparietal fascia flap.
[a] Terminal branch of the posterior lateral nasal artery of the sphenopalatine artery.

is composed of a thin mucosa layer. Nevertheless, the flap is good for reconstruction of small (smaller than 1 cm) transphenoidal and anterior cranial fossa defects. The second is the palatal flap. In theory, this flap can reach all areas of the skull base given its 3-cm pedicle, but dissection of the palatine canals is difficult and clinical experience is limited. This flap is a last-line vascular tissue option because of surgical inexperience as well as potential oral cavity donor site morbidity.

EVIDENCE-BASED QUESTION: HOW DOES ENDOSCOPIC COMPARE WITH OPEN RECONSTRUCTION OF THE SKULL BASE?

A review of the published literature was undertaken to critically and systematically collate the data available on endoscopic endonasal techniques to reconstruct large skull base defects. The nature of such surgical innovation is likely to be reported in case series, retrospective cohorts, or case-control studies rather than higher-level evidence. A systematic review is essential to assess the perioperative outcomes associated with endoscopic reconstructive techniques.

A search strategy was designed to include articles describing any endoscopic endonasal reconstruction of the skull base to search EMBASE (1980–December week 1 2010), Medline (1950–December week 1 2010), Cochrane Collaboration database, and NHS Evidence Health Information Resources database (**Box 1**). A title search was then performed on these articles to select those relevant to clinical or basic science of an endoscopic approach. A subsequent abstract search selected those articles describing any defect other than simple CSF fistula, sella-only defects,

Box 1
Search strategy

1. Nasal.mp. or Nasal Cavity/
2. nose.mp. or Nose/
3. paranasal sinus.mp. or Paranasal Sinuses/
4. (transnas$ or trans-nas$).mp.
5. (sinonasal or sino-nasal).mp.
6. endoscop$.mp.
7. Endoscopes/
8. Endoscopy/
9. (endonas$ or endosin$).mp.
10. or/1–9
11. Surgical Flaps/ or Reconstructive Surgical Procedures/ or Suture Techniques/
12. reconstruct$.mp.
13. defect.mp.
14. repair.mp.
15. closure.mp.
16. sealing.mp.
17. Cerebrospinal Fluid/su [Surgery]
18. Dura Mater/su [Surgery]
19. or/11–18
20. Ethmoid Sinus/ or Ethmoid Bone/ or ethmoid.mp.
21. Sphenoid Sinus/ or Sphenoid Bone/ or sphenoid.mp.
22. (clivus or clival).mp.
23. anterior cranial fossa.mp. or Cranial Fossa, Anterior/
24. middle cranial fossa.mp. or Cranial Fossa, Middle/
25. posterior cranial fossa.mp. or Cranial Fossa, Posterior/
26. (transethm$ or transsphen$ or transcliv$ or transplan$).mp. [mp = title, original title, abstract, name of substance word, subject heading word, unique identifier]
27. (trans-ethm$ or trans-sphen$ or trans-cliv$ or trans-plan$).mp. [mp = title, original title, abstract, name of substance word, subject heading word, unique identifier]
28. Craniotomy/ or craniotomy.mp.
29. craniectomy.mp.
30. Skull Base/ or skull base.mp. or skullbase.mp.
31. Brain Neoplasms/ or Pituitary Neoplasms/ or Skull Neoplasms/
32. Sella Turcica/ or Sella Turcica.mp.
33. or/20–32
34. 10 and 19 and 33
35. limit 34 to English language

Table 2
Characteristics of included studies by endoscopic reconstruction type (vascular flap or mixed)

Study	Year	Study Focus (Flap or Pathology)	n	n (With Defect)	Repair Type	Age (SD or Range)	Gender (% Female)	Defect Size (Longest Axis mm)	Defect Location	Lumbar Drain Use (Days)	Prior Radio-Therapy
El-Sayed[24]	2008	Local Flap -Posterior Septal	30	20	Vascular flap	52 (18–86)	50%	1.86 cm^2	E,P,C,ITF	55% (4)	4
Fortes[9,17]	2007	Local Flap - ITPF	4	4	Vascular flap	52.8 (4)	50%	NR	C,P	NR	—
Fortes[9,17]	2007	Regional Flap - TPF	2	2	Vascular flap	NR	NR	NR	C	NR	2
Hackman[25]	2009	Regional Flap - Palatal	1	1	Vascular flap	70	100%	NR	C	NR	1
Hadad[3]	2006	Local Flap - Posterior Septal	43	43	Vascular flap	Range 22–74	28%	NR	F,E,P,C	NR	NR
Harvey[13,26]	2009	Local Flap - Septal and ITF	30	30	Vascular flap	45.5 (20.2)	43%	24.9 mm	E,P,C,O	0%	NR
Horiguchi[27]	2010	Local Flap - Posterior Septal	21	14	Vascular flap	58 (20–78)	43%	NR	P,C	7%	NR
Kassam[6]	2008	Local Flap - Posterior Septal	75	55	Vascular flap	47 (4–80)	37%	NR	E,P,C,ITF,O	100% (4)	NR
Luginbuhl[28]	2010	Mixed benign and malignant neoplasms, CSF leak	16	16	Vascular flap	NR	NR	17 mm	E,P,C	44% (7)	NR
Madhok[29]	2010	Rathke Cysts	35	3	Vascular flap	34 (12–67)	NR	NR	P	NR	NR

Study	Year	Tumor			Flap	Age					
Nyquist[30]	2010	Mixed benign neoplasms	5	5	Vascular flap	56.4 (31–72)	60%	NR	P,C	20% (1)	NR
Patel[16]	2010	Regional Flap - Pericranial	10	10	Vascular flap	NR	NR	NR	E,P	NR	3
Shah[5]	2009	Local Flap - Posterior septal pediatric	6	6	Vascular flap	13 (2.5)	NR	NR	E,P	NR	NR
Stamm[31]	2008	Craniopharyngioma	4	4	Vascular flap	23.4 (16.3)	25%	NR	E,P,C	0%	NR
Zanation[7,8,15]	2009	Local Flap - Posterior septal	70	70	Vascular flap	NR	NR	>20 mm in 60%	E,P,C	93% (3)	16
Greenfield[37]	2010	Mixed benign and malignant neoplasms, CSF leak	44	33	Mixed	55.4 (17–85)	61%	NR	F,E,P	NR	NR
Ceylan[33]	2009	Mixed benign and malignant neoplasms	13	13	Mixed	47 (12.3)	62%	NR	E,P,C	31%	NR
Cavallo[32]	2009	Craniopharyngioma	22	22	Mixed	49.4 (18–80)	32%	NR	P	NR	27%
Folbe[36]	2009	Olfactory Neuroblastoma	23	19	Mixed: 1 flap 18 free	56.6 (15–79)	30%	NR	E,P	NR	NR
de Divitiis[34]	2008	Meningioma	11	11	Mixed: 3 flap 8 free	56.1 (44–80)	64%	29.8 mm	E,P	NR	NR
Dehdashti[35]	2008	Chordoma	12	9	Mixed: 5 flap 7 free	49.4 (15.8)	33%	40.3 mm	C	NR	25%

Abbreviations: AD, adenoma; C, transclival; Ch, chordoma; CP, craniopharyngioma; CSF, cerebrospinal fluid; E, trans-ethmoid/cribriform; F, transfrontal; ITPF, inferior turbinate pedicled flap; ITF, transpetrous, ptyergoid or infratemporal fossa; Men, meningioma; NR, not reported; P, transplanum; RC, Rathke cyst; TPF, temporoparietal flap.

meningocele, or simple case report. The articles selected were subjected to a full text review to extract data sets on perioperative outcomes for endoscopic skull base reconstruction.

From the search, 4770 articles were initially selected. A title search found 416 articles of skull base surgery. An abstract search found 190 articles directly relating to endoscopic skull base repair or the management of conditions in which reconstruction would be required. Full-text analysis produced 38 studies with extractable endoscopic skull base reconstruction data. These articles included the following: 12 vascularized reconstructions, 17 free graft repairs, and 9 mixed reconstructions. Three of these had mixed data levels in clearly defined patient groups that could be used for meta-analysis.[3,5–7,9,16,17,24–31] The other 6 are described only.[32–38]

CSF leak rates were routinely reported with other perioperative morbidity inconsistently noted. There were 609 patients collectively included in the review. Of these included patients, 326 underwent a free graft reconstruction and 283 had a vascularized reconstruction. The overall rate of CSF leak was 11.5% (70/609). This was represented as 15.6% (51/326) for free grafts and 6.7% (19/283) for the vascularized reconstruction ($\chi^2 = 11.88$, $P = .001$). The included studies with vascularized reconstructions are listed in **Table 2**. The vascularized reconstruction group compares favorably with the published rates in the International Collaborative Study on Craniofacial Surgery (6.5%–25.0%).[38]

Most of the publications were case series (level 4) and several case-control studies (level 3b). Thus, a grade C recommendation could be made on the expected outcomes of vascularized endoscopic skull base reconstruction with regard to the published rates in open surgery. It is unlikely that direct comparison studies will be made between open and endoscopic approaches, but collective reports of similar techniques suggest reconstructive outcomes are comparable.

SUMMARY

Advancements in endoscopic skull base reconstruction must match the ever-increasing size and complexity of lesions that are approached and resected endoscopically. The principles of multilayer reconstructions and the routine use of vascularized flaps in expanded endonasal surgery have reduced postoperative CSF leak rates to less than 5%. Future advances will help us to understand and manage patients at high risk for a postoperative CSF leak, especially those who have been previously irradiated and/or require revision surgery.

EBM Question	Author's Reply
How does endoscopic compare to open reconstruction of the skull base?	Vascularized flap repairs are associated with a 6.7% CSF leak rate compared to free grafts (15.6%) for endoscopic reconstruction and compare favourably to open reconstruction (Level 3a Grade C).

REFERENCES

1. Neligan PC, Mulholland S, Irish J, et al. Flap selection in cranial base reconstruction. Plast Reconstr Surg 1996;98(7):1159–66.
2. Hegazy HM, Carrau RL, Snyderman CH, et al. Transnasal endoscopic repair of cerebrospinal fluid rhinorrhea: a meta-analysis. Laryngoscope 2000;110(7): 1166–72.

3. Hadad G, Bassagasteguy L, Carrau RL, et al. A novel reconstructive technique after endoscopic expanded endonasal approaches: vascular pedicle nasoseptal flap. Laryngoscope 2006;116(10):1882-6.
4. Pinheiro-Neto CD, Prevedello DM, Carrau RL, et al. Improving the design of the pedicled nasoseptal flap for skull base reconstruction: a radioanatomic study. Laryngoscope 2007;117(9):1560-9.
5. Shah RN, Surowitz JB, Patel MR, et al. Endoscopic pedicled nasoseptal flap reconstruction for pediatric skull base defects. Laryngoscope 2009;119(6): 1067-75.
6. Kassam AB, Thomas A, Carrau RL, et al. Endoscopic reconstruction of the cranial base using a pedicled nasoseptal flap. Neurosurgery 2008;63(1 Suppl 1): ONS44-52 [discussion: ONS52-3].
7. Zanation AM, Snyderman CH, Carrau RL, et al. Prospective evaluation of 70 nasoseptal flaps for endoscopic reconstruction of high flow intraoperative CSF leaks during endoscopic skull base surgery. Am J Rhinol Allergy 2009;23(5): 518-21.
8. Zanation AM, Carrau RL, Snyderman CH, et al. Nasoseptal flap takedown during endoscopic skull base surgery. Laryngoscope 2011;121(1):42-6.
9. Fortes FS, Carrau RL, Snyderman CH, et al. The posterior pedicle inferior turbinate flap: a new vascularized flap for skull base reconstruction. Laryngoscope 2007;117(8):1329-32.
10. Padgham N, Vaughan-Jones R. Cadaver studies of the anatomy of arterial supply to the inferior turbinate. J R Soc Med 1991;84:728-30.
11. Hadar T, Ophir D, Yaniv E, et al. Inferior turbinate arterial bloody supply: histologic analysis and clinical implications. J Otolaryngol 2005;34:46-50.
12. Murakami CS, Kriet D, Ierokomos A. Nasal reconstruction using the inferior turbinate mucosal flap. Arch Facial Plast Surg 1999;1:97-100.
13. Harvey RJ, Sheahan PO, Schlosser RJ. Inferior turbinate pedicle flap for endoscopic skull base defect repair. Am J Rhinol Allergy 2009;23(5):522-6.
14. Prevedello DM, Carrau RL, Snyderman CH, et al. Posterior pedicled middle turbinate flap for endoscopic skull base reconstruction. Laryngoscope 2009;119(11): 2094-8.
15. Zanation AM, Snyderman CH, Carrau RL, et al. Minimally invasive endoscopic pericranial flap: a new method for endonasal skull base reconstruction. Laryngoscope 2009;119(1):13-8.
16. Patel MR, Shah RN, Snyderman CH, et al. Pericranial flap for endoscopic anterior skull-base reconstruction: clinical outcomes and radioanatomic analysis of preoperative planning. Neurosurgery 2010;66(3):506-12 [discussion: 512].
17. Fortes FS, Carrau RL, Snyderman CH, et al. Transpterygoid transposition of a temporoparietal fascia flap: a new method for skull base reconstruction after endoscopic expanded endonasal approaches. Laryngoscope 2007;117(6):970-6.
18. Moore KL, Dalley AF. Clinically oriented anatomy. 5th edition. Baltimore (MD): Lippincott Williams and Wilkins; 2006. p. 788-98.
19. Pinar YA, Govsa F. Anatomy of the superficial temporal artery and its branches: its importance for surgery. Surg Radiol Anat 2006;28:248-53.
20. Casoli V, Dauphin N, Taki C, et al. Anatomy and blood supply of the subgaleal flap. Clin Anat 2004;17:392-9.
21. David SK, Cheney SL. An anatomic study of the temporoparietal fascial flap. Arch Otolaryngol Head Neck Surg 1995;121:1153-6.
22. Oliver CL, Hackman TG, Carrau RL, et al. Palatal flap modifications allow pedicled reconstruction of the skull base. Laryngoscope 2009;118(12):2102-6.

23. Patel MR, Shah RN, Snyderman CH, et al. How to choose? Endoscopic skull base reconstructive options and limitations. Skull Base 2008;18(6):385–94.
24. El-Sayed IH, Roediger FC, Goldberg AN, et al. Endoscopic reconstruction of skull base defects with the nasal septal flap. Skull Base 2008;18(6):385–94.
25. Hackman TG, Chicoine MR, Uppaluri R. Novel application of the palatal island flap for endoscopic skull base reconstruction. Laryngoscope 2009;119(8): 1463–6.
26. Harvey RJ, Nogueira JF Jr, Schlosser RJ, et al. Closure of large skull base defects after endoscopic transnasal craniotomy: clinical article. J Neurosurg 2009;111(2): 371–9.
27. Horiguchi K, Murai H, Hasegawa Y, et al. Endoscopic endonasal skull base reconstruction using a nasal septal flap: surgical results and comparison with previous reconstructions. Neurosurg Rev 2010;33(2):235–41 [discussion: 241].
28. Luginbuhl AJ, Campbell PG, Evans J, et al. Endoscopic repair of high-flow cranial base defects using a bilayer button. Laryngoscope 2010;120(5):876–80.
29. Madhok R, Prevedello DM, Gardner P, et al. Endoscopic endonasal resection of Rathke cleft cysts: clinical outcomes and surgical nuances. J Neurosurg 2010; 112(6):1333–9.
30. Nyquist GG, Anand VK, Singh A, et al. Janus flap: bilateral nasoseptal flaps for anterior skull base reconstruction. Otolaryngol Head Neck Surg 2010;142(3): 327–31.
31. Stamm AC, Vellutini E, Harvey RJ, et al. Endoscopic transnasal craniotomy and the resection of craniopharyngioma. Laryngoscope 2008;118(7):1142–8.
32. Cavallo LM, Prevedello DM, Solari D, et al. Extended endoscopic endonasal trans-sphenoidal approach for residual or recurrent craniopharyngiomas. J Neurosurg 2009;111(3):578–89.
33. Ceylan S, Koc K, Anik I. Extended endoscopic approaches for midline skull-base lesions. Neurosurg Rev 2009;32(3):309–19 [discussion: 318–9].
34. de Divitiis E, Esposito F, Cappabianca P, et al. Endoscopic transnasal resection of anterior cranial fossa meningiomas. Neurosurg Focus 2008;25(6):E8.
35. Dehdashti AR, Karabatsou K, Ganna A, et al. Expanded endoscopic endonasal approach for treatment of clival chordomas: early results in 12 patients. Neurosurgery 2008;63(2):299–307 [discussion: 307–9].
36. Folbe A, Herzallah I, Duvvuri U, et al. Endoscopic endonasal resection of esthesioneuroblastoma: a multicenter study. Am J Rhinol Allergy 2009;23(1):91–4.
37. Greenfield JP, Anand VK, Kacker A, et al. Endoscopic endonasal transethmoidal transcribriform transfovea ethmoidalis approach to the anterior cranial fossa and skull base. Neurosurgery 2010;66(5):883–92 [discussion: 892].
38. Ganly I, Patel SG, Singh B, et al. Complications of craniofacial resection for malignant tumors of the skull base: report of an International Collaborative Study. Head Neck 2005;27(6):445–51.

Training in Neurorhinology: The Impact of Case Volume on the Learning Curve

Carl H. Snyderman, MD[a,b,]*, Juan Fernandez-Miranda, MD[b],
Paul A. Gardner, MD[b]

KEYWORDS

• Neurorhinology • Surgical training • Learning curve
• Case volume • Skull base surgery

EBM Question	Level of Evidence	Grade of Recommendation
How many cases are needed to achieve proficiency in endoscopic endonasal skull base surgery?	4	C

Surgeons spend most of their professional life acquiring new surgical skills and learning new surgical procedures. There is a hierarchy of training outside of a structured residency program that usually commences with a course employing anatomic models or cadaveric dissection. Clinical learning progresses from observation/assisting to supervised surgery to independent surgery. The goal of this process is the attainment of surgical proficiency.

What is the definition of surgical proficiency? A proficient surgeon can be defined as one who is "competent or skilled in doing or using something." The road to proficiency is a progression through 5 stages: novice, advanced beginner, competent, proficient, and expert. Not all surgeons reach this level and few will achieve expert status. There are multiple potential obstacles to the achievement of proficiency by a surgical team.

[a] Department of Otolaryngology-Head and Neck Surgery, University of Pittsburgh Medical Center, 200 Lothrop Street, EEI Suite 500, Pittsburgh, PA 15213, USA
[b] Department of Neurosurgery, University of Pittsburgh Medical Center, 200 Lothrop Street, PUH 400, Pittsburgh, PA 15213, USA
* Corresponding author. Department of Otolaryngology-Head and Neck Surgery, University of Pittsburgh Medical Center, 200 Lothrop Street, EEI Suite 500, Pittsburgh, PA 15213.
E-mail address: snydermanch@upmc.edu

Otolaryngol Clin N Am 44 (2011) 1223–1228
doi:10.1016/j.otc.2011.06.014
0030-6665/11/$ – see front matter © 2011 Elsevier Inc. All rights reserved.

oto.theclinics.com

Of these, the volume of cases is probably the most important factor, and will establish the length of the learning curve.

LEARNING CURVE

Endoscopic endonasal surgery has a long learning curve that is attributable to multiple factors: unfamiliar endoscopic anatomy, lack of endoscopic skills, potential risk of neural and vascular injury, and reconstructive challenges. The learning curve must deal with issues of endoscopic anatomy, instrumentation, 2-dimensional visualization, team dynamics, and dealing with complications. An incremental training plan has been proposed that is applicable to both otolaryngologists and neurosurgeons performing endonasal skull base surgery (**Table 1**).[1] The levels are based on level of technical difficulty, potential risk of vascular and neural injury, and unfamiliar endoscopic anatomy. Levels I to III are extradural procedures. Most pituitary surgeons will be between levels III and IV. Levels IV and V are intradural procedures and require a greater level of anatomic knowledge, surgical finesse, and teamwork. Level IV is further divided into pathology that has a cuff of cortical brain tissue between the tumor and the cerebral vasculature (**Fig. 1**). Absence of a cortical cuff (**Fig. 2**) increases the risk of vascular injury and may prevent complete tumor removal. Mastery of each level is recommended before attempting procedures at a higher level.

Before examining the limited data regarding the learning curve for endonasal skull base surgery, it is instructive to review the extensive literature regarding the learning

Table 1
Incremental training levels for endoscopic endonasal skull base surgery

Level	Description	Examples
I	Sinus surgery	Endoscopic sphenoethmoidectomy Sphenopalatine artery ligation
II	Advanced sinus surgery Basic skull base surgery	Endoscopic frontal sinusotomy Cerebrospinal fluid leaks Lateral recess sphenoid Sella/pituitary (intrasellar) Medial orbital decompression
III	Extradural skull base	Sella/pituitary (extrasellar) Optic nerve decompression Transodontoid approach (extradural) Transclival approaches (extradural) Petrous apex (medial expansion)
IV	Intradural skull base 1. Cortical cuff 2. No cortical cuff	Petrous apex (exposure of carotid) Transplanum approach (intradural) Craniofacial resection Transclival approaches Transodontoid approach (intradural) Suprapetrous carotid approach
V	Coronal plane Vascular dissection	Infrapetrous carotid approach Parapharyngeal space Aneurysms Vascular malformations Highly vascular tumors

Adapted from Snyderman C, Kassam A, Carrau R, et al. Acquisition of surgical skills for endonasal skull base surgery: a training program. Laryngoscope 2007;117(4):701; with permission.

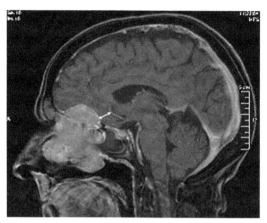

Fig. 1. Level IVA case. There is clear separation of the tumor from the cerebral vasculature (*double-ended arrow*).

curve for endoscopic cholecystectomy.[2] Following the application of laparoscopic techniques to gallbladder surgery, there was a large spike in complications such as common bile duct injury that gradually returned to baseline as the surgical community gained more experience. Possible predictors of surgical expertise included proficiency in traditional techniques, endoscopic experience with other procedures, duration of practice, and number of cases performing a specific procedure. Of these, only the number of cases performing a specific procedure was significant. Various investigators have suggested that the threshold of proficiency is 25 to 30 cases for laparoscopic fundoplication and 15 to 20 cases for laparoscopic cholecystectomy. Whether these numbers could be applied to other endoscopic procedures is not known.

In skull base surgery, one can also look at microscopic surgeries that require a similar level of expertise to gain insight about the learning curve. Moffat and colleagues[3] looked at facial nerve outcomes in vestibular schwannoma surgery. In 300 consecutive surgeries, postoperative facial nerve function was House grades I to III in 52% of the first 50 cases and 78% of the second 50 cases. Functional preservation continued to improve at a slower rate with 92% House grades I to III in the last 50 cases. Most of the learning curve was associated with the translabyrinthine approach.

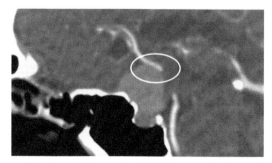

Fig. 2. Level IVB case. The tumor is in contact with the cerebral vasculature (*circle*).

EVIDENCE-BASED REVIEW

A PubMed review of the medical literature was performed using the search terms "learning curve, skull base" and "learning curve, cranial base." Article selection was restricted to the period 1996 to 2010. Guidelines established by the Oxford Center for Evidence-Based Medicine levels of evidence were used to grade the publications.[4]

Specific data regarding endoscopic endonasal skull base surgery is limited and deals primarily with pituitary surgery (**Table 2**). Most surgical teams have evaluated their experience as they transitioned from microscopic to endoscopic pituitary surgery. Sonnenburg and colleagues[5] investigated the learning curve in their first 45 endoscopic pituitary surgeries. The series of patients was divided into 3 cohorts of 15 patients each and outcomes such as complication rates, blood loss, length of stay, and histology within each group were compared [level of evidence: IV]. Because there was no difference between the groups, they concluded that there was "no learning curve." Their study, however, did not account for the complexity of cases, extent of resection, or experience of the neurosurgeon. In a study by Leach and colleagues,[6] patients undergoing endoscopic pituitary surgery were divided into two consecutive groups of 53 and 72 patients [level of evidence: IV]. A comparison of the two time periods demonstrated that outcome measures (operative time, improvement in vision, remission of Cushing disease, and length of stay) were better in the second group. There was no change in the incidence of postoperative hypopituitarism. This study would suggest that proficiency is achieved after approximately 50 surgeries.

A comparison of 25 endoscopic and 25 microscopic removals of pituitary adenomas by O'Malley and colleagues[7] looked at the incidence of intraoperative and postoperative complications, intraoperative cerebrospinal fluid leaks, gross total resection, and the need for multiple surgeries [level of evidence: IV]. Similar outcomes were noted, and they concluded that the learning curve was less than 17 cases. A similar study performed by Smith and colleagues[8] compared outcomes in a group of 51 patients undergoing endoscopic transsphenoidal skull base surgery with outcomes in a cohort of 46 patients undergoing microscopic transsphenoidal skull base surgery [level of evidence: IV]. Outcome measures included endocrine control of secretory pituitary tumors, incidence of intraoperative/postoperative cerebral spinal fluid leaks, postoperative diabetes insipidus, and length of stay. No significant differences were noted between treatment groups. The endoscopic group was further divided into 3 equal sequential cohorts of 17 patients; comparison of the first and third cohorts demonstrated a significant decrease in the incidence of cerebrospinal fluid leaks, operative time, and length of stay. This result suggests that proficiency is achieved after approximately 34 surgeries.

Table 2 Evidence-based medicine review of literature				
Publication	**Design**	**Results**	**Recommendation**	**EBM Level**
Sonnenburg et al[5]	Endo pit; 3 cohorts	No difference	No learning curve	IV
Leach et al[6]	Endo pit; 2 cohorts	Improved	>53 cases	IV
O'Malley et al[7]	Endo versus micro pit	No difference	<17 cases	IV
Smith et al[8]	Endo versus micro SB	No difference	—	—
	Endo SB; 3 cohorts	Improved	18–34 cases	IV

Abbreviations: EBM, evidence-based medicine; pit, pituitary; SB, skull base.

Imaging technology is frequently used during endoscopic sinus surgery and skull base to guide surgeons and avoid complications. Static preoperative computed tomography and magnetic resonance imaging may be combined with intraoperative navigation to identify key anatomic structures and the margins of the pathology. It is intuitive that such technological aids may compensate for the learning curve and narrow the differential between the novice and the expert surgeon. A study by Wise and colleagues,[9] however, demonstrated that image guidance technology was not a replacement for anatomic knowledge and surgical experience in novice skull base surgeons in a laboratory setting.

DISCUSSION

The published literature on endoscopic endonasal skull base surgery is limited by small series of patients, nonstandardized measures of the learning curve, and exclusion of relevant factors. Other issues to consider include the specialty of the surgeon, the region of the skull base, and the quality of the learning experience. Otolaryngologists and neurosurgeons differ in regard of prior endoscopic experience, volume of endoscopic cases unrelated to the skull base, necessary surgical skills, and exposure to high-risk skull base surgeries with potential for neurovascular injury. In comparison with the ventral skull base surgeon, the pituitary surgeon may lack anatomic knowledge of the skull base beyond the sella and may differ regarding prior surgical experience, frequency of nonsellar cases, and additional surgical skills needed. Finally, the quality of the learning experience is of paramount importance. What is the case mix of the learning experience with regard to histology, location, and extent of skull base pathology? The skull base novice needs to be exposed to situations that develop his or her surgical judgment and prepare him or her for rare events that are unlikely to be encountered in a small series of cases (eg, injury of the internal carotid artery).

Finally, surgical proficiency is more than just technical expertise. The skull base surgeon needs to become proficient in the management of patients with diseases of the skull base. This management includes good diagnostic acumen, the development of a rational treatment plan, sound surgical judgment in the operating theater, and thorough postoperative care. The number of cases needed to achieve proficiency will depend on the level of training, surgical specialty, past surgical experience, case mix, type of surgery, and extent of surgery.

RECOMMENDATIONS

Current recommendations in the literature for volume of cases to achieve surgical proficiency are based on inadequate data and fail to consider relevant factors that affect the learning curve. The current grade of recommendation based on evidence-based medicine guidelines is "C." To improve the level of evidence, a precise definition of surgical proficiency with well-defined and validated measures is needed. It is naïve to claim that there is no learning curve or to assume that the learning curve is minimal because of an uneventful early experience. The learning curve will depend on the demands of the particular pathology and will not be the same for all individuals. In the absence of good data, can one nevertheless make reasonable recommendations? One proposal is to adopt the 5-stage training program previously submitted,[1] and suggest that surgeons should perform a minimum volume of cases (ie, 20–30) at each level before proceeding to the next level. Ideally, proficiency would be assessed using objective measures at each stage before progressing to the next stage.

The learning curve is not static and will change as new knowledge is gained and technologies change. The next generation of skull base surgeons will need a strong foundation in endoscopic skull base anatomy, and exposure to emerging technologies in areas of imaging, navigation, robotics, biomaterials, and so forth. As surgical simulation devices mature and become more realistic, more of the learning curve will occur outside the operating room in the simulation laboratory.

EBM Question	Author's Reply
How many cases are needed to achieve proficiency in endoscopic endonasal skull base surgery?	A minimum volume (20 to 30 cases) at each level of a 5-stage training program is likely to be required for endonasal skull base surgery proficiency (Level 4 Grade C).

REFERENCES

1. Snyderman C, Kassam A, Carrau R, et al. Acquisition of surgical skills for endonasal skull base surgery: a training program. Laryngoscope 2007;117(4):69–705.
2. Gibbs VC, Auerbach AD. Learning curves for new procedures—the case of laparoscopic cholecystectomy. Chapter 19, Making health care safer: a critical analysis of patient safety practices. Evidence Report/Technology Assessment: Number 43. AHRQ Publication No. 01-E058, July 2001. Agency for Healthcare Research and Quality, Rockville (MD). Available at: http://www.ahrq.gov/clinic/ptsafety/. Accessed June 19, 2011.
3. Moffat DA, Hardy DG, Grey PL, et al. The operating learning curve and its effect on facial nerve outcome in vestibular schwannoma surgery. Am J Otol 1996;17(4): 643–7.
4. OCEBM Levels of Evidence Working Group. The Oxford 2011 Levels of Evidence. Oxford Centre for Evidence-Based Medicine. Available at: http://www.cebm.net/index.aspx?o=5653. Accessed June 3, 2011.
5. Sonnenburg RE, White D, Ewend MG, et al. The learning curve in minimally invasive pituitary surgery. Am J Rhinol 2004;18(4):259–63.
6. Leach P, Abou-Zeid AH, Kearney T, et al. Endoscopic transsphenoidal pituitary surgery: evidence of an operating learning curve. Neurosurgery 2010;67(5): 1205–12.
7. O'Malley BW Jr, Grady MS, Gabel BC, et al. Comparison of endoscopic and microscopic removal of pituitary adenomas: single-surgeon experience and the learning curve. Neurosurg Focus 2008;25(6):E10.
8. Smith SJ, Eralil G, Woon K, et al. Light at the end of the tunnel: the learning curve associated with endoscopic transsphenoidal skull base surgery. Skull Base 2010; 20(2):69–74.
9. Wise SK, Harvey RJ, Goddard JC, et al. Combined image guidance and intraoperative computed tomography in facilitating endoscopic orientation within and around the paranasal sinuses. Am J Rhinol 2008;22:635–41.

Index

Note: Page numbers of article titles are in **boldface** type.

Otolaryngol Clin N Am 44 (2011) 1229–1234
doi:10.1016/S0030-6665(11)00169-1
0030-6665/11/$ – see front matter © 2011 Elsevier Inc. All rights reserved.

oto.theclinics.com

Moving?

Make sure your subscription moves with you!

To notify us of your new address, find your **Clinics Account Number** (located on your mailing label above your name), and contact customer service at:

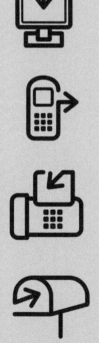

Email: journalscustomerservice-usa@elsevier.com

800-654-2452 (subscribers in the U.S. & Canada)
314-447-8871 (subscribers outside of the U.S. & Canada)

Fax number: 314-447-8029

**Elsevier Health Sciences Division
Subscription Customer Service
3251 Riverport Lane
Maryland Heights, MO 63043**

*To ensure uninterrupted delivery of your subscription, please notify us at least 4 weeks in advance of move.

United States Postal Service

Statement of Ownership, Management, and Circulation
(All Periodicals Publications Except Requester Publications)

1. Publication Title	2. Publication Number	3. Filing Date
Otolaryngologic Clinics of North America	4 6 6 - 5 5 0	9/16/11

4. Issue Frequency	5. Number of Issues Published Annually	6. Annual Subscription Price
Feb, Apr, Jun, Aug, Oct, Dec	6	$310.00

7. Complete Mailing Address of Known Office of Publication (Not printer) (Street, city, county, state, and ZIP+4®)

Elsevier Inc.
360 Park Avenue South
New York, NY 10010-1710

Contact Person: Stephen Bushing
Telephone (Include area code): 215-239-3688

8. Complete Mailing Address of Headquarters or General Business Office of Publisher (Not printer)

Elsevier Inc., 360 Park Avenue South, New York, NY 10010-1710

9. Full Names and Complete Mailing Addresses of Publisher, Editor, and Managing Editor (Do not leave blank)

Publisher (Name and complete mailing address)

Kim Murphy, Elsevier, Inc., 1600 John F. Kennedy Blvd. Suite 1800, Philadelphia, PA 19103-2899

Editor (Name and complete mailing address)

Joanne Husovski, Elsevier, Inc., 1600 John F. Kennedy Blvd. Suite 1800, Philadelphia, PA 19103-2899

Managing Editor (Name and complete mailing address)

Barton Dudlick, Elsevier, Inc., 1600 John F. Kennedy Blvd. Suite 1800, Philadelphia, PA 19103-2899

10. Owner (Do not leave blank. If the publication is owned by a corporation, give the name and address of the corporation immediately followed by the names and addresses of all stockholders owning or holding 1 percent or more of the total amount of stock. If not owned by a corporation, give the names and addresses of the individual owners. If owned by a partnership or other unincorporated firm, give its name and address as well as those of each individual owner. If the publication is published by a nonprofit organization, give its name and address.)

Full Name	Complete Mailing Address
Wholly owned subsidiary of	4520 East-West Highway
Reed/Elsevier, US holdings	Bethesda, MD 20814

11. Known Bondholders, Mortgagees, and Other Security Holders Owning or Holding 1 Percent or More of Total Amount of Bonds, Mortgages, or Other Securities. If none, check box ☐ None

Full Name	Complete Mailing Address
N/A	

12. Tax Status (For completion by nonprofit organizations authorized to mail at nonprofit rates) (Check one)
The purpose, function, and nonprofit status of this organization and the exempt status for federal income tax purposes:
☐ Has Not Changed During Preceding 12 Months
☐ Has Changed During Preceding 12 Months (Publisher must submit explanation of change with this statement)

PS Form 3526, September 2007 (Page 1 of 3 (Instructions Page 3)) PSN 7530-01-000-9931 PRIVACY NOTICE: See our Privacy policy in www.usps.com

---

13. Publication Title	14. Issue Date for Circulation Data Below
Otolaryngologic Clinics of North America	June 2011

15. Extent and Nature of Circulation			Average No. Copies Each Issue During Preceding 12 Months	No. Copies of Single Issue Published Nearest to Filing Date
a. Total Number of Copies (Net press run)			2117	2100
b. Paid Circulation (By Mail and Outside the Mail)	(1)	Mailed Outside-County Paid Subscriptions Stated on PS Form 3541. (Include paid distribution above nominal rate, advertiser's proof copies, and exchange copies)	833	742
	(2)	Mailed In-County Paid Subscriptions Stated on PS Form 3541 (Include paid distribution above nominal rate, advertiser's proof copies, and exchange copies)		
	(3)	Paid Distribution Outside the Mails Including Sales Through Dealers and Carriers, Street Vendors, Counter Sales, and Other Paid Distribution Outside USPS®	523	483
	(4)	Paid Distribution by Other Classes Mailed Through the USPS (e.g. First-Class Mail®)		
c. Total Paid Distribution (Sum of 15b (1), (2), (3), and (4))		►	1356	1225
d. Free or Nominal Rate Distribution (By Mail and Outside the Mail)	(1)	Free or Nominal Rate Outside-County Copies Included on PS Form 3541	116	108
	(2)	Free or Nominal Rate In-County Copies Included on PS Form 3541		
	(3)	Free or Nominal Rate Copies Mailed at Other Classes Through the USPS (e.g. First-Class Mail)		
	(4)	Free or Nominal Rate Distribution Outside the Mail (Carriers or other means)		
e. Total Free or Nominal Rate Distribution (Sum of 15d (1), (2), (3) and (4))		►	116	108
f. Total Distribution (Sum of 15c and 15e)		►	1472	1333
g. Copies not Distributed (See instructions to publishers #4 (page 83))		►	645	767
h. Total (Sum of 15f and g)		►	2117	2100
i. Percent Paid (15c divided by 15f times 100)			92.12%	91.90%

16. Publication of Statement of Ownership

☐ If the publication is a general publication, publication of this statement is required. Will be printed in the October 2011 issue of this publication. ☐ Publication not required.

17. Signature and Title of Editor, Publisher, Business Manager, or Owner	Date
Stephen R. Bushing – Inventory/Distribution Coordinator	September 16, 2011

I certify that all information furnished on this form is true and complete. I understand that anyone who furnishes false or misleading information on this form or who omits material or information requested on the form may be subject to criminal sanctions (including fines and imprisonment) and/or civil sanctions (including civil penalties).

PS Form 3526, September 2007 (Page 2 of 3)

Printed and bound by CPI Group (UK) Ltd, Croydon, CR0 4YY

03/10/2024

01040449-0002